ACSM'S GUIDELINES FOR THE TEAM PHYSICIAN

ACSM'S GUIDELINES FOR THE TEAM PHYSICIAN

edited by

ROBERT C. CANTU, M.D., F.A.C.S.M.

Chairman, Department of Surgery
Chief, Neurosurgical Service
Director, Service of Sports Medicine
Emerson Hospital
Concord, Massachusetts

LYLE J. MICHELI, M.D., F.A.C.S.M.

Director, Division of Sports Medicine
Children's Hospital
Boston, Massachusetts

LEA & FEBIGER   Philadelphia • London • 1991

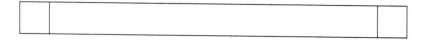

Lea & Febiger
200 Chester Field Parkway
Malvern, Pennsylvania 19355-9725
U.S.A.
(215) 251-2230

Cover Photo courtesy of Cleveland Clinic Foundation, Tom Merce photographer.

Library of Congress Cataloging-in-Publication Data

American College of Sports Medicine's guidelines for the team
  physician / edited by Robert C. Cantu and Lyle J. Micheli.
      p.   cm.
    Includes index.
    ISBN 0-8121-1370-5
      1. Sports medicine—Handbooks, manuals, etc. I. Cantu, Robert C.
II. Micheli, Lyle J., 1940–   . III. American College of Sports
Medicine. IV. Title: Guidelines for the team physician.
    [DNLM: 1. Athletic Injuries. 2. Sports Medicine. QT 260 A5113]
RC1210.A44   1991
617.1'027—dc20
DNLM/DLC
for Library of Congress   91-10089
                                                                CIP

Printed in the United States of America

Print number: 5   4   3   2   1

ACKNOWLEDGMENTS

The editors wish to thank the 28 authors who contributed the 29 chapters that comprise this book. Without their efforts this important College project would not have been possible. Furthermore, we wish to acknowledge the Continuing Medical Education Committee who served a critical review function as did several other prominent College members. Finally, we wish to thank Mark D. Robertson for his tireless assistance and the production staff at Lea & Febiger for their expeditious handling of this project.

FOREWORD

Beginning in 1989, the American College of Sports Medicine has presented a highly successful, well-attended post-graduate course specifically for the team physician. Now, ACSM offers a text authored by 28 experienced experts in their respective fields. The text encompasses the three-part course content. This premier resource for the team physician covers the topics a team physician requires to provide optimal care.

Guidelines for the prevention, diagnosis, treatment, and rehabilitation of injuries, as well as medical and administrative problems incurred by both amateur and professional athletes are clearly and succinctly presented. In addition to musculoskeletal injuries, topics receiving special emphasis include:

- physiologic and metabolic response to exercise
- pre-participation evaluation
- environmental medicine
- legal aspects of administering care
- identification and management of nutritional, psychological, and drug problems
- development of conditioning and training programs
- injury prevention and rehabilitation
- criteria for returning to participation after injury

Based on a solid foundation in medical and scientific research, *ACSM's Guidelines for the Team Physician* is an authoritative text providing the clinician with clear, concise illustrations and easily understood recommendations to assist in discharging the unique responsibilities of the team physician.

John A. Bergfeld, M.D., F.A.C.S.M.
Head, Section of Sports Medicine
Cleveland Clinic Foundation
Team Physician
Cleveland Browns Football Club
Cleveland Cavaliers Basketball Team
Cleveland, Ohio

CONTRIBUTING AUTHORS

BRUCE E. BAKER, M.D., F.A.C.S.M.
Team Physician and Orthopedist
Syracuse University
Syracuse Irving Medical Center
Syracuse, NY

DONNA B. BERNHARDT, Ed.D., P.T., A.T.C.
Director, Program in Athletic Training
Assistant Professor
Boston University
Sargent College of Allied Health Professions
Boston, MA

GEORGE A. BROOKS, Ph.D., F.A.C.S.M.
Professor, Director Exercise Physiology Laboratory
University of California
Berkeley, CA

ROBERT C. CANTU, M.A., M.D., F.A.C.S., F.A.C.S.M.
Chief, Neurosurgical Service
Chairman, Department of Surgery
Director, Service of Sports Medicine
Emerson Hospital, Concord, MA
Medical Director, National Center for Catastrophic Sports
    Injury Research
Chapel Hill, NC

NANCY CLARK, M.S., R.D.
Nutritionist, Sports Medicine Brookline
Brookline, MA

E. RANDY EICHNER, M.D.
Professor of Medicine
Hematology Section, Department of Medicine
University of Oklahoma Health Sciences Center
Oklahoma City, OK

JACK HARVEY, M.D., F.A.C.S.M.
Director, Sports Medicine
Orthopaedic Center of the Rockies
Fort Collins, CO

DAVID L. HERBERT, Esq.
Senior Partner
Herbert, Benson & Scott
Attorneys-at-Law
President, Professional Reports Corporation
Canton, OH

WILLIAM G. HERBERT, Ph.D., F.A.C.S.M.
Professor and Director of Laboratory for Exercise Sport and
  Work Physiology
Virginia Tech
Blacksburg, VA

STANLEY A. HERRING, M.D., F.A.C.S.M.
Puget Sound Sports Physicians
Clinical Assistant Professor
Department of Rehabilitation
University of Washington
Clinical Assistant Professor
Department of Orthopedics
University of Washington
Seattle, WA

ELLIOTT B. HERSHMAN, M.D., P.C.
New York, NY

BRUCE H. JONES, M.D., MPH
Chief, Occupational Medicine Division
U.S. Army Research Institute of Environmental Medicine
Natick, MA

W. BEN KIBLER, M.D., F.A.C.S.M.
Medical Director
Lexington Clinic Sports Medicine Center
Lexington, KY

JOHN A. LOMBARDO, M.D., F.A.C.S.M.
Professor and Chairman
Department of Family Medicine
The Ohio State University
Columbus, OH

**DOUGLAS B. McKEAG, M.D., M.S., F.A.C.S.M.,
F.A.B.F.P.**
Professor of Family Practice
Coordinator of Sports Medicine
College of Human Medicine
Michigan State University
East Lansing, MI

LYLE J. MICHELI, M.D., F.A.C.S.M.
Director, Division of Sports Medicine
Boston Children's Hospital
Associate Clinical Professor of Orthopaedic Surgery
Harvard Medical School
Boston, MA
Immediate Past President
American College of Sports Medicine

SHANE M. MURPHY, Ph.D.
United States Olympic Committee
Colorado Springs, CO

JAMES C. PUFFER, M.D.
Associate Professor and Chief
Division of Family Medicine
UCLA School of Medicine
Los Angeles, CA

PETER B. RAVEN, Ph.D., F.A.C.S.M.
Professor of Physiology
Texas College of Osteopathic Medicine
Fort Worth, TX

E. LEE RICE, D.O., F.A.A.
San Diego Sports Medicine Center
San Diego, CA

WILLIAM O. ROBERTS, M.D.
Medical Director, Twin Cities Marathon
MINHEALTH, P.A.
White Bear Lake, MN

BRIAN J. SHARKEY, Ph.D., F.A.C.S.M.
Human Performance Laboratory
University of Montana
Missoula, MT
President
American College of Sports Medicine

ARTHUR J. SIEGEL, M.D., F.A.C.P.
Medical Director
Hahnemann Hospital
Boston, MA
Assistant Professor of Medicine
Harvard Medical School
Boston, MA

ANGELA D. SMITH, M.D.
Head, Section of Pediatric Orthopaedics
Mt. Sinai Medical Center
Cleveland, OH

RICHARD H. STRAUSS, M.D., F.A.C.S.M.
Associate Professor of Preventive Medicine and Internal
    Medicine
Team Physician, Athletic Department
The Ohio State University
Columbus, OH

MELVIN H. WILLIAMS, Ph.D., F.A.C.S.M.
Director, Human Performance Laboratory
Department of Health, Physical Education, and Recreation
Old Dominion University
Norfolk, VA

PRESTON M. WOLIN, M.D.
Associate Professor of Orthopaedic Surgery
Rush Medical College
Team Physician
DePaul University and Loyola University
Chicago, IL

JACK E. YOUNG, M.D., Ph.D.
Medical Director
Health/Fitness Institute and Emergency Services
Doctors' Hospital
Associate Team Physician
University of Miami
Coral Gables, FL

CONTENTS

SECTION I: PRECOMPETITION PHASE

1. EXERCISE PHYSIOLOGY
Peter B. Raven   3

2. METABOLIC RESPONSE TO EXERCISE
George A. Brooks   24

3. TRAINING FOR SPORT
Brian J. Sharkey   34

4. SPECIAL MEDICAL CONDITIONS
E. Randy Eichner   48

5. NUTRITION: PRE-, INTRA-, AND POSTCOMPETITION
Nancy Clark   58

6. ERGOGENIC AIDS
Melvin H. Williams   66

7. PREPARTICIPATION EXAMINATION
John A. Lombardo   71

8. ORGANIZATIONAL ASPECTS
James C. Puffer   95

9. ENVIRONMENTAL PHYSIOLOGY AND MEDICINE
Peter B. Raven   101

10. MEDICAL-LEGAL ISSUES
David L. Herbert and William G. Herbert   118

11. BRACING, SPLINTING, AND TAPING TECHNIQUES
Bruce E. Baker   127

SECTION II: COMPETITION PHASE	

12. LIFE-THREATENING EMERGENCIES
Jack E. Young and Robert C. Cantu — 143

13. TRANSPORTATION/IMMOBILIZATION
Robert C. Cantu — 151

14. LIMB-THREATENING EMERGENCIES
Preston M. Wolin — 153

15. FIRST AID OF INJURIES IN SPORTS
Jack Harvey — 159

16. INJURY RECOGNITION AND EVALUATION: UPPER EXTREMITY
Lyle J. Micheli and Angela D. Smith — 163

17. INJURY RECOGNITION AND EVALUATION: LOWER EXTREMITY
Lyle J. Micheli and Angela D. Smith — 172

18. INJURY RECOGNITION AND EVALUATION: FOOT AND ANKLE
Elliott B. Hershman — 185

SECTION III: POSTCOMPETITION PHASE	

19. REHABILITATION
Stanley A. Herring and W. Ben Kibler — 191

20. CRITERIA FOR RETURN TO COMPETITION AFTER MUSCULOSKELETAL INJURY
Douglas B. McKeag — 196

21. CRITERIA FOR RETURN TO COMPETITION AFTER HEAD OR CERVICAL SPINE INJURY
Robert C. Cantu — 205

22. OVERTRAINING
W. Ben Kibler — 209

SECTION IV: SPECIAL MEDICAL CONCERNS

23. GENDER SPECIFIC: FEMALE ATHLETE
Arthur J. Siegel   215

24. THE MEDICAL BAG
E. Lee Rice   223

25. THE CHILD ATHLETE
Lyle J. Micheli   228

26. THE PHYSICALLY CHALLENGED ATHLETE
Donna B. Bernhardt   242

27. BEHAVIORAL CONSIDERATIONS
Shane M. Murphy   252

**28. MEDICAL MANAGEMENT OF ENDURANCE EVENTS:
INCIDENCE, PREVENTION, AND CARE OF CASUALTIES**
Bruce H. Jones and William O. Roberts   266

29. DRUG USE AND ABUSE
Richard H. Strauss   287

30. OVERUSE INJURIES
Angela D. Smith   297

INDEX   307

PRECOMPETITION PHASE

C H A P T E R 1

EXERCISE PHYSIOLOGY

Peter B. Raven

Physiology is a science dedicated to the study of the function of living organisms and the organ systems involved in maintaining life. Exercise physiology is a branch of physiology concerned with the functions associated with skeletal muscle action. As depicted in Figure 1–1, skeletal muscle activity in humans requires the coordinated function of various physiologic and metabolic systems. The purpose of this chapter is to describe concisely the physiologic responses to acute exercise and the adaptations to exercise training.

ENERGY METABOLISM

Muscle action can be described as shortening or contracting (concentric), lengthening or extension (eccentric), and static (or isometric). All three types of action require increased muscle tension and result from an integration of neural signals that produce a chain of biochemical reactions resulting in free energy transformation. These reactions transform potential chemical energy to the mechanical energy of muscle action.

ATP REGENERATION

Free energy is stored in the body as adenosine triphosphate (ATP). Release of stored energy (E) occurs when one of the three phosphates is broken (hydrolyzed) away from the ATP molecule.
Energy Release:

or

$$\left.\begin{array}{l} (1)\ ATP = ADP + Pi + E \\ (2)\ ADP = AMP + Pi + E \end{array}\right\} \quad AMP + 2\ Pi + 2\ Energy$$

3

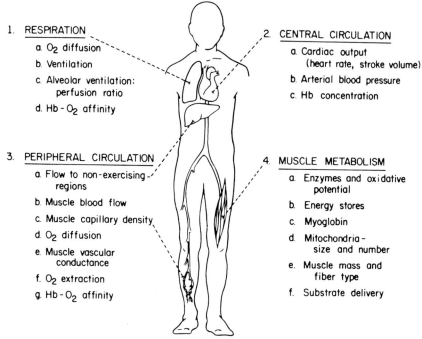

1. RESPIRATION
   a. O_2 diffusion
   b. Ventilation
   c. Alveolar ventilation: perfusion ratio
   d. Hb - O_2 affinity

2. CENTRAL CIRCULATION
   a. Cardiac output (heart rate, stroke volume)
   b. Arterial blood pressure
   c. Hb concentration

3. PERIPHERAL CIRCULATION
   a. Flow to non-exercising regions
   b. Muscle blood flow
   c. Muscle capillary density
   d. O_2 diffusion
   e. Muscle vascular conductance
   f. O_2 extraction
   g. Hb - O_2 affinity

4. MUSCLE METABOLISM
   a. Enzymes and oxidative potential
   b. Energy stores
   c. Myoglobin
   d. Mitochondria - size and number
   e. Muscle mass and fiber type
   f. Substrate delivery

FIG. 1–1. A cartoon summarizing possible limitations to oxygen consumption during exercise. See text for discussion. (Adapted from Saltin and Rowell, 1980, In Rowell LB: *Human Circulation: Regulation during Physical Stress.* New York: Oxford University Press, 1986.)

Reaction (1) occurs more easily than reaction (2) and therefore is the more prevalent reaction for energy production during exercise. Unfortunately, the body stores of ATP are very small (Table 1–1), necessitating continuous replacement via the reversal of the foregoing reactions. Replacement or regeneration of ATP can occur anaerobically (i.e., without oxygen) or aerobically (with oxygen). The two primary anaerobic reactions are:

1. Phosphocreatine breakdown

$$PC + ADP \rightarrow ATP + C$$

2. Breakdown of glycogen or glucose to lactate

$$Glucose + 2\ ADP + 2\ Pi \rightarrow 2\ ATP + Lactate$$

5

TABLE 1–1. Relative Energy Content of the Human

| | Energy/
Mole
(Cal) | Total Energy | |
		mmol/kg Wet Muscle (Cal)	75 kg Body Wt (Cal)
ATP	10	5	1
Phosphocreatine	10.5	17	3.8
Glycogen	700	80	1,100
Fat	2,400	—	75,000

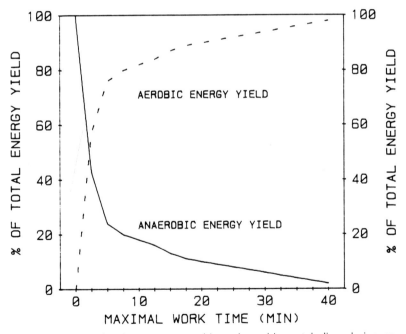

FIG. 1–2. Interaction between anaerobic and aerobic metabolism during exercise. Note energy to perform short-term high-intensity exercise comes primarily from anaerobic sources, whereas energy for muscular contraction during prolonged work comes from aerobic metabolism. (Redrawn from McArdle W, Katch F and Katch V: *Exercise Physiology*. Philadelphia: Lea & Febiger, 1986.)

The aerobic production of ATP requires the presence of oxygen to link the citric acid (Krebs) cycle with the respiratory electron transport chain to generate 36 ATP per molecule of glucose metabolized:

$$Glucose + 6\ O_2 + 36\ ADP + 36\ Pi \rightarrow 6\ H_2O + 6\ CO_2 + 36\ ATP$$

Exercise requires both the aerobic and the anaerobic production of free energy, and different exercises are regarded as "anaerobic" or "aerobic" based on the extent to which their energy requirements are met by one or the other of the energy systems. A key factor is the ability of the oxygen delivery system to provide active muscles with the oxygen needed by the aerobic system. As shown in Figure 1–2, the contribution of aerobic metabolism to total energy requirement is greater with longer-duration, lower-intensity activities. The contribution of energy obtained from anaerobic metabolism is proportional to the intensity of the activity. At the start of exercise, a greater proportion of energy production is obtained from anaerobic metabolism because oxygen uptake kinetics lag behind the total energy demand placed on the system. As indicated in Figure 1–3, this lag produces a so-called "oxygen deficit."

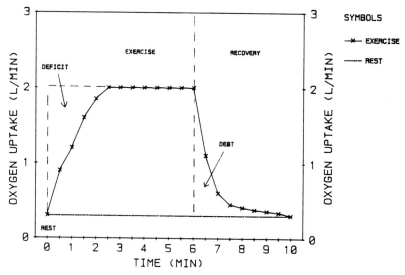

FIG. 1–3. Oxygen uptake dynamics at onset and offset of exercise. (Redrawn from McArdle W, Katch F and Katch V: *Exercise Physiology*. Philadelphia: Lea & Febiger, 1986.)

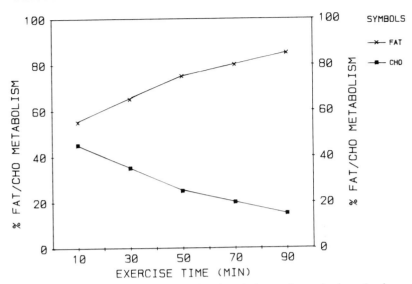

FIG. 1–4. Alterations in substrate utilization during prolonged submaximal exercise. CHO, Carbohydrate. (Data from Powers S, Riley W and Howley E: Comparison of fat metabolism between trained men and women during prolonged aerobic work. *Res Q Exerc Sport,* 51:427, 1980 *In* American College of Sports Medicine: *Resource Manual for Guidelines for Exercise Testing and Prescription.* Philadelphia: Lea & Febiger, 1986.)

SUBSTRATE UTILIZATION

The substrates for energy metabolism are primarily carbohydrates and fats; in malnourished individuals, however, including those with anorexia, protein can be used as an energy source. In general, carbohydrates are used preferentially at the beginning of exercise and during high-intensity exercise (>70–85% $\dot{V}_{O_{2max}}$). During lower-intensity exercise fat is the primary energy source, and during prolonged exercise (>30 minutes) fat makes an increasing contribution as duration increases (Fig. 1–4).

MAXIMAL AEROBIC POWER $\dot{V}_{O_{2max}}$

One's ability to sustain exercise is determined by the availability of oxygen in the working muscles. A measure of the functional state of the oxygen delivery system is the maximal aerobic power (or $\dot{V}_{O_{2max}}$). Maximal aerobic power is the greatest rate of oxygen utilization during exercise; it reflects the rate at which oxygen can be transported by the cardiorespiratory system to the active muscles.

A cycle ergometer or a motor-driven treadmill can be used to measure $\dot{V}_{O_{2max}}$ in the laboratory. Power output on the cycle ergometer is adjusted by changing the resistance required to move the pedals, and on the treadmill the power output is adjusted by changing the treadmill's speed and/or its incline. Measures of oxygen uptake are made at rest and at increasing workloads on a breath-by-breath basis and a minute-by-minute average (Fig. 1–5). The relationship between rate of oxygen uptake and power output is linear until the subject's maximal oxygen uptake ($\dot{V}_{O_{2max}}$) is achieved, when the measured oxygen uptake plateaus (i.e., fails to increase with increasing power output). Exercise above the level of $\dot{V}_{O_{2max}}$ requires greater anaerobic metabolism with consequent marked increases in lactate production. Anaerobic processes, in combination with $\dot{V}_{O_{2max}}$, provide sufficient energy sources for brief periods of exercise at "supramaximal" workloads. Sustained supramaximal activity is impossible because of the progressive accumulation of lactate and other metabolites that interfere with the contractile process in muscle.

The measurement of maximal aerobic power is an accepted, objective means of determining an individual's level of cardiorespiratory or "aerobic" fitness. It is, in fact, an assessment of the organism's cardiorespiratory reserves. A review of some basic expressions of cardiopulmonary physiology will identify the interrelationships among some key parameters.

$$\text{Maximal Aerobic Power} = \text{Cardiac Output} \qquad (1)$$
$$\dot{V}_{O_{2max}} \qquad \dot{Q}_{max}$$
$$\times \text{ Arteriovenous Oxygen Difference}$$
$$a - \dot{V}_{O_{2max}}$$

$$\text{Cardiac Output} = \text{Heart Rate} \times \text{Stroke Volume} \qquad (2)$$
$$\dot{Q}_{max} \qquad HR_{max} \qquad SV_{max}$$

Equation 1 is the basic Fick equation. Measurement of $\dot{V}_{O_{2max}}$ provides a direct indication of the maximal capacity of the cardiorespiratory system and is linked directly to the capacity for endurance exercise. Like height and weight, $\dot{V}_{O_{2max}}$ is a reproducible characteristic of the individual showing insignificant day-to-day variation. $\dot{V}_{O_{2max}}$ is used as a means of scaling cardiovascular responses in different individuals.

CARDIORESPIRATORY RESPONSES TO ACUTE EXERCISE

PHYSIOLOGIC CONTROL THEORY

The cardiovascular system and the respiratory system are endowed with many control systems that tend to maintain oxygen delivery to the peripheral tissues at a level adequate for tissue function. In this regard, exercise may be considered a disturbance to these control systems. Exercise causes an increase in oxygen usage by the working muscle and, therefore, an increase in oxygen demand. The increase in oxygen usage by the working muscles causes, for a short period of time, a large error signal between oxygen delivery to the tissues and oxygen usage by the tissues. Considering the entire cardiorespiratory system as a negative feedback system, this error signal is detected and command signals generated within the central nervous system bring about a response of many components of the system. All these various system responses operate to reduce the error signal, i.e., to increase oxygen delivery to the tissues to match the oxygen usage by the tissues.

Responses to the command signals include: (1) a reduction in the vascular resistance of the working muscle; (2) an increased pumping action by the heart with an increased cardiac contractility and an increase in heart rate; and (3) an increase in pulmonary ventilation. The remarkable aspect of this regulation is the strong relationship between exercise-induced demand for oxygen and the cardiovascular and ventilatory responses required to deliver the oxygen to the working tissues.

CARDIOVASCULAR RESPONSES TO EXERCISE

Cardiac Output ($\dot{Q}$). Cardiac output increases linearly with oxygen uptake ($\dot{V}O_2$) with a slope of 5 L/min per L/min $\dot{V}O_2$. Maximal recorded and believable cardiac output = 42 L/min (see Figure 1–6).

Stroke Volume (SV). This parameter decreases approximately 40% when an individual stands upright from supine rest. The heart (stimulated during exercise) in conjunction with the muscle pump returns the upright exercising stroke volume to a level equivalent to supine rest values rapidly, which then remains constant up to the level of $\dot{V}O_{2max}$ in moderately active individuals. Endurance-trained athletes, however, seem able to further increase stroke volume slightly at maximal effort. Athletes have very high resting and exercise stroke volumes (mechanism remains unknown). In general, cardiac disease reduces pump function and therefore stroke volume (Fig. 1–5).

Heart Rate (HR). The heart rate rises linearly with increasing rate of oxygen uptake. The slope of the rise in HR is inversely related to the individual's V_{O_2max}. Maximal heart rates range from 190 to 196 beats/min and depend on age ($220 - Age = HR_{max}$). The range of HR change during exercise is related to the resting heart rate. Some athletes have resting heart rates lower than 40 beats/min and therefore have a greater range than the unfit sedentary individual, who has a HR at rest of 70 to 80 beats/min.

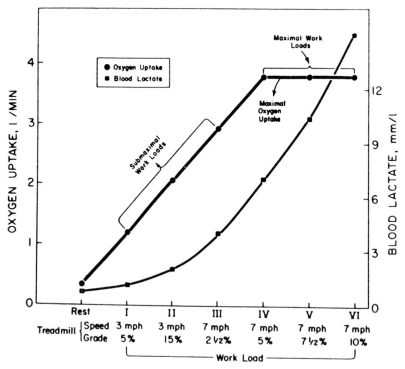

FIG. 1–5. Determination of maximal oxygen uptake in liters/minute on a motor-driven treadmill. (Reprinted with permission of the *New England Journal of Medicine* from Mitchell JH and Blomqvist G: Maximal oxygen uptake. *N Engl J Med* 284:1018–1022, 1971.)

Arteriovenous Oxygen Difference (a − $\bar{V}O_2$). This measures oxygen extraction of the working tissues; it widens with increasing overall rate of oxygen uptake. At rest, a − $\bar{V}O_2$ = 4 to 5 ml O_2/100 ml or 25% extraction; at $\dot{V}O_{2max}$, the arteriovenous oxygen difference increases to 15 to 17 ml/100 ml or 80 to 85% extraction (Fig. 1–6).

Regulation of the Cardiovascular Response to Exercise.

Heart Rate. The initial increase in heart rate with exercise from rest to 100 to 110 beats/min is primarily a result of vagal withdrawal; cardiac acceleration above 100 to 110 beats/min is predominantly due to increases in sympathetic activity (Fig. 1–7).

Stroke Volume. Changes in stroke volume are regulated by factors that are both extrinsic and intrinsic to the heart. The extrinsic factors are: (1) changes related to venous return or preload, which elicit the classic Frank-Starling mechanism, i.e., for an increase in end-diastolic volume there is an increase in stroke volume; (2) changes in afterload, i.e., systolic blood pressure. The intrinsic factors that affect stroke volume are those that alter contractility or inotropy. These are: (1) increases in heart rate increase calcium ion release, which increases contractility—Treppe effect; (2) increases in sympathetic drive via central command as feedback from the muscle or peripheral baroreceptors increase contractility; (3) general sympathetic activation resulting in release of epinephrine from the adrenal gland increases contractility.

Arterial Blood Pressure and Total Vascular Conductance. Arterial pulse (systolic BP-diastolic BP) increases with maximal exercise and this is primarily due to increasing systolic pressure (Fig. 1–8). Mean blood pressure rises only moderately (approximately 25 mm Hg). Conductance or blood flow through the working muscles rises directly with cardiac output. The increase in blood flow is brought about by increased cardiac output and preferential redistribution of blood flow to the working muscles and away from non-exercising areas (e.g., the splanchnic bed). This increase in blood flow is pulsated in phase with the muscle contraction through a dilated working muscle vascular bed (Fig. 1–9). Local released metabolites, particularly adenosine, result in vasodilation of the vessels of the muscle.

Systemic Arteriovenous Difference. Arterial O_2 content depends on hemoglobin concentration, O_2 binding capacity, alveolar PO_2, pulmonary diffusion capacity, and alveolar ventilation.

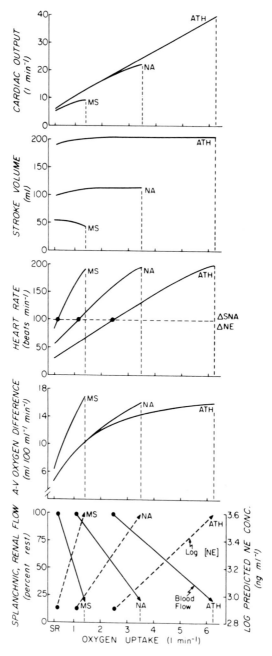

FIG. 1–6.

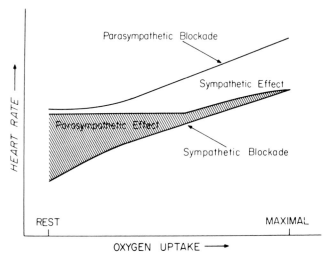

FIG. 1–7. Relative contribution of sympathetic and parasympathetic nervous systems to the rise in heart rate during exercise. The hatched region shows that the relative magnitude of vagal withdrawal (parasympathetic effect) predominates at low levels of exercise; the initial cardioacceleration is due almost entirely to this mechanism. At higher levels of exercise the sympathetic effect predominates (shown by open region). Comparisons were made from subjects with blockade of parasympathetics alone, sympathetics alone, and blockade of both. (Adapted from Robinson et al., 1966, In Rowell LB: *Human Circulation: Regulation during Physical Stress.* New York: Oxford University Press, 1986.)

FIG. 1–6. Representative cardiovascular responses to graded dynamic exercise in three groups of individuals whose levels of $\dot{V}o_2$ max are very low (patients with "pure" mitral stenosis [MS]), normal (normally active subjects [NA]), or very high (elite endurance athletes [Ath]). The four determinants of $\dot{V}o_2$ max are plotted versus oxygen uptake in the first four panels with vertical dashed lines at the end of each curve showing the $\dot{V}o_2$ max of each group. Note the marked differences in maximal cardiac outputs and stroke volumes and the similarity in maximal heart rates and systemic arteriovenous oxygen differences. In the third panel the dashed horizontal line at heart rate 100 and the solid circles show the points at which plasma norepinephrine concentration (ΔNE) and sympathetic nervous activity (ΔSNA) increase. These solid circles are transferred to the splanchnic and renal blood flow and the norepinephrine-oxygen uptake axes in the bottom panel. They show that in each group splanchnic and renal flows begin to fall when heart rate reaches 100 beats min^{-1}, and that plasma norepinephrine concentration also begins to rise rapidly at this heart rate. This panel shows that the three groups decrease regional flows and raise norepinephrine concentration similarly but over very different ranges of total oxygen uptake. (From Rowell LB: *Human Circulation: Regulation during Physical Stress.* New York: Oxford University Press, 1986.)

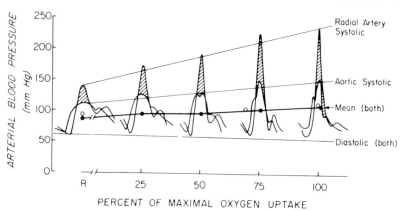

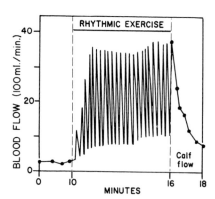

FIG. 1–8. Simultaneously measured radial arterial and aortic pressure during rest (R) and upright exercise. Note the similarities in mean aortic pressure at a given percent of $\dot{V}O_{2max}$ from two studies on subjects whose absolute values of $\dot{V}O_{2max}$ varied widely (Åstrand et al., 1964, open circles; Rowell et al., 1968, closed circles). Peripheral wave amplification caused large increases in radial arterial pulse pressure. Pressure wave forms were traced from direct simultaneous recordings from a representative subject (Rowell et al., 1968. In Rowell LB: *Human Circulation: Regulation during Physical Stress.* New York: Oxford University Press, 1986.)

FIG. 1–9. Effects of muscle exercise on blood flow in the calf of a leg during strong rhythmic contraction. The blood flow was much less during contraction than between contractions. (From Barcroft and Dornhorst: *J Physiol 109*:402, 1949.)

Arterial O_2 content is well maintained during exercise, although saturation may drop from 96 to 93% because of the Bohr effect (rightward shift of O_2/desaturation curve) due to a decrease in pH and an increased temperature. Hemoglobin concentration, and hence its effective O_2 carrying capacity, rises 10% because of fluid shifts out of the vascular compartment. Venous O_2 content decreases to approximately 2 ml/100 ml in venous blood draining from the active musculature, whereas mixed venous blood may decrease to 3 or 4 ml/100 ml. This is due to increased O_2 extraction by the working muscle and regional vasoconstriction of resting organs.

Abnormal Cardiovascular Responses. Typical values at $\dot{V}_{O_{2max}}$ for a young, normal sedentary subject, a champion long-distance runner, and a patient with moderately severe left ventricular heart disease are shown in Fig. 1–10. The reduction in stroke volume with heart disease during submaximal and maximal workloads was probably due to a decreased ability of the myocardium to

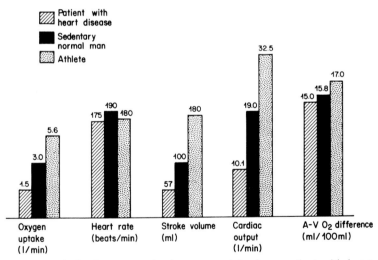

FIG. 1—10. Typical values at maximal oxygen uptake for a patient with heart disease, a sedentary normal man, and an endurance athlete. (Reprinted with permission from Blomqvist G: Exercise physiology related to diagnosis of coronary artery disease. In *Coronary Heart Disease: Prevention, Detection, Rehabilitation with Emphasis on Exercise Testing* Edited by SM Fox III. Denver: Department of Professional Education, International Medical Corporation, 1974, pp. 2-1 through 2-26.)

contract during systole. The ejection fraction (EF), which is the ratio of the stroke volume (SV) to the end-diastolic volume (EDV),

$$EF = SV/EDV \times 100$$

increases during exercise in normal subjects because of a decreased end-systolic volume and an increased end-diastolic volume. In patients with heart disease, the ejection fraction decreases during submaximal exercise because of significant increases in end-systolic volume.

VENTILATORY RESPONSES TO EXERCISE

Ventilation volume ($\dot{V}$) is the amount of air passing in and out of the lungs in 1 minute. Physiologically the inspired minute volumes ($\dot{V}_I$) equal the expired minute volume ($\dot{V}_E$). Because of gas exchange at the alveolar surfaces measured, $\dot{V}_I$ does not equal $\dot{V}_E$, yet corrections can be made to account for these differences. $\dot{V}_E$ is expressed in liters of air (L/min). Because the volume of a given amount of gas is related to environmental conditions (Charles' and Boyle's gas laws), ventilatory volumes must be "corrected" to indicate the volume of the air under standardized conditions. Ventilatory volumes are usually corrected to either BTPS (body temperature and pressure, saturated with water vapor) or STPD (standard temperature 0° C) and pressure (760 mm Hg), dry). The STPD convention is employed when minute ventilation ($\dot{V}_E$) is to be used with respiratory gas analysis in the measurement of oxygen uptake.

Ventilation volume per minute ($\dot{V}_E$) increases linearly with increasing rate of oxygen uptake (1 L O_2/min uptake = 25 L/min $\dot{V}_E$) until approximately 50 to 70% $\dot{V}O_{2max}$. At this point, ventilation increases exponentially and 1 L O_2/min uptake = 35 L/min $\dot{V}_E$ (Fig. 1–11). Tidal volume (V_T) increases linearly with increasing workload up to two thirds of the vital capacity and then levels off as the workload increases up to maximum. Respiratory rate (RR) increases linearly with increasing workload up to a maximum rate of 35 to 50 breaths/min at maximal work at sea level altitude. The ventilatory response is the primary determinant of arterial blood gas and acid-base status during exercise.

Maximal ventilatory capacity is measured as the maximal voluntary ventilation (MVV) in 15 seconds ($MVV_{.25}$) expressed as liters/minute. Individual $MVV_{.25}$ ranges from 160 to 260 L/min depending on the size of the individual and respiratory muscle fitness.

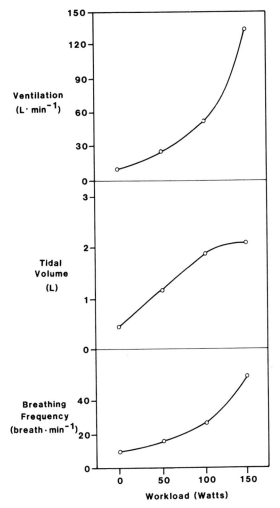

FIG. 1–11. Ventilatory responses to graded exercise. (From American College of Sports Medicine: *Resource Manual for Guidelines for Exercise Testing and Prescription.* Philadelphia: Lea & Febiger, 1986.)

Maximal exercise expired ventilation volumes ($\dot{V}_{Emax}$) range from 100 to 170 L/min (BTPS). In normal, healthy individuals, exercise exhaustion usually occurs at a $\dot{V}_E$ of approximately 70% of $MVV_{.25}$ (or $\dot{V}_{Emax}/MVV_{.25} = 70\%$). In some highly fit individuals, however, exercise exhaustion may occur at $\dot{V}_{Emax} = 90\%$.

Ventilatory Threshold. As noted previously (see Fig. 1–11), ventilation at higher intensities of exercise increases exponentially with increasing power output. The workload (or rate of oxygen consumption) at which the ventilatory response to graded exercise first departs from linearity is the ventilatory threshold (VT). Although the physiologic mechanism that underlies VT remains a matter of debate, VT occurs at a work rate that corresponds closely to the intensity at which lactic acid begins to accumulate in the blood. The rapid increase in ventilation that occurs at exercise intensities about VT may be a result of the bicarbonate buffer system that helps to maintain blood pH by buffering within the blood nonmetabolically produced carbon dioxide, and then via transportation to the lung excreting the excess carbon dioxide at the lung.

Most individuals who exercise regularly are able to perceive VT as the exercise intensity at which breathing becomes somewhat labored and talking becomes difficult. Because VT and blood lactic acid accumulation occur at similar exercise intensities in most persons, VT provides a convenient marker for the upper end of the exercise intensity range usually applied in "aerobic" training programs. At exercise intensities above VT, rapid accumulation of lactic acid in the muscle and blood result in cessation of exercise. Thus, prescribed aerobic exercise programs often employ an exercise intensity below VT.

ADAPTATIONS TO EXERCISE TRAINING

AEROBIC TRAINING

Exercise training significantly improves the oxygen transport system and increases $\dot{V}O_{2max}$ by increasing both the maximal cardiac output and the maximal arteriovenous oxygen difference. This change occurs primarily by improvements in central circulation and cardiac function, peripheral circulation, and skeletal muscle metabolism.

Pulmonary System. In the untrained individual, arterial oxygen tension is maintained at maximal workloads, demonstrating that pulmonary factors do not limit oxygen transport in normal individuals. Unfortunately, maximal oxygen transport through the lungs is not significantly improved by endurance training. Furthermore, in the untrained individual, the capacity for oxygen transport by respiration is greater than that by circulation. This mismatch is dramatically reduced, however, as the level of exercise training improves the cardiovascular capacity for oxygen transport. Oxygen saturation and content may begin to decrease near maximal work in elite endurance athletes. Therefore, it appears that in some elite athletes the pulmonary system may contribute to the limitation of $\dot{V}O_{2max}$ by reducing the amount of oxygen carried by the blood.

Cardiac Function and Central Circulation. Resting cardiac output is not altered, but maximal cardiac output can be twice as large in a well-trained endurance athlete as in an untrained subject of the same body size (Table 1–2). The ability of an individual to achieve a high maximal cardiac output is probably related to genetic factors and to a prolonged period of endurance training. Maximal heart rate is not affected by endurance training and is usually the same in highly trained athletes as in untrained subjects. The higher maximal cardiac outputs are exclusively a result of the heart's ability to eject a larger maximal stroke volume. The increased maximal stroke volume is a result of the following: (1) cardiac dimensions are increased; and (2) endurance-trained athletes have a significantly greater absolute left ventricular mass (eccentric hypertrophy) normalized to lean body mass than sedentary subjects. In addition, endurance training alters autonomic function, preload, and afterload. An augmented preload independently produces an increase in stroke volume by the Frank-Starling mechanism. Evidence suggests that preload is increased after endurance training by an increase in total blood volume consequent to an increase in plasma volume. In addition, the effective left ventricular diastolic compliance may be increased after endurance training, which also would enhance submaximal or maximal preload.

TABLE 1–2. Changes in Cardiovascular Variables Due to Endurance Exercise Training

Variables	Resting	Maximal Exercise
Oxygen consumption	No change	Increase
Cardiac output	Not clear	Not clear
Contractility	Not clear	Not clear
Heart rate	Decrease	No change
Stroke volume	Increase	Increase
Muscle blood flow	No change	Increase
Oxygen extraction	No change	Increase
Ventilation	No change	No change

(From the American College of Sports Medicine: *Resource Manual for Guidelines for Exercise Testing and Prescription.* Philadelphia: Lea & Febiger, 1986.)

Endurance-trained individuals have a reduced heart rate at rest and at any given level of submaximal exercise. The rising sinus bradycardia is attributable to a shift of autonomic balance in favor of the parasympathetic nervous system and a decrease in intrinsic heart rate, which is the rate obtained with complete blockade of the autonomic nervous system. Cardiac output is not significantly changed at submaximal workloads by endurance training; therefore, stroke volume is elevated at all levels of submaximal work. The changes in heart rate and stroke volume improve "efficiency" of the heart at submaximal workloads. The effect of endurance training on ventricular performance or contractility is far less certain. At maximal exercise little is gained from enhanced contractility. The enhanced preload, decreased afterload, and unaltered or slightly augmented contractility result in a dramatically increased maximal stroke volume.

Peripheral Vascular Resistance and Tissue Oxygen Extraction. Endurance training is associated with a reduction in total peripheral resistance, or afterload, during exercise. This reduction in peripheral resistance is a result of an increase in vascularity and enables the endurance athlete to achieve levels of cardiac output double those of a sedentary subject at similar arterial pressures during maximal exercise. The maximal tissue oxygen extraction (arte-

TABLE 1–3. Skeletal Muscle Adaptations to Training

Properties of Muscle	Type of Training		
	Endurance	Sprint	Strength
Fiber composition	+?*	+?	0?
Fiber area	0	+, −, 0	+
Enzyme activities			
Krebs cycle	+ + +	+ +	+, −, 0
Fatty acids	+ +	+	0
Glycolytic	+, −, 0 (type I)	+	+, 0
Myosin ATPase	+?	+?	0
Substrate storage			
ATP/CP	+	+	0
Glycogen	+	+, 0	0
Myoglobin content	+?	+?	0
Mitochondrial number	+ +	+	0
Capillary density	+	0?	0

* Symbols indicate relative changes: +, + +, + + + = small, medium, and large increases; − = decrease; 0 = no change; ? = unknown.

riovenous oxygen difference) increases after endurance training. This effect is brought about by an increase in the diffusion gradient for oxygen between the capillaries and the active skeletal muscle cells and the total myoglobin content of trained muscle. These changes within the skeletal muscle tissue enhance the diffusion capacity of oxygen at the tissue level. In addition, tissue oxygen extraction within the active muscle is enhanced by the increased capillary density that occurs with endurance training. The total number and the density (total number per gram of tissue) of capillaries increase. The increased capillary density results in an increased capillary diffusion surface area, which is advantageous for nutrient and metabolic byproduct exchange. The arterial tree also increases as a result of the opening of dormant collateral vessels. Endurance training also increases the degree of shunting of blood away from the splanchnic and renal circulations at maximal exercise. These changes improve redistribution of blood flow during exercise and act in concert with the increased tissue extraction to augment total body arteriovenous oxygen difference.

SKELETAL MUSCLE

The specific adaptations that occur within the skeletal muscle depend on the frequency, duration, and intensity of the contractions or on the amount of overload imparted for the specific action. Skeletal muscle adaptations to endurance, sprint, and weight training are summarized in Table 1–3.

Endurance Training. The general effects of endurance training are enhanced skeletal muscle oxidative capacity resulting in improvements in endurance performance, increased fatty acid utilization, and decreased glycogen utilization during prolonged exercise. Presumably, with an increased oxidative potential, less of a disturbance in homeostasis occurs for a given level of work, minimizing the accumulation of adenosine diphosphate (ADP) and activation of glycolysis, thereby sparing glycogen and enhancing fat utilization. Furthermore, the enhanced oxidative capacity of type I and type IIa fibers allows more work to be done before anaerobic glycolysis and type IIb fiber recruitment are required, minimizing or delaying the onset of lactic acid accumulation.

Sprint Training. Sprint training induces changes in enzymatic activities in skeletal muscle similar to those observed with endurance training (Table 1–3).

A change in fiber-type contractile properties can occur with sprint training. Repeated bouts of exercise at 90 to 100% of $\dot{V}O_{2max}$ can produce a decrease in the proportion of type I fibers and an increase in the proportion of type IIc fibers. Similar results were reported when endurance athletes were placed on an "anaerobic" training program, and a decrease in type I myofiber twitch time was observed after high-intensity training.

Strength Training. The primary adaptation of skeletal muscle to strength training is an increase in muscle bulk that results from hypertrophy of existing fibers. The cross-sectional area of the trained fibers, primarily the type IIa fibers, increases to accommodate additional sarcomeres formed parallel to the existing myofibrils. Fiber type conversion does not appear to occur. The contractility of the fibers, i.e., the maximal tension produced per square millimeter of muscle tissue and per crossbridge interaction, is not altered by strength training. In general, the overall gain in strength is proportional to the increase in cross-sectional area of the muscle. In the early stages of training, however, strength may increase more rapidly than muscle bulk because of increased motor unit recruitment and coordination. In addition, muscle bulk may increase more than strength if hypertrophy alters the attachment angle to bone and reduces the mechanical advantage of the lever arm. The cross-sectional area and strength of connective tissue also increase in response to muscle overload and strength training. Little or no change in muscle enzyme activities occurs with strength training. Traditional high-resistance isotonic training regimens do not appear to enhance oxidative or glycolytic enzyme activities.

LIGAMENTS AND BONE

More and more information is being obtained on the effects of endurance, sprint, and strength training on mineralized tissues (ligaments, bones, and cartilage). In all cases weight-bearing activities increase tensile strength and thickness of the specific tissues. Obviously, training of these tissues occurs in consort with skeletal muscle.

DETRAINING

When physical training ceases (i.e., detraining), the adaptations readjust backward as a result of the decreased training stimulus. In other words, many training-induced adaptations are reversed. The evidence suggests that the increases in $\dot{V}_{O_{2}max}$ produced by endurance training of low to moderate intensities and durations are totally reversed after several months of detraining. When people detrain after several years of intense training, they display large reductions (i.e., 5 to 15%) in stroke volume and $\dot{V}_{O_{2}max}$ during the first 12 to 21 days of inactivity. These declines do not indicate a deterioration of heart function, but instead are largely a result of reduced blood volume and the ability to return venous blood to the heart. The $\dot{V}_{O_{2}max}$ of endurance athletes continues to decline during the 21 to 56 days of detraining because of reductions in maximal arteriovenous O_2 difference. These reductions are associated with a loss of mitochondrial enzyme activity within the trained musculature, which declines with a half-time of approximately 12 days.

Well-trained endurance athletes, however, do not regress to levels displayed by individuals who never participated in exercise training. Levels of mitochondrial enzyme activity remain 50% higher than those in sedentary subjects, skeletal muscle capillarization is maintained at high levels, and $\dot{V}_{O_{2}max}$ and the maximal arteriovenous O_2 difference stabilize at a point 12 to 17% higher than untrained levels after 84 days of detraining. Whether this superior level of physiological function is maintained with continued detraining is not known. Similar detraining effects of the sprint- or weight-trained athlete are suspected, although relatively little information concerning the time of detraining effects is available.

CHAPTER 2

METABOLIC RESPONSE TO EXERCISE

George A. Brooks

The metabolic response to exercise is governed primarily by factors of intensity and duration. Superimposed on these, factors of training, immediate exercise and nutritional history, and environment play roles of secondary importance.

PRIMARY FACTORS

Intensity. For steady-state exercise, the O_2 consumption response is a linear function of power output (Fig. 2–1). Using the steady-state assumption that the O_2 consumption response represents the metabolic response to exercise, it is possible to conclude that the metabolic response to exercise is tightly coupled to the exercise power output. From the slope of the $\dot{V}O_2$-power relationship, the efficiency of muscular exercise can be estimated to be approximately 25%.

Based on urinary nitrogen and respiratory gas-exchange measurements ($R = \dot{V}CO_2/\dot{V}O_2$), it is estimated that in resting, postabsorptive individuals, amino acids supply 5 to 10% of energy to support metabolic processes, whereas a balance of carbohydrate (CHO) and lipid-derived fuels supply most of the remainder (Fig. 2–2). In the transition from rest to exercise, an immediate shift in the direction of carbohydrate-derived energy sources and a suppression of lipid utilization occur (Fig. 2–2A). Further, as exercise intensity progresses to maximum, dependency on carbohydrate increases. Thus, carbohydrate-derived fuels represent the main and essential sources of potential energy to support physical exercise.

Duration. Over the course of an exercise task at a given power output, the balance of substrate supplies change. As exercise progresses, the initial dependency on carbohydrate (muscle glyco-

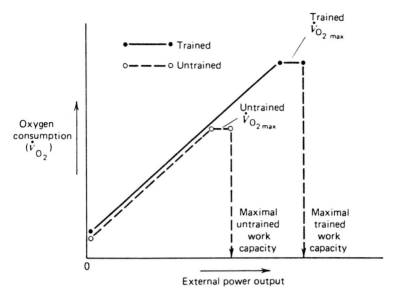

FIG. 2–1. Relationship between oxygen consumption ($\dot{V}O_2$) and external work rate (power output). In response to increments in power output, both trained and untrained individuals respond with an increase in $\dot{V}O_2$. The greater ability of trained individuals to sustain a high power output is largely due to a greater maximal O_2 consumption ($\dot{V}O_{2max}$). (Reprinted with permission of Macmillan Publishing Company from Brooks GA and Fahey TD: Fundamentals of Human Performance. New York: Macmillan, 1987. Copyright 1987 by Macmillan Publishing Company.)

gen) wanes and other substrates increase in importance. The fall in respiratory gas-exchange ratio (R) over time indicates an increasing utilization of blood-borne free fatty acids and intramuscular triglycerides. This shift is generally viewed as desirable because it retards the rate of muscle glycogen depletion and protects blood glucose homeostasis. Because the overall carbohydrate dependency remains, however, sustained exercise eventually results in muscle glycogen depletion and fatigue.

SECONDARY FACTORS

Training. Prior endurance training results in numerous peripheral (muscular) adaptations that increase the ability to utilize all energy sources, including lipids. The shift toward greater

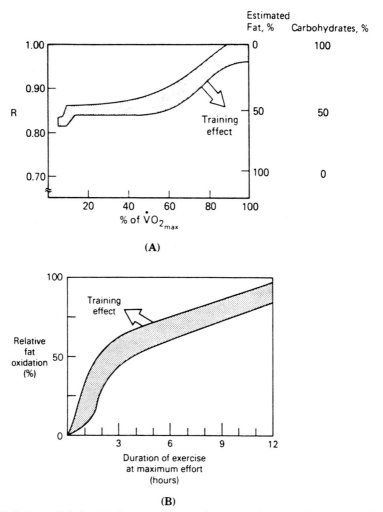

FIG. 2–2. A, Relationship between the ventilatory respiratory exchange ratio (R = $\dot{V}_{CO_2}/\dot{V}_{O_2}$) and relative exercise intensity in well-nourished individuals. Utilization of fat and carbohydrate can be estimated from the R. As relative exercise intensity increases, the proportional use of carbohydrate increases. Training shifts the curve to the right. (Based on tables of Zuntz and Schumberg and other sources.) B, Relationship between the relative utilization of fat and the duration of exercise. The utilization of fat was estimated from the R. As exercise duration increases, the relative utilization of fat increases. Training shifts the curve to the left. (Reprinted with permission of Macmillan Publishing Company from Brooks GA and Fahey TD: Fundamentals of Human Performance. New York: Macmillan, 1987. Copyright 1987 by Macmillan Publishing Company.)

lipid utilization is indicated by the arrows in Figure 2–2. The biochemical basis for this shift is the induction of a greater muscle mitochondrial mass. Superior mitochondrial respiratory control afforded by a larger mitochondrial reticulum (discussed later) allows a higher ATP/ADP ratio to be maintained within working muscle (Fig. 2–3). The higher ATP/ADP ratio serves to down-regulate phosphofructokinase and other enzymes of the glycolytic pathway, allowing increased oxidative utilization of lipid-derived energy sources.

Rest to Exercise Transition. The transition between resting and exercise steady states poses regulatory challenges. Similarly, exercises requiring maximal power output stress the muscles' capacity for energy transduction. Usually, the rest-exercise transition and all-out performance are understood in terms of the ability of skeletal muscle to be sustained by immediate, nonoxidative, and oxidative energy sources (Fig. 2–4).

Immediate Energy Sources. Adenosine triphosphate (ATP) and creatinine phosphate (CP) are high-energy energy storage forms in muscle cells. Adenosine triphosphate is used directly in the contraction process, and CP is used as the immediate source to restore ADP (the degradation product) to ATP. In turn, CP must be

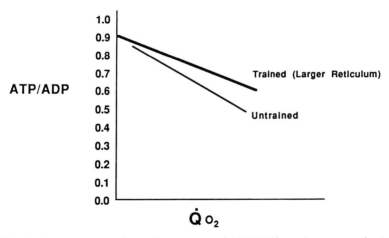

FIG. 2–3. Improvement in respiratory control (ATP/ADP) at given rates of mitochondrial O_2 consumption ($\dot{Q}_{O_2}$) associated with increasing the mitochondrial mass.

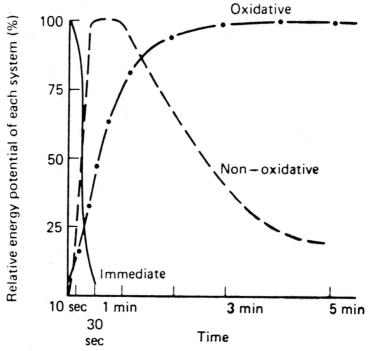

FIG. 2–4. Energy sources for muscle as a function of activity duration. Schematic presentation showing how long each of the major energy systems can endure in supporting all-out work. (Reprinted with permission of Macmillan Publishing Company from Brooks GA and Fahey TD: Fundamentals of Human Performance. New York: Macmillan, 1987. Copyright 1987 by Macmillan Publishing Company.)

restored by the nonoxidative and oxidative energy systems. Cellular reserves of ATP and CP are relatively small, and they are quantitatively insufficient (10 calories) to sustain intense activity for more than a few seconds. Therefore, the nonoxidative energy system provides the first backup mechanism to restore the high-energy phosphates used in contraction.

Not only is the energy capacity of the immediate energy sources and their related enzymes small, but also the capacity of this energy source does not appear to respond well to training. Although there is some controversy on the subject, it appears that if muscle cells increase the concentration of ATP and CP energy storage forms through training, the magnitude of change is small. An improvement in muscle mass through training is the most feasible means to increase stored levels of high-energy phosphates.

MUSCLE ENERGETICS

"Nonoxidative" Energy System.

The nonoxidative pathway involves the intracellular breakdown of stored carbohydrate (glycogen) and the use of blood sugar (glucose). The nonoxidative energy system is, then, comprised of two metabolic (enzymatic) pathways: (1) glycogenolysis, the degradation of glycogen; and (2) glycolysis, the dissolution of sugar. Sometimes these pathways are mistakenly termed "anaerobic." The nonoxidative energy system involves the conversion of muscle carbohydrate and sugar to lactic acid. The accumulation of lactic acid can cause sensations of distress and interfere with muscle contraction. Lactic acid accumulation from rapid glycogenolysis and glycolysis is, therefore, one of the causes of muscle fatigue.

The capacity of nonoxidative energy system approximates 15 calories. This value exceeds that of the immediate energy sources, but the difference is not all that great. As suggested in Figure 2-4, the nonoxidative pathways can sustain activities lasting from a few seconds to approximately 1 minute. Power activities are heavily dependent on the nonoxidative energy system. Lactic acid will be an inevitable product of this energy system, and so the performer must learn to tolerate and dispose of accumulated lactic acid. Issues of lactic acid metabolism will be discussed more thoroughly later in this chapter.

Enhancement of the capacity of nonoxidative energy systems is usually addressed by intense, interval training. In response to endurance training the levels of oxidative enzymes and cellular components of oxygen use will double. Training has not yet been shown to increase the levels of glycolytic or glycogenolytic enzymes, however, but probably enhances the capacity of nonoxidative energy metabolism by improving tissue oxidative capacity and blood flow so acidic products of contraction can be cleared.

In summary of the immediate and nonoxidative (anaerobic) energy systems, the following need to be emphasized. These mechanisms represent essential energy sources to sustain rapid and powerful muscular contractions as well as to make the transition from rest to submaximal exercise. The energy capacity of these pathways is limited, however, and recovery is an aerobic (oxidative) process.

Oxidative Energy System. As indicated in Figure 2–4, sustained muscular activity depends on oxidative metabolism. Energy capacity of the oxidative system not only far exceeds those of the nonoxidative systems, but oxidative metabolism also allows recovery of the immediate and nonoxidative energy sources. We can simplify our approach to describing the oxidative energy system by segmenting it into two components. The cardiovascular system transports oxygen to working muscle. The mitochondrial reticulum in skeletal muscle utilizes oxygen to restore ATP (and CP) degraded as the result of muscle contraction.

Mitochondrial Bases of Energy Transduction. Mitochondria are the cellular organelles in which the great preponderance of adenosine triphosphate (ATP) is produced from the combination of inorganic phosphate (Pi) and adenosine diphosphate (ADP). This combination (synthesis) involves the utilization of O_2. Traditionally, the mitochondria in muscle and other tissues were believed to be discrete, capsule-shaped organelles. Within muscle cells, mitochondria have been observed in two general regions: (1) immediately beneath the cell surface (i.e., the subsarcolemmal mitochondria); and (2) deep within the cell, among the contractile elements (i.e., the interfibrillar mitochondria) (Kirkwood et al., 1987; Brooks and Fahey, 1984). Serial sectioning of skeletal muscle and examination of mitochondria within individual muscle fibers (cells), however, indicate that the mitochondria interconnect to form a network, or reticulum (Kirkwood et al., 1986, 1987; Brooks and Fahey, 1984). This arrangement of the cell's oxidative machinery in a mitochondrial reticulum (as opposed to discrete units) favors the transport of O_2 and fuels of combustion from the muscle cell surface to the interfibrillar sites of utilization. Further, according to the chemiosmotic theory of oxidative phosphorylation, the presence of a mitochondrial reticulum allows for the cellular energy charge to be more evenly maintained, even when high rates of ATP utilization occur deep within muscle fibers during exercise.

The proliferation of mitochondrial material within muscle cells is induced by prolonged endurance exercise training (Holloszy, 1967; Davies et al., 1981). On the other hand, sprint training provides a minimal stimulus for mitochondrial proliferation (Davies et al., 1982). Results of some studies on laboratory animals indicate that the muscular content of mitochondrial enzymes doubles in response to endurance training. This large increase in muscle mitochondrial mass allows greater rates of combustion of derivatives of carbohydrates, fats, and amino acids in muscles of trained individuals. Further, mitochondrial proliferation allows pyruvic acid to be removed without incurring the accumulation of large amounts of lactic acid (described later).

Limits of Oxygen Utilization. The ability to transport O_2 from sites of pulmonary consumption to tissue mitochondrial utilization depends on the capacity of the cardiovascular system. Given that circulatory O_2 transport capacity (T_{O_2}) depends on the product of arterial O_2 content (Ca_{O_2}) and cardiac output ($\dot{Q}$) [$T_{O_2} = (Ca_{O_2})(\dot{Q})$], and that Ca_{O_2} is unaffected by training, then T_{O_2} depends on the maximal cardiac output.

Because the maximal capacity to transport oxygen (T_{O_2}) is determined by cardiac output, the maximal rate at which oxygen can be used is also related to cardiac output, not surprisingly. In cross-sectional studies on human subjects, the direct relationship between $\dot{V}_{O_{2max}}$ and $\dot{Q}_{max}$ is clearly seen (Brooks and Fahey, 1984). These factors are covered in other sections of this work.

Exercise Substrates. Muscle glycogen represents the major exercise fuel source. The precursor to muscle glycogen synthesis is blood glucose, and it is well documented that an individual's activity and nutritional history determine the muscle glycogen content. Under aerobic conditions, glycogen breaks down during contraction with the end products being pyruvate (for intracellular oxidation) and lactate, which represents a metabolic intermediate for exchange among tissues (described later).

Blood glucose represents another major carbohydrate energy source for exercise. By comparison with muscle glycogen reserves, however, the blood glucose (and liver glycogen) pool is small, and its rate of use increases relatively little during exercise. For instance, resting blood glucose turnover approximates 1.8 mg/kg/min. This will double during exercise to 50% $\dot{V}_{O_2}$ max, but the rates of O_2 consumption and total carbohydrate combustion may increase 10 and 15 times, respectively.

It is now becoming recognized that through the "lactate shuttle" mechanism the body possesses a previously unknown means of distributing carbohydrate energy sources. Under the influences of epinephrine and contraction-induced factors, the rate of intracellular glycogen catabolism exceeds the rate of pyruvate entry into the mitochondrial oxidative pathways. The excess glycolytic flux is converted to lactate, which represents a metabolic intermediate that can be released into the interstitium and vasculature. By this means of shuttling through the extracellular lactate pool, glycogen reserves in particular cells and tissues become available for utilization as fuel at anatomically distributed sites and gluconeogenic precursors in the liver and kidneys.

The uptake of free fatty acids from the blood by contracting muscle depends on arterial concentration, blood flow, capillarity, and mitochondrial density. For these reasons, highly perfused cells containing an elaborate mitochondrial reticulum possess advantages in terms of lipid utilization during exercise. Muscle glucose uptake increases during exercise, but circulating insulin falls. The fall in insulin is thought to restrain an exercise-induced *rise in blood glucose utilization*, thereby leaving sufficient glucose available for CNS function. Recent studies have indicated that contracting muscle possesses insulin-independent mechanisms of glucose uptake, which, along with the insulin-mediated mechanisms, direct blood glucose reserves to the active musculature.

So far as is known, muscle lactic acid uptake is not mediated by insulin or any other factor. Lactic acid uptake is mediated through a lactic acid carrier protein that is sensitive to concentration and hydrogen ion gradients. Thus, lactate exchange is from high to low concentration and from low to high pH. This orientation promotes the shuttling of lactic acid from production to removal sites.

Endocrine Factors. During exercise insulin falls, whereas glucagon and catecholamines rise. These changes promote hepatic glycogenolysis and gluconeogenesis as well as muscle glycogenolysis. Thus, the endocrine response to exercise can be viewed as one to spare blood glucose by directing it to active tissues and to those with essential glucose requirements, maintaining blood glucose concentration (through glycogenolysis and gluconeogenesis), and providing alternatives to blood glucose (lactate and free fatty acids).

Mobilization of Lipid Energy Stores. Adipose triglycerides are mobilized by elevations in circulating epinephrine and growth hormone and by a fall in the insulin/glucagon ratio. A fall in the insulin/glucagon ratio also is thought to be important in the activation of the type H, lipoprotein lipase that causes hydrolysis of intramuscular triglycerides. Mobilization of both blood-borne and intramuscular lipids results in a coordinated physiologic response to sustained exercise.

SUMMARY

The oxygen consumption response during exercise is tightly coupled to the exercise power output. In contrast, glycolytic carbon flux can be regulated over a wide range to supply oxidizable substrates with cells, as well as to provide material (lactate) in the circulation. In this way a source of fuel and a gluconeogenic precursor can be shared among cells and tissues. Endurance exercise training causes a proliferation of the mitochondrial reticulum. A greater muscle mitochondrial mass increases the sensitivity of respiratory control ($\uparrow$ ATP/ADP) during high rates of O_2 consumption. An effect of better respiratory control is a retardation of the glycolytic rate and a sparing of muscle glycogen. Because carbohydrate-derived energy sources represent the main substrates for exercise, retardation of glycogen usage through use of alternatives (mainly lipids) increases the time that submaximal exercise can be endured.

RECOMMENDED READING

Blomqvist CG and Saltin B: Cardiovascular adaptations to physical training. *Annu Rev Physiol* 45:169–189, 1983.

Brooks GA: Lactate: Glycolytic end product and oxidative substrate during sustained exercise in mammals—The "lactate shuttle." In *Comparative Physiology and Biochemistry—Current Topics and Trends*, Vol. A: Respiration-Metabolism-Circulation. Edited by R Gilles. New York, Springer-Verlag, 1985, pp. 208–218.

Brooks GA and Fahey TD: *Exercise Physiology: Human Bioenergetics and Its Applications.* New York: Macmillan, 1984.

Davies KJA, Packer L, and Brooks GA: Biochemical adaptation of mitochondria, muscle, and whole animal respiration to endurance training. *Arch Biochem Biophys* 209:539–559, 1981

Davies KJA, Packer L, and Brooks GA: Exercise bioenergetics following sprint training. *Arch Biochem Biophys* 215:260–265, 1982.

Holloszy JO: Biochemical adaptations in muscle. *J Biol Chem* 242:2278–2282, 1967.

Hultman E: Physiological role of muscle glycogen in man, with special reference to exercise. In *Physiology of Muscular Exercise*. Monograph 15. New York: American Heart Association, 1967, pp. I99–I112.

Kirkwood SP, Munn EA and Brooks GA: Mitochondrial reticulum in skeletal muscle. *Am J Physiol* (Cell Physiol) 20:C395–C402, 1986.

Kirkwood SP, Packer L and Brooks GA: Effects of endurance training on a mitochondrial reticulum in limb skeletal muscle. *Arch Biochem Biophys* 255:80–88, 1987.

Mazzeo RS, Brooks GA, Schoeller DA and Budinger TF: Disposal of [1-^{13}C]-lactate during rest and exercise. *J Appl Physiol* 60:232–241, 1986.

Scheuer J and Tipton CM: Cardiovascular adaptations to physical training. *Annu Rev Physiol* 39:221–251, 1977

Stanley WC, Wisneski JA, Gertz EW, Neese RA and Brooks GA: Glucose and lactate interrelations during moderate intensity exercise in man. *Metabolism* 37:850–858, 1988.

C H A P T E R 3

TRAINING FOR SPORT*

Brian J. Sharkey

Sports conditioning or training has been described as a gentle pastime in which we coax subtle changes from the body. This chapter presents proved physiologic principles and practices that help athletes achieve improvements in performance while avoiding overuse injuries and illness. It outlines steps for the development of energy sources and pathways (energy fitness) and provides prescriptions for the achievement of muscular fitness. It also includes important principles of training so you can understand the bases on which successful programs are constructed.

Training Principle #1: Adaptation
Training induces subtle changes as the body adapts to added demands. Day-to-day changes are often so small as to be unmeasurable. It takes weeks, months, and years of patient work to achieve high levels of performance. Rush the process and you risk injury, illness, or both. Many adaptations to training are reversible when training stops.

Energy fitness involves the ability to store and use fuels to power muscular contractions. I use the term energy fitness to describe the training of specific aerobic and anaerobic energy systems and to focus on the target organ of training, *skeletal muscle*.

Muscular fitness includes flexibility, strength, muscular endurance, power, and speed. It also involves the nervous system that controls muscular contractions, so muscular fitness training cannot be separated from neuromuscular or skill training. When training programs are properly developed, they follow the principle of specificity, so energy and muscular fitness support the skills involved in the sport.

---

*Adapted with permission of the publisher from Sharkey BJ: Fitness for sport. In *Successful Coaching* by R Martens. Champaign, IL: Human Kinetics, 1990.

Training Principle #2: Specificity
The adaptations to training are specific in regard to muscle fibers, energy pathways, and the mode of training. Endurance training develops aerobic enzymes and pathways, with little effect on strength. Strength training leads to increases in contractile protein, with little effect on aerobic fitness. You get what you train for. (Of course, every rule has an exception. Specificity does not mean one should avoid training opposite, adjacent, or accessory muscles. Other muscles should be trained to avoid imbalances that predispose the athlete to injury.)

ENERGY FITNESS

Energy fitness is the ability to store and use fuels efficiently to provide the power for muscular contractions. It also involves important adaptations in supply and support systems (respiratory, cardiovascular, hormonal) that deliver oxygen and fuels to muscles and carry off carbon dioxide and other wastes. To achieve energy fitness it is important to know the major energy pathways used in the sport, how muscles use the energy available to them, and how to avoid the inefficient use that hastens fatigue.

ENERGY PATHWAYS

The energy muscles use to contract comes from two pathways: aerobic (with oxygen) and anaerobic (without oxygen). Which pathway is used depends on several factors. Anaerobic energy sources are used at the beginning of exercise, before the respiration and circulation adjust to the effort and supply oxygen to the muscles. Most of the energy comes from carbohydrate (glycogen) stored in the muscles. Aerobic sources are used for steady-state efforts, such as running, with most of the energy coming from the oxidation of fat and carbohydrate (and some coming from the metabolism of protein). In low-intensity effort fat is the principal fuel, but as intensity increases, stored glycogen becomes the major source of energy. When the activity becomes very intense and the energy demands outstrip the ability of the aerobic or oxidative pathways, some of the energy for muscular contractions comes from the anaerobic or nonoxidative breakdown of muscle's glycogen to lactic acid.

Fueling muscles anaerobically is a less efficient way to use energy than using the aerobic pathway. For example, when muscle glycogen is used aerobically, it produces 39 molecules of energy in the form of high-energy adenosine triphosphate (ATP). When glycogen is used anaerobically it only produces 3 ATP molecules. Furthermore, the inefficient anaerobic pathway produces more lactic acid, a metabolic intermediate that can interfere with the contractile process and hinder energy production, causing fatigue and poor performance. In short, when athletes exercise at a level of intensity that demands anaerobic energy production, they quickly deplete limited supplies of muscle glycogen, produce excess lactic acid, and hasten fatigue. Fortunately, the muscles can be trained to work much more efficiently, to use more fat and less glycogen, even at higher intensities. How athletes best train for energy fitness is the next topic of discussion.

ENERGY TRAINING

Energy training should follow a systematic process, beginning with the development of a strong aerobic base (Fig. 3–1). Training progresses in intensity until the athlete is ready for peak performances.

Aerobic Foundation. Aerobic fitness, the ability to *take in, transport, and utilize oxygen*, is necessary for athletes in all sports. Training for aerobic fitness helps toughen ligaments, tendons, and connective tissue, reduces the risk of injury, and provides the endurance needed for more intensive training. It provides the foundation on which all future practices and performances are built. Even in football, where the average play lasts but a few seconds, aerobic fitness helps athletes recover faster between plays and allows more effective practice before fatigue sets in.

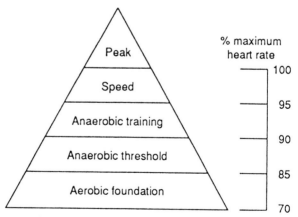

FIG. 3–1. The training pyramid. (From Sharkey BJ: *Training for Cross-Country Ski Racing.* Champaign, IL: Human Kinetics, 1984, p. 88.)

Good aerobic training consists of:
1. Low-intensity, long-duration activity (e.g., distance running, swimming, or cycling).
2. Natural intervals (medium distance with occasional periods of increased intensity).
3. Hills or a similar resistance effort once a week.

Aerobic fitness training leads to improved mitochondrial mass and increases in aerobic enzyme concentration and activity, along with improvements in blood volume, stroke volume, and cardiac output. As endurance grows, aerobic overload can be increased with more distance and/or greater intensity of effort. Remember, the intensity should not be so great that the muscles rely on the anaerobic energy pathway. It is far more efficient to use oxygen, so get all you can from the aerobic pathways before moving on to more intense training. Start slowly, use gradual progression, overload the system with distance and then intensity.

Training Principle #3: Progression
Progression implies gradual increases in training intensity, duration, and frequency. Modern training programs utilize training cycles to ensure progression as well as time for recovery. A typical 4-week endurance training cycle calls for 3 weeks of progressive increases in training load, followed by a week of reduced load.

Provide variation in training (e.g., cross-train to reduce the risk of overuse injuries), but increase specificity as the season approaches.

Training Principle #4: Variation
Vary the program to avoid boredom and overuse injuries. Alternate hard with easy, work with rest. Successive sessions of hard work without adequate time for rest and recovery are certain to hinder progress.

Young Athletes. Immature children differ from young adults in several respects. Whereas their aerobic fitness is not low, they are less efficient and are less able to withstand high temperatures. So intense aerobic training can be more difficult, especially when temperatures are high. Moreover, training is less effective for young athletes, so minimize hard training until the youngsters reach puberty. It will help them avoid the early "burnout" that often accompanies excessive training.

Anaerobic Threshold. As shown in Figure 3–1, the next stage of training is designed to raise the anaerobic (or lactate) threshold. The threshold marks the level of exertion at which an athlete produces more lactic acid than is being removed. It designates the upper limit of efficient aerobic energy production. Work above the threshold demands involvement by less oxidative muscle fibers with greater anaerobic energy production. Fortunately, the threshold can be raised with appropriate training, such as:

1. Four to six extended (over 2-minute) work intervals at or near threshold.
2. Fartlek (speed play) over natural terrain.
3. Pace training (e.g., 1 km at race pace).

How does an athlete know when he or she is at or near the threshold? One way is to conduct a laboratory or field lactate test. With practice, however, the athlete can learn what the threshold *feels* like. When breathing begins to become difficult, when sustained effort begins to become doubtful, the athlete is approaching the threshold. He or she should back off a bit and hold that pace. Some coaches use heart rate monitors to guide training intensity. The threshold is usually about 85 to 90% of the maximum heart rate (estimated max HR = 220 − age). Four to six weeks of twice-weekly threshold training will raise the threshold and the velocity that can be sustained at the threshold, presumably by improving the oxidative capacity of fast twitch muscle fibers. With appropriate training, the lactate threshold (as a percentage of the maximal oxygen intake) continues to rise even after the maximal oxygen intake has reached a plateau.

Young Athletes. Threshold training is difficult for all ages and should only be used once or twice a week during the preseason. Young athletes are less able to utilize muscle glycogen and to produce lactic acid, so threshold training does not yield results until the athlete is more mature. It seems unnecessary to subject young athletes to much of this training. Use some to help the athlete achieve relaxation and efficiency at this level of exertion. Too many strenuous threshold workouts will lead to fatigue, burnout, and loss of interest.

Anaerobic Training. Anaerobic energy pathways are trained when they are overloaded in short, intense bouts of exercise. Anaerobic training is achieved through progressive increases in speed, with decreases in distance or duration of effort. This method of training, called *interval training*, consists of an exercise interval followed by a period of *active* rest, such as easy jogging. The active rest maintains circulation and employs muscular contractions (muscle pump) to remove waste products and hasten recovery.

TABLE 3–1. Interval Training Suggestions

Interval	Use	Work Duration	Rest Duration	Work/ Rest Ratio	Reps	% of Maximum Speed	% of Maximum Heart Rate
Long	Anaerobic threshold training	2–5 min	2–5 min	1:1	4–6	70–80	85–90
Medium	Anaerobic Training	60–90 sec	120–180 sec	1:2	8–12	80–90	95
Short	High energy training (anaerobic)	30–60 sec	90–180 sec	1:3	15–20	95	100
Sprint	Speed (anaerobic)	10–30 sec	30–90 sec	1:3	25+	100	100

Reps, Repetitions.

Use Table 3–1 to guide the development of an interval training program. Identify intervals in Table 3–1 that most closely approximate the intensity of the sport. According to the principle of specificity, some part of the training should mimic that intensity (e.g., race pace). The intermittent nature of interval training allows a greater volume of training at high intensity before athletes become fatigued. Young athletes should not participate in more than two high-intensity workouts per week (count games or competition as high-intensity workouts). I recommend 4 to 6 weeks of anaerobic training, followed by a taper period prior to the most important competition of the season. If the timing is correct, the athletes will peak for the important competition. Too much anaerobic training can lead to chronic fatigue, staleness, illness, or injury.

Young Athletes. The effects of anaerobic training on adults are subtle at best, but with young athletes the benefits, if any, are too small to measure. The anaerobic capabilities of children are lower than for young adults. Glycogen stores, anaerobic enzymes, and lactic acid levels are all lower. With young athletes, the development of anaerobic capacity seems to be related more to age than to training. So it seems unnecessary to subject young athletes to large amounts of this strenuous effort. Do some to achieve neuromuscular skill, mechanical efficiency, and psychological toughness, but wait until athletes reach puberty to do more demanding interval training programs.

Speed Training. When athletes are new to a sport they should follow the training pyramid to prepare them for high-speed training and peak performances. Experienced athletes are able to do some speed training throughout the season. Speed is partially inherited and partially learned. The inherited part is due to fast twitch muscle fibers and biomechanical factors. Even if an athlete did not inherit a lot of fast twitch fibers or a biomechanical advantage, however, he or she can be taught to run, swim, or cycle faster. Some improvement in speed comes when athletes learn to relax and become more efficient. More comes when they engage in speed drills supplemented with weight training.

Speed training usually involves sprints. If your sport requires speed, try some of these:

1. Acceleration sprints—start easy then speed up (safest kind).
2. Hollow sprints—fast at start and finish, easier in middle.
3. Starts—if needed for track, swimming, football.

For skill sports such as basketball, the most specific speed work is on the court (line drills), using the ball (fast break drills). I say more about speed training later in this chapter.

Peaking. The training pyramid shows how the various forms of training build toward a competitive peak (Fig. 3–1). If stages of training are omitted the result is certain to be less successful, and it may lead to an injury. As practice progresses so does the intensity of training. Athletes should not attempt to achieve peak performances in the early season. instead, they should use early contests to build training, sharpen skills, and do necessary speed work. By midseason the athletes should be at a competitive peak that can be maintained until the last competition of the season. If athletes peak too early they may slump before the season ends.

Training Seasons. Figure 3–2 illustrates how the different types of training fit into the overall training program. If possible, schedule at least 1 month for each season of training. If athletes train in the off season, before regular practices begin, more than 1 month should be spent on aerobic training. If they come to practice without the aerobic foundation, they should spend time developing an endurance base before moving to intense anaerobic effort.

Each season has an emphasis. The athlete must maintain the improvements achieved in one season as he or she moves to the next, however. Each weekly training plan will include training activities to enhance the seasonal emphasis, as well as activities designed to maintain previous gains (in aerobic fitness, anaerobic threshold, speed, etc.).

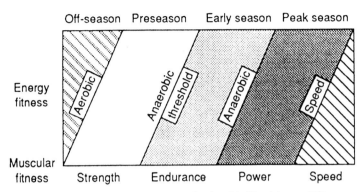

FIG. 3–2. Seasonal training goals. From Sharkey BJ: *Physiology of Fitness*, 3rd Ed. Champaign, IL: Human Kinetics, 1990, p. 244.)

Taper. The taper is a period of reduced training prior to important competitions. It allows recovery from the rigors of training, optimal energy storage, and time to repair any minor injuries. Some coaches train right up to early competitions, then provide a taper before the conference championship. The length of taper differs according to the sport, the event (e.g., sprint versus distance), and the difficulty of the training buildup. Some taper for a few days; others prefer a week or more. The length probably depends on the volume of training, with a longer taper for greater volumes.

Training Principle #5: Individual Response
Athletes respond differently to the same training for many reasons. Among them are inherited differences, maturity, nutrition, level of fitness, environmental factors, sleep and rest, illness, injury, readiness, and motivation. Training programs should be individualized to account for individual differences.

MUSCULAR FITNESS

Muscular fitness includes strength, endurance, power, and speed. In Figure 3–2 you see how these components of athletic performance can be woven into the training program. Young athletes and newcomers are best started with endurance training, using less resistance and more repetitions, but experienced athletes usually do off-season strength training to build muscle size and force, then proceed to add endurance, power, and speed, as required in the sport.

Muscle strength, endurance, and power can be enhanced with resistance training, where a body part is moved against a resistance. High resistance and few repetitions build strength, whereas low resistance and more repetitions build muscular endurance. Resistance can be applied with free weights, with machines that use stack weights, and with hydraulic and electronic apparatus. Weight machines may provide constant or variable resistance. Space does not permit complete coverage of this expanding area, so I suggest you consult an authoritative text on the subject for more information.

STRENGTH

Strength is the maximal ability to exert force. Athletes need adequate strength for their sport. If the sport demands more strength than the athlete has, then strength training is needed. If, however, they do not need additional strength, they should move on to endurance, power, or speed work.

Strength improves when the muscle is overloaded. A weight that can only be lifted a few times is sufficient to overload the muscle and cause adaptation. Adaptations to strength training include increased contractile proteins, thickened connective tissue, increased ability to recruit muscle fibers, and reduced inhibitions. Male athletes quickly show increased muscle size (hypertrophy), whereas females become stronger, with somewhat less hypertrophy. Gradual progression using free weights, weight machines, or even resisted calisthenics will improve strength when you follow this basic prescription.

1. Set the amount of weight so the maximum number of repetitions is 6 to 10.
2. Do 3 sets of 6 to 10 repetitions for each muscle group.
3. Increase the resistance when the athlete can do more than 10 repetitions in each set.
4. Lift every other day, 3 times per week.

With this prescription for strength, athletes will improve at the rate of 1 to 3% per week. When they have achieved an adequate level of strength for the sport, they should move to the next stage of muscular fitness training. They should continue to include at least one set of high-resistance training exercises each week to maintain strength, however.

Training Principle #6: Overload
The body adapts to increased training loads (overload). Training must exceed typical daily demands to elicit the desired adaptations. As the body responds to the increased load, more should be added.

Young Athletes. Young athletes gain strength with resistance training, but before puberty there is little increase in muscle size. This suggests that the increases in strength are due to neuromuscular changes, including a learned ability to exert force more effectively, and reduced inhibitions. The strength prescription leads to improvements with little risk of injury. Special care should be taken however, to warm up and to lift properly with spotting or supervision. Heavy free weights should be avoided and training apparatus should be scaled to fit the young athlete. Because significant strength and muscle development depend on maturation and hormonal support, it may be possible to achieve the neuromuscular benefits of resistance training with lighter weights or fewer sets, thereby minimizing the risk of injury to the immature skeleton.

MUSCULAR ENDURANCE

Swimmers only need a certain amount of strength to move arms against the resistance of water. If they are capable of exerting at least 2.5 times the force required in the average pull, they probably have enough strength for the sport. Thereafter they will need the muscular endurance required to maintain stroke tempo and form. There are several types of muscular endurance. In Table 3–2 you can see how different numbers of training repetitions produce a strength or different types of endurance, ranging from short-

TABLE 3–2. The Strength-Endurance Continuum

	Strength	Short-Term Endurance	Intermediate Endurance	Long-Term Endurance
Goal	Maximum force	Persistence with heavy load	Persistence with intermediate load	Persistance with light load.
Prescription	6–10 RM	15–25 RM	30–50 RM	Over 100 repetitions
	3 sets	3 sets	2 sets	1 set
	3 times/week	3 times/week	3 times/week	3 times/week
Improves	Contractile protein (actin and myosin)	Some strength and anaerobic metabolism (glycolysis)	Some endurance and anaerobic metabolism	Aerobic enzymes
	Connective tissue		Slight strength improvement	Mitochondria
				Oxygen and fat utilization
Does not improve	Oxygen intake	Oxygen intake		Strength
	Endurance			

RM, Repetitions maximum.
(Modified from Sharkey BJ: *Physiology of Fitness*, 3rd Ed. Champaign, IL: Human Kinetics, 1990, p. 91.)

term (anaerobic) endurance to the long-term type needed by the endurance athlete.

As I have said, training should be specific to the sport; if short-term (anaerobic) endurance is required for 1 to 2 minutes of effort, use that prescription. If long-term endurance is essential, follow that prescription. When sports involve some of each, use several types of muscular endurance training in a circuit training program. Endurance exercises should be specific to the way the muscles will be used in the sport. Use free weights, weight machines, calisthenics, or other methods (e.g., rubber tubing) to achieve results. Endurance is extremely trainable. Athletes can go from 20 to over 200 push-ups, or more. Often these dramatic improvements in endurance are associated with increases in performance.

POWER

Power, the rate of doing work, can be described as:

$$\text{Power} = \frac{\text{Force} \times \text{Distance}}{\text{Time}}$$

As such, it involves the components of strength (force) and speed (distance divided by time). Power is an essential ingredient in such sports as football, baseball, ice hockey, and many others. Training for power usually involves strength training. To improve jumping ability in basketball or volleyball, coaches prescribe squats to build strength in thigh muscles. Squats are slow and somewhat nonspecific for the neuromuscular skill of jumping, however. Therefore, training must progress to power exercises, where force and speed are combined in a sport-specific movement.

Power can be developed by following the power prescription:

Resistance:	30–60% RM—as *fast* as possible
Repetitions:	15–25
Sets:	3
Frequency:	3 times/week

Best results are achieved when the resistance can be moved at a moderate speed, neither too fast nor too slow. So select a resistance somewhere between 30 and 60% of maximum strength and do as many fast repetitions as possible. When you can do more than 25 repetitions in each set it is time to increase the resistance.

Barbells are not well suited for this type of training. Some types of weight machines are better, but the best approach is to use iso-kinetic or variable-resistance devices that allow some control of resistance and the speed of contraction. With these devices, you can use the resistance and speed you need to conduct the program safely. Avoid soreness by starting with less resistance and slower contractions; then work up to the prescription during a 2-week period of adjustment (Delayed-onset muscle soreness is caused by an overly vigorous effort in the early season or by lowering a heavy weight, i.e., contracting a lengthening muscle in an eccentric contraction.)

Plyometrics. This calisthenic-like exercise is used to develop power. When used in conjunction with strength training, these explosive exercises (e.g., the Indian hop) build strength and the elastic recoil that provides more power for jumping and other activities. Because body weight is about 33% of maximum leg strength, plyometrics fit the power prescription. Start gradually to avoid injury and stop if the legs get sore. Do all training on grass, dirt, or a softer surface. Work up to 3 sets of 25 exercises, then increase resistance by adding a more difficult exercise, by working uphill, or by wearing a weighted vest. Plyometrics will increase strength, improve elastic recoil, and increase the muscle's short-term energy stores. They may also teach the efficient use of power.

Young Athletes. Although power does not develop rapidly in young athletes, some power training will be useful to develop the neuromuscular skill of moving quickly against resistance. Do not overdo power training, however, especially plyometrics; these exercises can be hard on young knees.

SPEED

You may have heard that sprinters are born and not made, and that is essentially true, because the proportion of fast muscle fiber is inherited to some extent. All athletes can use specific training to improve the components of speed, reaction time, and movement time, however. Reaction time is the time it takes to initiate a movement, whereas movement time is the interval from the start to the end of the movement. Both components can be improved with practice and training.

Fast reactions are taught in practice drills. The knowledgeable coach speeds reactions by narrowing the choices athletes must make and then drilling the proper reaction (e.g., if the defensive end comes at the option quarterback he pitches the ball; if not he runs). In track and swimming there is but one choice: when the gun goes so does the athlete. The fewer the choices the faster the reaction.

Movement time can be enhanced via a program that includes stretching, along with strength and power training, form training, and specific speed training. A recent book on speed training suggests the following speed training program:

Basic training	Aerobic and muscular fitness
Functional strength/power	Explosive movements with 55 to
Ballistics	85% resistance
Plyometrics	Explosive movements
Sprint loading	Explosive jumping/throwing
Sport speed/speed endurance	movements
Overspeed	Resisted sprinting
	Participation and extended sprints
	Exceeding maximum speed

Adapted from Dintiman and Ward (1988).

Overspeed or assisted speed training involves the athletes' being pulled by an elastic cord, running downhill, or otherwise causing them to move faster than their maximum speed. In time they relax and become comfortable, skilled, and efficient at higher speeds. To build speed endurance, gradually increase sprint length while decreasing the rest interval between each sprint. A wise coach once said, "Speed is an environment, and one must become acclimated to it." Use sport-specific training to improve the speed of your athletes.

Training Principle #7: Warm-up and Cool-down
The warm-up increases the body temperature. It should also include stretching and skill rehearsal. The warm-up helps guard against muscle, tendon, and ligament strains. The cool-down hastens the removal of waste products that increase soreness and prolong recovery.

Training Principle #8: Long-term Training
It takes years of effort to approach the level of training needed to achieve high-level performances. Long-term dedication to training allows gradual adaptation and the development of neuromuscular skills, along with normal growth and development. As a general rule, neither weekly nor annual training loads should be increased faster than 10 to 15%.

SUMMARY

Training is a gradual process that cannot be rushed. Too much training exceeds the body's ability to respond with protein synthesis and other adaptations. Excess training (overtraining) leads to illness and injury. Immune and hormonal systems that respond favorably to moderate activity may be suppressed or exhausted by overtraining. The well-designed training program follows the principles of training, providing progression, overload, variation, and time for rest and recovery. In other words, it is faithful to the final principle of training.

Training Principle #9: Moderation
This principle applies to training and to other aspects of life; too much of anything can be bad for your health. Temper dedication with judgment and moderation. Train too hard, too long, or too fast, and the body begins to deteriorate. Practice moderation in all things, including training for sport.

RECOMMENDED READING

Dintiman G and Ward R: *Sport Speed*. Champaign, IL: Human Kinetics, 1988.

Fleck S and Kraemer W: *Designing Resistance Training Programs*. Champaign, IL: Human Kinetics, 1987.

Sharkey BJ: *Sport Physiology*. Champaign, IL: Human Kinetics, 1986.

Sharkey BJ: Specificity of exercise. In *Resource Manual for Guidelines for Exercise Testing and Prescription*. Edited by S Blair et al. Philadelphia: Lea & Febiger, 1988.

Sleamaker R: *Serious Training for Serious Athletes*. Champaign, IL: Leisure Press, 1989.

| C | H | A | P | T | E | R | 4 |

SPECIAL MEDICAL CONDITIONS

E. Randy Eichner

Athletes are susceptible to diverse medical conditions related to their sport. The special medical conditions covered in this chapter include anemia, gastrointestinal problems, renal abnormalities, environmental hazards, and exercise-induced asthma.

ANEMIA

Compared with the general population, athletes—especially endurance athletes—tend to have slightly lower hemoglobin concentrations. In other words, athletes seem to be slightly anemic. This has often been called "sports anemia."

Sports anemia is a poor term, however, both imprecise and a misnomer. Most commonly, the lower hemoglobin concentration in an athlete is a false anemia, caused by dilution of the red blood cells by an increased volume of plasma. The increase in plasma volume is a beneficial adaptation that enhances athletic performance. The resultant hemoglobin concentration, often at least 1 g/dl below "normal," causes no symptoms and calls for no treatment.

Athletes can also develop true anemia, however, most commonly caused by iron deficiency. The early symptoms include a decline in all-out athletic performance, undue dyspnea, heavy sweating, and, from rapid accumulation of lactic acid, heavy limbs, "tying up," nausea, and even retching.

Does athleticism, per se, cause iron deficiency? Probably it does not. Over the past decade, many reports on iron deficiency in athletes have implied that: (1) up to 80% of elite female endurance athletes, for example, are deficient in iron; (2) athletes are uniquely susceptible to iron-deficiency anemia; and (3) a low serum ferritin, even in the absence of anemia, impairs athletic performance. All three of these implications are wrong.

Recent research, in fact, suggests that athletes, as a group, have serum ferritin values similar to those of nonathletes and that athletes do not necessarily lose more iron than nonathletes. The notion that a low serum ferritin alone curtails performance is also ill founded. Recent studies agree that low ferritin curbs performance only in the presence of anemia.

But what is true anemia for an athlete? Clinically, anemia is defined as a hemoglobin value subnormal for the subject at hand. An athletic woman with a hemoglobin of 13 g/dl, then, is anemic if her usual hemoglobin level is 15 g/dl. In other words, even though her hemoglobin level is within the broad range of "normal," for her she is anemic.

If the "usual" hemoglobin level for a given athlete is unknown, one has to use guidelines. In general, hemoglobin levels among healthy female athletes are often under 14 g/dl, commonly under 13 g/dl, rarely under 12 g/dl, and almost never under 11 g/dl. The corresponding values for male athletes are 1 to 2 g/dl higher.

Although a low ferritin level alone does not impair athletic performance, anemia, even very mild anemia, does. When in doubt, then, the wise course is a trial of iron therapy. Give ferrous sulfate, 325 mg, 3 times daily for 2 months. A rise in hemoglobin level (of at least 1 g/dl) proves that the anemia was due at least in part to iron deficiency.

Iron deficiency can be prevented in most athletes by directing more attention to diet. To increase iron intake, one should: (1) eat more lean red meat or dark meat of chicken; (2) improve iron absorption from bread and cereal by avoiding coffee or tea with meals and drinking instead a source of vitamin C, such as orange juice; (3) cook occasionally in cast-iron skillets and pans; and (4) eat poultry or seafood with dried beans or peas—the animal protein here increases the absorption of the iron in the vegetables.

GASTROINTESTINAL PROBLEMS

Vigorous or prolonged exercise can cause gastrointestinal (GI) problems. Generally, these problems are distressing, but not disabling. Exercise has also been linked with GI bleeding that ranges from occult to major. With the recent boom in endurance races, more and more athletes are seeking medical advice about GI symptoms.

Many runners and triathletes, for example, occasionally experience lower GI tract symptoms during their sport. These symptoms, termed "runner's trots," include cramping, bloating, and loose bowel movements, sometimes mixed with a little blood. Such symptoms, which seem to be more common in women than men and in younger athletes than older ones, tend to flare up during a rapid increase in training or a race.

What to do about "runner's trots?" Most athletes learn to cope. Practical tips: (1) wait 3 to 4 hours after eating—for digestion and for bowel movements—before working out; (2) cut down on foods that can cause diarrhea: caffeine, fiber, dairy products (in those who cannot digest lactose; yogurt is an exception), some sugar substitutions (especially sorbitol, in breath mints and "sugarless" gum), vitamin C tablets; and (3) cut back on "gassy" foods: apples, bananas, citrus fruits, beans, bran, carrots, cabbage, cucumber, raisins, and others.

GI bleeding also occurs in some runners, cyclists, and triathletes. How common is it? In a survey of 700 marathoners, 2% had a bloody stool occasionally or frequently. A similar figure is cited for triathletes. Occult bleeding, of course, is more common. In 6 studies of runners, the average rate of occult blood in the stool after a distance race was 20%.

How important is GI bleeding in athletes? Most of the time, it is minor and brief. In our research with runners and cyclists over a season, occult GI bleeding occurred sporadically in half the athletes, correlated more with racing then training, and always disappeared in a day or two.

In some runners, at least, however, GI bleeding seems to cause anemia. Several reports, for example, document exercise-related GI bleeding as a cause of iron-deficiency anemia in women runners. The preponderance of women in such reports is intriguing, but may be an artifact of case finding. Compared with men (who have greater iron stores), it takes less bleeding in women to cause iron-deficiency anemia.

What is the site of the GI bleeding? Sometimes, despite endoscopies, no site is found. Sometimes, the stomach is the site, i.e., erosive gastritis is the cause. Occasionally, the cause is proximal hemorrhagic colitis. Rarely, the site is the rectum, i.e., an unmasking of ulcerative proctitis. Finally, in theory, the site can be the esophagus. In a recent study, working out caused esophageal reflux in some healthy runners and, to a lesser extent, in some cyclists and weight lifters.

How does exercise cause GI bleeding? We are not certain. The gastritis may stem in part from the stress and high cortisol secretion associated with rigorous training and racing. The colitis may be ischemic, in that all-out exercise can reduce visceral blood flow by up to 80%. In some cases, aspirin or other drugs may play roles.

Finally, all-out exercise, by enhancing fibrinolysis, or by other mechanisms, may impair hemostasis.

Practical management tips: (1) the risk of GI bleeding seems to correlate with the intensity of exercise, so gradual conditioning may help prevent it; (2) if symptoms point to an upper GI source (gastritis, ulcer), antacids or H_2 blockers may help; (3) aspirin, which adversely affects both gastric mucosa and platelet function, should be avoided for a few days before a race; (4) attribute GI bleeding to athleticism only after excluding treatable GI lesions.

RENAL ABNORMALITIES

For more than 100 years, we have known that vigorous exercise can cause hematuria, proteinuria, and, rarely, hemoglobinuria. Generally, these renal abnormalities are brief and benign. Together, they can be thought of as a "pseudonephritis." Unwise exercise, however, can also cause renal nephritis—acute renal failure. Athleticism, then, can provoke a wide range of renal abnormalities, from benign to lethal.

Proteinuria, for example, is almost invariable during strenuous exercise. Occurring in a wide variety of sports (running, rowing, swimming, cycling, skiing, boxing, lacrosse, football, baseball, and others), proteinuria is part of the "athletic pseudonephritis," first reported in football players, that is also characterized by hematuria and red-cell casts. These abnormalities, which disappear with rest, are thought to be benign.

Proteinuria, the most common renal abnormality of exercise, is thought to be physiologic, not pathologic. Most pronounced in runners, it usually clears within 1 to 2 days after a marathon. For practical diagnosis, then, if proteinuria can be temporally related to athleticism, it needs no further investigation.

If, in contrast, proteinuria persists in the supine position, and if the urinalysis yields no diagnostic clues, one should consider an intravenous pyelogram (IVP) and collect a 24-hour urine sample for creatinine clearance, total protein, and protein electrophoresis, to look for chronic renal disease, the nephrotic syndrome, or tubular interstitial disease.

Hematuria, usually microscopic, is less common than proteinuria. Up to 20% of marathoners, for example, have hematuria immediately after the race. Like proteinuria, microscopic hematuria usually clears within 2 days after the marathon.

The mechanism and source of exertional hematuria are debated.

Some studies suggest a glomerular source; others suggest the source is the lower urinary tract. Consider gross hematuria, for example, Much rarer than microscopic hematuria, gross hematuria is more common in male than female athletes. Some men, usually after long runs in the heat, void bloody urine, sometimes with clots. they may note discomfort in the glans penis or perineum. In one study, of 18 such patients in whom no upper tract lesion was found, 8 had bladder contusions on cystoscopy, presumably from the posterior wall of the empty bladder banging into the trigone.

Similarly, male cyclists have reported painless gross hematuria after bumpy rides, presumably from trauma to the perineum. Rarely, the gross hematuria can be from sickle cell trait. Gross hematuria occurs sooner or later in 4% of persons with sickle trait. Usually, it is spontaneous; rarely, it occurs after sports. When it occurs after sports, however, it is usually a contact sport, e.g., boxing or football, suggesting that the cause is not exercise, but trauma.

Indeed, most experts think that sickle cell trait does not increase the risk of exercise-related hematuria, and that an episode of hematuria in an athlete with sickle trait should not bar him or her from returning to the sport.

Practical management tips: Hematuria that, with rest, persists beyond 2 days merits investigation. One approach is to begin with a urine culture, and treat any urinary-tract infection. If the culture is negative, check the serum creatinine and exclude sickle cell trait. Next, obtain an IVP and/or cystoscopy. If both are normal, measure the creatinine clearance and the 24-hour urine protein excretion, and consult a nephrologist to consider other studies.

When managing an athlete with sickle cell trait and gross hematuria, attribute the hematuria to sickle trait only by exclusion. After all, an athlete with sickle trait, just like anyone else, can have hematuria from a renal stone or acute glomerulonephritis. In addition, the hematuria may stem not from the sickle trait, but from coincidental inheritance of von Willebrand's disease. In such patients, infusing cryoprecipitate stops the bleeding.

Gross hematuria from "jogger's bladder" can be prevented by better hydration and by not voiding just before running. Bicycle-seat hematuria can be prevented by lowering the nose of the saddle, using a special seat cover, and rising off the saddle when cycling over railroad tracks and other bumps.

Exertional acute renal failure is rare, but potentially lethal. In fact, it is the cause of the exercise deaths in sickle cell trait. How does it happen? Who gets it? How can it be prevented? The sickle trait story serves as an example.

The pattern of exercise death in sickle cell trait is severe exertional rhabdomyolysis (usually with heat stress), cardiovascular collapse, shock, acute renal failure, acidosis, hyperkalemia, and death within 1 to 2 days. This catastrophic illness is not unique to sickle cell trait; indeed, it is the well-known syndrome of exertional myoglobinuria. Heat and poor fitness play predisposing roles, especially among military recruits. Altitude, viral illness, and/or heroic exercise regimens also contribute, especially among athletes.

Athletes with sickle trait may or may not be at increased risk for collapse from exertional rhabdomyolysis, but they seem to be at increased risk of death if they do collapse, presumably because shock and acidosis trigger widespread sickling. Certainly, however, exertional rhabdomyolysis, often with acute renal failure, if not death, has occurred in athletes lacking the sickle trait. This disorder has occurred, in fact, after football, basketball, wrestling, karate, conga drumming, ice skating, mountain climbing, marathon running, and other sports.

Most cases of exertional renal failure have clear-cut predisposing factors: improper training, prerace infection, crash dieting, vomiting or diarrhea, as well as foolhardy attempts to continue exercising despite heat exhaustion, muscle pain, dark urine, vomiting, and even confusion. The keyword, then, is prevention.

Practical tips for prevention: (1) athletes should select a sport suitable for their age and physical condition; (2) they should train wisely, not charge recklessly into heroic regimens, especially when at a new altitude; (3) when sick, they should rest, not work out; and (4) they must avoid dehydration and heat stress.

HEAT STRESS

Heat illness develops when dehydration coincides with excessive heat production from exercise, the environment, or both. Factors predisposing to heat stress include obesity, poor fitness, lack of acclimatization, infection, salt and water depletion, potassium deficiency, skin disorders that impair sweating, and certain drugs, e.g., diuretics, anticholinergics, phenothiazines, antihistamines, and alcohol.

Heat cramps are brief, intermittent, excruciating muscular cramps, as in the gastrocnemius. They tend to occur in heat-acclimatized athletes (runners, tennis players) who play long and hard, drink copious amounts of water, but fail to replace losses of salt. The higher the sweat rate, the more sodium is lost, and, although the mechanism of heat cramps is unclear, some experts think that hyponatremia plays a role. If heat cramps are the only symptom of heat stress, sufficient treatment is rest, oral fluids, cooling, stretching, and deep muscle massage.

Heat exhaustion, the most common disorder of athletes in the heat, stems from salt and water depletion. Symptoms vary, but often include headache, fatigue, malaise, myalgias or cramps, dizziness, nausea, mild confusion, and piloerection ("gooseflesh"). These symptoms can mimic "summer flu." At this stage of heat stress, the athlete may have lost, through sweating, 3 to 5% of body weight, and the core temperature may range up to 105° F. Treatment consists of cooling and rapid fluid replacement by mouth or intravenously.

Heat stroke, the extreme, potentially lethal form of heat stress, involves profound dehydration and a rise in core temperature to the range of 105 to 110° F. It is more common in men than women and most common in runners and football players. Symptoms include all the foregoing, as well as delirium, ataxia, and collapse in shock and coma. Therapy involves rapid cooling, using cool water, fanning, and ice packs to major arteries, e.g., carotid, maxillary, femoral, and popliteal, along with rapid intravenous rehydration with 5% dextrose and normal saline or equivalent. Comatose patients need attention to ventilation and fast transit to the hospital.

Ultraendurance athletes (triathletes, ultramarathoners) who drink mainly water are at risk, late in the event, of hyponatremia, with attendant delirium and seizures. This can be prevented by drinking one of the sports drinks, which provides adequate fluid plus some sodium to replace sweat loss and some sugar to enhance energy in the final third of the race. So long as the concentration of sugar in the drink is no more than 6 to 8%, GI absorption is rapid and efficient. In fact, especially in the summer, one can recommend sports drinks (instead of only water) for any workout or event that lasts 1 hour or more.

Other practical tips to avoid heat stress: (1) slowly acclimatize by graded training in the heat for weeks before the race; (2) during the summer, boost dietary salt intake (do not use salt pills) and drink ample fluids; (3) do not drastically alter one's customary diet the week before the race; (4) wear white, cotton, or mesh clothing and dress lightly; (5) during the race, drink early and often: 1 pint of water 15 minutes before the start and at least half a cup of water or sports drink every 15 minutes thereafter; and (6) begin the race slowly, do not try to speed up at the end, and know when to stop, get in the shade, and seek help.

A final word on diagnosis: Do not rely on oral or axillary temperatures: they are often falsely low and, in fact, can lead to a wrong diagnosis of hypothermia when hyperthermia is present. Use rectal thermometers.

HYPOTHERMIA

Athletes—joggers, hikers, skiers, skaters, swimmers—can fall prey to hypothermia when they tire after long exercise in the cold. Predisposing factors include lack of subcutaneous fat, alcohol use, inadequate clothing, getting wet, and facing a strong wind. Physical fitness, too, is a key variable, because those most fit can work the hardest and longest and thereby produce the most metabolic heat. Consider, for example, the paradox of opposite environmental hazards during a cool-weather marathon. The winners tend to finish the race hyperthermic; the stragglers tend to finish hypothermic. Why? The winners make more heat than they lose; the stragglers, vice versa.

Initial symptoms of hypothermia include shivering, lethargy, weakness, and confusion The mildly hypothermic athlete, however, may remain alert, with stable vital signs. The key to diagnosis, then, is an awareness that the given athlete is at risk for hypothermia, and the use of a rectal thermometer to measure core temperature.

Treatment for mild hypothermia is active rewarming with blankets, hot water bottles, or a water bath at 40° C and intravenous infusion of normal saline warmed to 32.2° C (90° F). For severe hypothermia, use peritoneal lavage with warmed saline.

Practical tips to avoid hypothermia: (1) respect Mother Nature; (2) wear clothing with multiple layers: an inner layer (e.g., polypropylene or cotton) to wick moisture away from the body, a middle layer (e.g., goose down) to insulate, and an outer layer (e.g., Goretex) to ward off wind and water; (3) wear a cap (e.g., wool) and gloves, and protect the ears, nose, digits, and penis from frostbite; (4) run home with the wind, not against it; (5) find an exercise buddy; and (6) after finishing, quickly get into dry clothes and a warm environment.

ASTHMA

Exercise-induced asthma (EIA) is defined as acute, reversible, self-limited airway obstruction that occurs during or after exercise. Like asthma in general, EIA seems to be on the increase and probably now occurs in 12 to 15% of the general population.

The cardinal feature of EIA is breathlessness, but cough and/or wheezing can also occur. Severity varies according to several factors. Brief exercise, i.e., under 6 minutes, may not provoke EIA. In general, the more strenuous the exercise, the more likely it will provoke EIA. Type of exercise is another factor: running is the most likely to provoke EIA, swimming the least, and cycling intermediate. Climate, too, plays a role: cold, dry air is more likely to cause EIA than is warm, humid air. Air pollutants, e.g., sulfur dioxide, can also exacerbate EIA.

What provokes EIA? Ventilation increases 20- to 30-fold during all-out exercise, and this large volume of air, especially cold, dry air, constricts the lower airways, apparently by vagal reflex and/or the release of mediators from mast cells. EIA typically has a "refractory period" of 30 to 90 minutes, perhaps owing to temporary depletion of mediators, during which further exercise causes little or no airway obstruction.

Diagnosis usually hinges on a history of asthma and the typical clinical features of EIA. Up to one third of athletes with EIA, however, are unaware they have it. If so, diagnosis requires provoking asthma via an exercise test and reversing it with a bronchodilator. In other words, the forced expiratory volume in 1 second (FEV_1) should increase by at least 15% after administration of the bronchodilator.

Any athlete with EIA should be encouraged to stay with his or her sport. Many asthmatics (Jim Ryun, Nancy Hogshead, Jackie Joyner-Kersey) have become champions. At the 1988 Olympic Summer Games in Seoul, South Korea, for example, 15% of the 667 United States competitors had confirmed or suspected EIA.

Practical tips for management of EIA: (1) further conditioning may help prevent it, because less effort will then be needed for a given event; (2) the drug of choice is a beta-adrenergic agonist by metered-dose inhaler: two puffs of albuterol, for example, 15 minutes before exercising; (3) if albuterol alone does not suffice, cromolyn sodium by metered-dose inhaler is a good addition; (4) second-line drugs include theophylline, ipratropium bromide, and corticosteroids; (5) athletes with allergies may need desensitization; and (6) a race-day tactic is to provoke EIA during the warm-up and race during the ensuing refractory period.

RECOMMENDED READING

Eichner ER: *Sports Hematology: 1988 Year Book of Hematology*. Chicago: Year Book Medical Publishers, 1988, pp. 65–70.

Eichner ER: Anemia in female athletes. *Your Patient and Fitness* 3:3–11, 1989.

Eichner ER: Gastrointestinal bleeding in athletes: a review. *Phys Sportsmed* 17:128–140, 1989.

Eichner ER: Renal abnormalities in athletes. *IM—Intern Med Specialist* 7:245–252, 1987.

Eichner ER: Sickle cell trait and the young athlete. *Your Patient and Fitness* 2:9–16, 1990.

Hiller WDB: Dehydration and hyponatremia during triathlons. *Med Sci Sports Exerc* 21:S219–S221, 1989.

Katz RM: Coping with exercise-induced asthma in sports. *Phys Sportsmed* 15:101–110, 1987.

Knochel JP: Heat stroke and related heat stress disorders. *DM* 35:306–337, 1989.

Pate RR: Special considerations for exercise in cold weather. *Sports Sci Exchange* (Gatorade Sports Science Institute) 1:1–4, 1988.

NUTRITION: PRE-, INTRA-, AND POSTCOMPETITION

Nancy Clark

PRECOMPETITION

The goals of the precompetition meal are:
1. To help prevent hypoglycemia with the symptoms of light-headedness, blurred vision, needless fatigue, and indecisiveness, all of which can interfere with top performance.
2. To abate hunger feelings, help settle the stomach, and absorb some of the gastric juices.
3. To provide energy for the muscles.
4. To provide adequate fluids to fully hydrate the body.

In preparation for competition, an athlete should make a special effort to eat a 60 to 70% carbohydrate rich diet and drink additional fluids both on the *day prior to* the event and on the *day of* the event, in combination with tapering of exercise to allow the muscles the opportunity to store the carbohydrates as glycogen.

- Athletes participating in endurance sports that last for longer than 90 minutes, such as marathoning or long-distance bike racing, should reduce exercise and emphasize carbohydrates for 3 days prior to the event.
- Athletes participating in events shorter than 90 minutes' duration can store adequate glycogen with 1 or 2 days of rest and a carbohydrate-rich diet.

Because a single precompetition meal cannot compensate for a poor training diet, athletes should eat a carbohydrate-rich sports diet *every day* to enhance daily muscle glycogen storage. The precompetition meal should be simply an extension of the tried-and-true daily training diet. The primary focus of the precompetition preparation should be to reduce exercise so the athlete's muscles can store the carbohydrates and optimally replenish depleted glycogen stores.

Although an athlete may want to know exactly when, what, and how much to eat, specific recommendations are hard to make because of metabolic differences from person to person. For example, some runners can eat within an hour of racing; others avoid food to reduce the risk of gastrointestinal (GI) distress. Some gymnasts want a little food to absorb gastric juices; others are so nervous they feel sick and unable to eat. Precompetition food preferences also vary from sport to sport. For example, cyclists are likely to eat more than runners, who fear GI problems related to the jostling that occurs with running. Because each athlete has unique food preferences and aversions, it is impossible to recommend a single food or meal that will ensure top performance.

Although many athletes have traditionally competed on an empty stomach, current research supports the benefits of precompetition food eaten within 4 hours of the event. Contrary to popular belief, food eaten within 4 hours of exercise *is* used for fuel. In one study (Jandrain et al., 1984), 5 males who consumed 400 calories of sugar 3 hours before running to 4 hours (45% $\dot{V}O_{2max}$) oxidized 68% of the glucose. In another study, (Ravussin et al., 1979), cyclists who consumed 400 calories of sugar 1 hour before cycling for 2 hours (35% $\dot{V}O_{2max}$) oxidized 41% of the sugar.

Precompetition food is especially important before morning events and in low-body-weight athletes (i.e., boxers, wrestlers). Athletes who enter competition after an overnight fast have depleted their liver glycogen stores; they are likely to have less stamina and endurance than when exercising after having eaten a light snack/meal that replenishes the liver glycogen stores and helps maintain normal blood sugar levels. Some popular food choices include a bagel, toast, cereal, fruit, and/or juice, about 100 to 400 calories as tolerated.

Meal Timing. When planning the time of the precompetition meal, the athlete should allow adequate time for the food to empty from the stomach, so he or she can exercise comfortably without nausea or gastrointestinal upset. Because high-calorie meals take longer to leave the stomach than lighter snacks, the general rule of thumb is for an athlete to allow:

- 3 to 4 hours for a large meal to digest.
- 2 to 3 hours for a smaller meal.
- 1 to 2 hours for a blended or liquid meal.
- Less than an hour for a light snack.

Because fatty foods delay gastric emptying, the meal should focus on carbohydrates; small portions of lean protein are also appropriate as an accompaniment, such as spaghetti with a little bit of very lean hamburger in the tomato sauce, or a turkey sandwich with thickly sliced bread and a thin layer of turkey.

The night before *morning events*, athletes should eat a hearty, high-carbohydrate dinner and bedtime snack. That morning, they should eat a light snack/breakfast to abate hunger feelings, to replenish liver glycogen stores, and to absorb some of the gastric juices. For example, a runner who is going to participate in a 10 AM road race will want only a light breakfast (such as a small bowl of cereal with low-fat milk, about 300 calories), because the primary fueling was done 10 to 72 hours before by the hearty carbohydrate-rich dinner. Before *afternoon events*, athletes should plan a hearty carbohydrate-rich dinner and breakfast, to be followed by a light lunch. A runner racing at noon can enjoy a heartier breakfast (such as 4 or 5 pancakes, about 600 calories), than when he or she races earlier in the day. Before *evening events*, athletes should plan a hearty carbohydrate-rich breakfast and lunch, followed by a light snack 1 to 2 hours prior to the event. In addition to focusing meals on carbohydrates, athletes should also consume an additional glass of fluid with each meal, as well as between meals, to ensure complete hydration. Water and juices are the recommended choices, although the less-nourishing soft drinks and sports drinks are also popular and acceptable choices.

Some athletes who are overly nervous, stressed, or have sensitive stomachs may prefer to abstain from food the day of competition. They should make a special effort to eat extra food the day prior to the event, to be well fueled for competition. They may want to experiment the day of the event with simple liquids, such as apple juice, canned liquid diets, or sports drinks.

Liquid Meals. Because liquid foods leave the stomach faster than solid foods, the athlete may want to experiment with blenderized meals to determine whether they offer any advantage. In one research study (Brouns et al., 1987), a 450-calorie meal of steak, peas, and buttered bread remained for 6 hours in the stomach. A blenderized version of the same meal emptied from the stomach in 4 hours. Before converting to blenderized meals, the athlete should keep in mind anecdotal reports that too much liquid may "slosh" in the stomach and contribute to a nauseous feeling. Hence, any new meal should be experimented with *during training* to determine whether it settles well and test timing a liquid meal.

Pre-Exercise Sugar. Historically, athletes have been advised to stay away from sugary foods prior to exercise, with the belief that the "sugar high" will trigger a rebound hypoglycemic effect that will hinder performance. More recent studies suggest that pre-competition sugar may actually enhance stamina and endurance. Sherman et al. (1988) report that cyclists who ate about 1200 calories of carbohydrates 3 hours prior to 95 minutes of intermittent exercise improved their performance. Gleeson et al. (1986) similarly report that subjects who ate about 280 calories of carbohydrate 45 minutes prior to hard exercise (73% $\dot{V}_{O_{2max}}$) improved their time to exhaustion by 12%.

For some athletes, pre-exercise sugar does result in a negative hypoglycemic feeling with lightheadedness, confusion and fatigue. Hence, athletes who perceive themselves as sugar sensitive should abstain from concentrated sweets and rely more on hearty meals than sugary snacks for energy.

The best advice regarding pre-exercise sugar is to *avoid the need* for a quick energy fix by having appropriately timed meals prior to the event. The high school athlete who craves a sugary quick-energy fix before an afternoon event could remedy the need for quick energy by having a wholesome breakfast and lunch, rather than skimping on those meals and then looking for a last-minute energizer. Not only would this pattern promote better performance but also better nutrition, and it would eliminate the risk of possibly hurting performance because of rebound hypoglycemia.

Psychological Value of Food. Precompetition food may have beneficial effects both physiologically and psychologically. If an athlete firmly believes that a specific food/meal (such as the traditional steak and eggs) enhances performance, then it probably does. The mind has a powerful effect on the body's ability to perform at its best. Athletes who believe in a "magic food" that ensures competitive excellence should take special care to be sure this food/meal is available before an event. This is particularly important for athletes who travel. They should bring along tried-and-true pre-competition foods, such as a favorite cereal, muffin, or sandwich. By doing this, the athlete will be worry free about what he or she is going to eat and will be better able to focus on performance.

Practice Precompetition Eating. Experience has shown that each athlete has to learn through trial and error during training and competitions what foods work best for his or her body, when they should be eaten, and in what amounts. Food preferences vary depending on the type of exercise, level of intensity, and time of day. Hence the foregoing guidelines regarding precompetition eating should be viewed as simply considerations to be pondered and experimented with *during training*. The bottom line is that each athlete has to experiment to learn which combinations of food work best for his or her body.

EATING DURING EXERCISE

Athletes who exercise for more than 90 minutes will have greater stamina and enhanced performance if they consume carbohydrates during the event. These carbohydrates help to maintain a normal blood sugar level as well as to provide a source of energy for the exercising muscles. Research suggests that trained cyclists (who weigh about 150 pounds) can metabolize about 1 gram carbohydrate per minute; this equals 240 calories of carbohydrates per hour of endurance exercise. This breaks down into 60 calories per 15 minutes (about 8 ounces of sports drink)—much more than most athletes are likely to consume.

The harder an athlete exercises, the less likely she or he is to want to consume food. During intense exercise ($>70\%$ $\dot{V}O_{2max}$), the stomach may get only 20% of its normal blood flow. This slows the digestive process; any food in the stomach may feel uncomfortable or may be regurgitated. Sports drinks or sugar solutions (5 to 7%) tend to be most readily accepted. Other popular choices include diluted juices, tea with honey, and defizzed Coke diluted with water.

Although blood flow is 60 to 70% of normal during moderate-intensity exercise, the athlete can still digest food. Hence, the solid food snacks, such as bananas, fig bars, and bagels, that recreational skiers, cyclists, and ultrarunners eat during exercise are digested and do contribute to lasting energy during long-term moderate-intensity events.

Because some athletes can tolerate food/fluids during exercise better, it is important to experiment during training with different snacks to determine what works best, and how much is tolerated.

POSTCOMPETITION EATING: RECOVERY FOODS

Many of the same athletes who carefully select a high-carbohydrate diet prior to competition neglect their recovery diet. Because muscles are most receptive to replacing muscle glycogen within the first 2 hours after a hard workout, a low-carbohydrate post-event diet can hinder optimal recovery. This, in turn, limits an athlete's readiness to compete again, particularly important in the case of repeated events on the same day, such as with swimming

or track meets. A poor recovery diet can also delay the athlete's ability to return to intense training.
  A carbohydrate-deficient recovery diet is commonly selected by athletes who eat:

- Too much protein, such as may happen at a post-event dinner that focuses on steak as a change from the precompetition pasta meal.
- Too many greasy foods, such as cheeseburgers and French fries, which are popularly eaten by athletes who frequent fast-food restaurants.
- Too many "sweets," when the "sweets" are actually fat-laden cookies, ice cream, and brownies that get at least half their calories from butter or margarine.
- Too few calories, such as may happen with diet-conscious athletes who skimp on carbohydrates (thinking that carbohydrates are fattening) and instead sustain themselves on protein-rich cottage cheese, tuna fish, and chicken.

To optimize the recovery process after a hard workout, an athlete should eat 200 to 400 calories of carbohydrates within 2 hours of the exercise bout, then repeat this another 2 hours later. This "dose" comes to about 0.5 gram carbohydrates per pound of body weight, and for a 150-pound person would be the equivalent of 300 calories of carbohydrates in a postexercise snack (such as juice) followed by a carbohydrate-rich meal after having stretched, showered, and recovered form the workout. Examples of 300-calorie snack/meals include:

- 2 Cups (16 ounces) of orange juice and a banana.
- An average-sized bowl of cereal with fruit for breakfast.
- A dinner with generous servings of starch and vegetables.

For those who report that exercise "kills their appetite," juices can provide adequate carbohydrates, as well as quench the thirst and supply fluids. The popularly advertised carbohydrate supplements are generally unnecessary after exercise, because a hungry athlete can easily consume the recommended amount of carbohydrates, and benefit from the nutritional value of wholesome foods, as compared to the empty calories of the supplements.
  In addition to replacing carbohydrates, the athlete should be careful to replace fluids lost through sweat. Carbohydrate-containing fluids, such as juices, replace both muscle glycogen and water losses; they are the best choice from a vantage point of both overall health and performance. Although many athletes may be tempted to drink sports drinks after an event, commercial fluid replacers are a poor

choice because they tend to be very dilute and thereby are poor sources of carbohydrates. For example, an athlete may have to drink 48 ounces of a commercial fluid replacer when he or she could more easily (and less expensively) ingest the same amount of carbohydrates in 16 ounces of cranapple juice.

To determine how much fluid an athlete needs to replace, she or he can be weighed before and after the event. Because each pound lost represents 2 cups of sweat losses, the athlete should drink enough to cover those losses, plus more. Thirst inadequately signals dehydration; an athlete may not feel thirsty but can still be dehydrated. The better way to monitor hydration is to pay attention to patterns of urination. An athlete is adequately hydrated if the urine is clear and voluminous. Dark urine is still concentrated with metabolic wastes.

Although beer is a popular postexercise "recovery drink," its alcohol content has a dehydrating effect. Hence, athletes who drink beer tend to frequent the bathroom, where they flush valuable fluids down the toilet, rather than replace sweat losses. Alcohol also has a depressant effect and, when consumed on an empty stomach (as commonly happens after an event), can quickly negate the more invigorating "natural high" that comes after hard exercise.

Although many athletes are concerned about replacing the sodium and potassium lost in sweat, few athletes are at risk of depleting their body stores. Athletes can easily replace these minerals with the foods and fluids they eat after an event without special supplements. Based on the assumption that athletes who exercise a lot also eat a lot, the healthy athlete who has concerns about electrolyte replacement can be assured that he or she will consume more than enough sodium, potassium, and other minerals in subsequent meals.

SUMMARY

The carbohydrate-rich foods that an athlete eats before, during, and after an event should be an extension of the daily 60 to 70% carbohydrate training diet. During training, the athlete should experiment to determine the foods and fluids that settle best and contribute to top performance. Coaches and exercise leaders should cautiously make specific food recommendations, because each athlete has individual tolerances and preferences that have to be self-determined.

RECOMMENDED READING

Brouns F, Saris W, and Rehrer N: Abdominal complaints and gastro-intestinal function during long-lasting exercise. *Intl J Sports Med 8:*175–189, 1987.

Evans W and Hughes V: Dietary carbohydrates and endurance exercise. *Am J Clin Nutr 41:*1146–1154, 1985.

Gleeson M, Maughan R, and Greenhaff P: Comparison of the effects of pre-exercise feedings of glucose, glycerol and placebo on endurance and fuel homeostasis in man. *Eur J Appl Physiol 55:*645–653, 1986.

Ivy J: Muscle glycogen synthesis after exercise and effect of time on carbohydrate ingestion. *J Appl Physiol 64:*1480–1485, 1988.

Jandrain B, Krzentowski G, Pirnay F, et al: Metabolic availability of glucose ingested three hours before prolonged exercise in humans. *J Appl Physiol 56:*1314–1319, 1984.

Ravussin L, Pahus P, Dorner A, et al: Substrate utilization during prolonged exercise preceded by ingestion of 13C-glucose in glycogen depleted and control subjects. *Pflugers Arch 382:*197–202, 1979.

Sherman W, Simonsen J, Wright D, and Dernbach A: Effect of carbohydrate in four hour pre-exercise meals. *Med Sci Sports Exerc 20:*S157, 1988

SPORTS NUTRITION BOOKS

American Dietetic Association: *Sports Nutrition: A Manual for Professionals Working with Active People.* Chicago, 1986. (PO Box 10960, Chicago, IL 60610-0960.)

Clark N: *Nancy Clark's Sports Nutrition Guidebook.* Champaign, IL: Leisure Press, 1990.

Clark N: *The Athlete's Kitchen.* Boston: New England Sports Publications, 1981. (Available by mailorder only through New England Sports Publications, PO Box 252, Boston MA 02113 ($7).

Coleman E: *Eating for Endurance.* Palo Alto: Bull Publishing Co., 1987.

Williams M: *Nutritional Aspects of Human Physiology and Performance.*Springfield, IL: Charles C Thomas, 1985.

| C | H | A | P | T | E | R | 6 |

ERGOGENIC AIDS

Melvin H. Williams

Although proper physiologic, psychological, and biomechanical training is the key to success in sports, athletes at all levels of competition are constantly searching for a means to obtain a competitive edge over their opponents. Often these means include substances, techniques, or equipment known as ergogenic aids, ergogenic meaning to enhance performance by improving energy production, energy control, or energy efficiency during exercise. For purposes of this discussion, five different categories of ergogenic aids are covered: mechanical or biomechanical, psychological, nutritional, physiologic, and pharmacologic. This categorization is arbitrary, however, because some agents, such as caffeine, may exert effects in each category.

MECHANICAL ERGOGENIC AIDS

Mechanical and biomechanical ergogenic aids are used to decrease the resistance to movement and include modifications in the weight and shape of the human body, sportswear, or sports equipment. Losing excess body fat will improve performance in a wide variety of sports, such as distance running, gymnastics, and high jumping, whereas increasing body weight as muscle mass may contribute to success in other sports dependent on the generation of maximal strength and power. The use of lighter running shoes and aerodynamic clothing are two examples of sportswear design that may enhance performance. Significant improvements in performance also result from improved equipment design. The phenomenal achievement of Greg Lemond in the final stage of the 1989 Tour de France was partially attributed to his aerodynamic clothing, helmet, and handlebar design.

PSYCHOLOGICAL ERGOGENIC AIDS

Psychological ergogenic aids, most of which are psychotherapeutic techniques, involve mental training. They are designed to optimize psychological energy As applied to sport, the inverted U theory suggests that an optimal amount of anxiety is needed for maximal performance; depending on the nature of the event, too much or too little anxiety could impair performance. Psychological energizers (analogous to pharmacologic stimulants) are techniques used to increase or focus energy levels, whereas psychological tranquilizers (analogous to pharmacologic depressants) may be helpful to eliminate negative psychological energy. Such techniques as hypnosis, goal setting, visual-motor behavioral rehearsal, and stress management may help to improve sports performance by helping the athlete achieve an optimal level of psychological readiness. The available research suggests that such methods are somewhat better than no intervention at all.

NUTRITIONAL ERGOGENIC AIDS

As noted elsewhere in this book, optimal nutrition is essential to help athletes optimize energy supplies, regulate human energy systems, and maximize growth of body tissues. Certain nutritional practices, such as carbohydrate loading in prolonged endurance events, may be ergogenic. In general, however, a balanced and adequate intake of calories, carbohydrates, fats, proteins, vitamins, minerals, and water satisfies the nutrient needs of most athletes. Nevertheless, numerous products are marketed as potential nutritional ergogenic aids for the athlete. Unfortunately, few experimental scientific data exist to support the efficacy of such purported ergogenic foods, nutrients, or pseudonutrients as amino acid supplements, bee pollen, carnitine, inosine, octacosanol, pangamic acid (vitamin B_{15}), or wheat germ oil. On the other hand, available data are conflicting regarding the ergogenic effect of aspartate salts and phosphate salts; several studies have shown improvements in physiologic functions or performance in aerobic endurance tests. More research is needed to support these preliminary findings.

PHYSIOLOGIC ERGOGENIC AIDS

Physiologic ergogenic aids, particularly alkaline salts and blood doping, have been utilized to directly improve specific physiologic processes important to sports performance. Alkaline salts, such as sodium bicarbonate, may increase the alkaline reserve and may help to buffer lactic acid in the muscle cell by facilitating the efflux of hydrogen ions. These salts are theorized to improve athletic performance in anaerobic-type events dependent primarily on anaerobic glycolysis. Approximately 50% of the studies support the efficacy of alkaline salts. These salts increase the serum pH and have been shown to improve time to exhaustion in high-intensity exercise tasks in the laboratory, as well as performance in anaerobic-type track and swim events. On the other hand, equally well-designed studies have evidenced no beneficial effects in short-term anaerobic or more prolonged aerobic-type events, but performance did not decrease either. In general, the data appear to support an ergogenic effect of alkaline salts, although one possible disadvantage is the associated diarrhea in some subjects.

Blood doping involves the removal of an athlete's blood and its storage in a frozen state for at least 6 to 8 weeks prior to infusion back into the athlete. In some cases, cross-matched blood from other individuals has been used. The purpose of blood doping is to increase RBC and hemoglobin levels with an accompanying increase in oxygen transport. Blood doping is also known as blood boosting or induced erythrocythemia. The results of carefully controlled studies reveal that blood doping is an effective ergogenic aid. It significantly increases hemoglobin concentration and maximal oxygen uptake, resulting in highly improved performance in aerobic-type events. Both laboratory and field studies support its effectiveness. At the present time, no test is available to detect the utilization of blood doping by an athlete.

PHARMACOLOGIC ERGOGENIC AIDS

Known as doping, pharmacologic ergogenic aids have been used to improve both physiologic and psychological functions deemed important to sports performance. The International Olympic Committee (IOC) originally developed its antidoping legislation to counter the prevalent use of drugs by athletes and even banned the use of medications prescribed for medical use if the medication contained a banned drug. Over the years, many drugs have been used by athletes, including stimulants such as amphetamines and caffeine, depressants such as alcohol and beta-blockers, tissue-growth enhancers such as anabolic steroids and human growth hormone, and miscellaneous agents such as diuretics. The IOC has an extensive list of banned ergogenic aids, ranging from potent anabolic steroids to Nyquil nighttime cold medicine. Research with stimulants, depressants, anabolic steroids, and diuretics is briefly summarized in the next few paragraphs.

A variety of stimulants have been used in attempts to enhance athletic performance, but the most researched are amphetamines and caffeine. These stimulants may favorably effect changes in a number of physiologic functions at rest, such as cardiac output, but these effects seen at rest appear to be abrogated by the natural sympathetic response during exercise. Nevertheless, actual physical performance in certain endeavors, particularly prolonged endurance tasks, may be improved by adequate dosage of stimulants. This performance-enhancing effect is believed due to improved psychological functions, leading to increased work output or tolerance to fatigue.

Depressants generally have been used to suppress pain to enable an injured athlete to continue to play. Depressants such as alcohol and beta-blockers have also been used for potential ergogenic effects, however. Research has shown that, for some athletic endeavors, depressants, at best, exert little effect on performance, but they actually impair performance in some sports. For example, alcohol has been shown repeatedly to adversely affect skill in tasks involving decision-making in response to rapidly changing stimuli, whereas beta-blockers have significantly decreased aerobic endurance performance in highly trained athletes. On the other hand, in sports such as archery and pistol and rifle shooting, depressants have been used to help reduce muscle tremor, to induce bradycardia, and to decrease the blood-pressure response to the anxiety of competition. In a recent study, beta-blockers improved pistol shooting performance by 13%.

Athletes have used anabolic steroids for a variety of reasons, but the most prevalent is to increase protein synthesis for increased body weight and muscle mass, ideally leading to increased strength and power. The general results of the well-controlled studies have shown that anabolic steroids may help increase body weight and lean body mass in humans. The average gains were 2 to 3 kilograms in body weight, but the percentage of increased muscle mass versus nonmuscle tissue and body water is not clear. Case studies of individuals self-administering anabolic steroids reveal substantially greater weight gains. Analysis of the well-controlled studies with anabolic steroids and strength reveals that in approximately 50% of the studies with humans, the subjects did have significant strength gains compared to the placebo group. The gains averaged 8 kilograms in the bench press and 11 kilograms in the squat. In general, experienced lifters increased significantly more than inexperienced lifters. Individual case studies support these laboratory findings.

Diuretics normally are used by athletes who must meet specific body weight standards, such as wrestlers and boxers. If these athletes are unable to rehydrate adequately prior to competition, their performance may be impaired, particularly if an aerobic endurance component is involved. For example, diuretics significantly decreased the plasma volume and performance of runners in distances ranging from 1.5 to 10 kilograms. Contrarily, because diuretics do not appear to impair strength or power, performance may be enhanced in events characterized by rapid power development to move the body weight, such as high jumping. Recent research has shown that vertical jumping ability increased significantly following a diuretic-induced body water loss.

ETHICAL ISSUES

One of the major concerns with the use of ergogenic aids is the ethical issue. It would appear that if an ergogenic aid were legal within the rules of the athletic governing body, such as the IOC or NCAA, and if it posed no health risk to the athlete, then it would not be unethical to use it. Such is the case for most biomechanical, psychological, and nutritional aids, and some physiologic aids, although some medical risks may be associated with excessive amounts of some nutritional and physiologic aids. Most pharmacologic aids that may theoretically enhance performance are banned, and hence it is illegal and unethical for athletes to use them; moreover, many drugs used as ergogenic aids may pose significant health risks to the athlete.

RECOMMENDED READING

American College of Sports Medicine: Position stand on the use of anabolic-androgenic steroids in sports. *Med Sci Sports Exerc* 19:534–539, 1987.

American College of Sports Medicine: Position stand on blood doping as an ergogenic aid. *Med Sci Sports Exerc* 19:540–543, 1987.

Morgan WP: *Ergogenic Aids and Muscular Performance.* New York: Academic Press, 1972.

Wadler G, and Hainline B: *Drugs and the Athlete.* Philadelphia: F.A. Davis, 1989.

Williams MH: *Ergogenic Aids in Sport.* Champaign, IL: Human Kinetics, 1983.

Williams MH: *Beyond Training: How Athletes Enhance Performance Legally and Illegally.* Champaign, IL: Leisure Press, 1989.

Williams MH: Drugs and sports performance. In *Sports Medicine.* Edited by A Ryan and F Allman. New York: Academic Press, 1989.

C H A P T E R 7

PREPARTICIPATION EXAMINATION*

John A. Lombardo

Every athlete has the right of a "thorough preseason history and medical evaluation" according to the American Medical Association Committee on Medical Aspects of Sports. As the area of sports medicine has developed, the preparticipation evaluation has also progressed from the "locker room lineup" to a sophisticated system of physical examination and performance assessment. There is no continuity of content, timing, frequency or type of examination, however. Various activity classifications and guidelines for participation exist. Agreement on these issues by the various state high school athletic associations and medical organizations would be a valuable asset to physicians administering this traditional ritual.

OBJECTIVES

The preparticipation evaluation should:

1. Determine the general health of the athlete
2. Detect any conditions that might limit participation
3. Detect conditions that might predispose the athlete to injury (untreated injuries or illness, lack of conditioning, or congenital or developmental problems)
4. Assess level of maturity
5. Evaluate fitness level
6. Afford an opportunity for physician-athlete contact to counsel about health and answer health-related questions
7. Meet legal and insurance requirements

* Portions of this chapter and Figures 7–1 to 7–12 are borrowed from Smith N: For the Practitioner: Orthopedic Screening Examination for Preparticipation in Sports. Columbus, OH: Ross Laboratories, 1981; that publication, in turn, contains material borrowed from the American Orthopaedic Society for Sports Medicine and coordinated with the American Academy of Pediatrics.

TIMING OF EXAMINATION

Six weeks prior to the season is the ideal time for the preparticipation physical examination. This allows for correction and/or rehabilitation of problems prior to the season.

FREQUENCY OF EXAMINATION

The three alternative frequencies used include:

1. Annual complete examination
2. Entry level (high school, college, etc.) with annual history
3. Prior to every season

A reasonable alternative would be an entry-level complete history and physical with a limited history and physical examination annually.

TYPE OF EXAMINATION

Evaluation in the primary-care physician's office has the advantage of:

1. Physician-patient familiarity
   a. complete history and medical records
   b. opportunity for discussion of sensitive issues
2. Continuity of care

The other type of examination is the station-type mass examination (Table 7–1). These have the advantages of:

1. Inclusion of more specialized personnel (sports-oriented physicians, athletic trainers, physical therapist, dietitians, exercise physiologists)
2. Time and cost efficiency
3. Ability to offer performance testing

The advantages of both can be obtained by including the local primary-care physicians in the station-type examination and providing a private room for the evaluation.

MEDICAL HISTORY

The medical history is the keystone of any medical examination. The areas of importance in the history include:

TABLE 7–1. Station Examination

1. Sign in	Athletic director or coach
2. Review history	Physician
3. Height and weight	Coach
4. Visual acuity	Coach, nurse
5. Vital signs	Nurse
6. Medical examination	Physician
7. Orthopedic examination	Physician
8. Review and reassessment	Physician
9. Body composition	Physiologist
10. Flexibility	Therapist or trainer
11. Strength	Therapist, coach, athletic trainer
12. Speed	Coach
13. Agility	Coach
14. Power	Coach
15. Balance	Coach
16. Endurance	Coach

1. Hospitalizations/surgery
2. Medication
3. Allergies
4. Tetanus status
5. Cardiovascular system
6. Family history of cardiovascular problems
7. Musculoskeletal system
8. Neurologic system
9. Dermatologic system
10. Heat problems
11. Other medical problems
12. Menstrual history

A sample history form is shown in Table 7–2.

Because athletes' completion of their medical history does not often agree with their parents' more thorough completion, it is very important that history forms are made available to the athletes prior to the day of the examination so their parents can assist in completing the form.

PHYSICAL EXAMINATION

The physical examination is a screening examination that emphasizes the evaluation of the areas of greatest concern and the areas identified as problems in the history. Included in the examination are:

TABLE 7–2. History Form

Name _____   Data of Birth _____
Address _____   Class _____
Parents _____   Phone # _____
Physician _____
Sports _____   _____

Fill in details of "YES" answers in space below:

	Yes	No
1. Have you ever been hospitalized?	___	___
Have you ever had surgery?	___	___
2. Are you currently taking medication?	___	___
3. Do you have any allergies (medicines, bees)?	___	___
4. Have you ever passed out during exercise:	___	___
Have you ever been dizzy during exercise?	___	___
Have you ever had chest pain?	___	___
Do you tire more quickly than your friends during exercise?	___	___
Have you ever had high blood pressure?	___	___
Have you ever been told you have a heart murmur?	___	___
Have you ever had racing of your heart or skipped beats?	___	___
Has anyone in your family died of heart problems or a sudden death before age 40?	___	___
5. Do you have any skin problems? (itching, moles, breaking out)	___	___
6. Have you ever had a head injury?	___	___
Have you ever been knocked out?	___	___
Have you ever had a seizure?	___	___
Have you ever had a stinger or burner?	___	___

7. Have you ever injured (sprained, dislocated, fractured, etc.):

___ Hand	___ Shoulder	___ Thigh
___ Wrist	___ Neck	___ Knee
___ Forearm	___ Chest	___ Shin/Calf
___ Elbow	___ Back	___ Ankle
___ Arm	___ Hip	___ Foot

	Yes	No
8. Have you ever had heat cramps?	___	___
Have you ever been dizzy or passed out in the heat?	___	___

9. Have you ever had:

___ Mononucleosis	___ Diabetes
___ Hepatitis	___ Headaches (frequent)
___ Asthma	___ Eye injuries
___ Tuberculosis	___ Stomach ulcer

10. Do you use special pads or braces?	___ ___
11. When was your last tetanus shot?	_____
12. When was your first period?	_____
When was your last period?	_____

Explain YES answers here:

_____
_____
_____
_____
_____
_____
_____
_____

Parent's signature: _____

Height
Weight
Visual acuity
Cardiovascular
  Blood pressure—130/75 < 10 years old
  140/85 > 10 years old
  Pulses—radial, femoral
  Heart—rhythm, murmurs, size
Musculoskeletal Appendix II
Abdominal—organomegaly
Skin—impetigo, acne, scabies, herpes, nevi
Genitalia—single or undescended testicle, testicular mass
Maturity—Tanner staging

In the musculoskeletal examination, a complete examination is performed on any area flagged on the history or identified as a problem on the physical examination. The examiner may wish to perform a more thorough examination of the part of the musculoskeletal system maximally stressed by an activity, e.g., the shoulder in baseball and swimming (see sample physical form, Table 7–3).

This examination should be performed upon entry to school (middle school or high school) with yearly cardiovascular examinations, (BP, pulse, heart exam) skin examination and maturity evaluation along with any area which is flagged by history (see Table 7–3).

PERFORMANCE TESTING

Measuring certain fitness parameters can help the athlete to optimize performance and also may (although never proved) help to prevent injuries. These tests can be performed in a general fashion or in a more directed sports-specific fashion. An example of sports-specific testing would be the evaluation of flexibility and strength of the shoulders of throwers. This sports-specific directing of performance testing is the ideal way of approaching this part of the preparticipation physical. The areas to be evaluated include:

Body composition	skin folds
	underwater weighing
Flexibility	sit and reach
	goniometric
Strength	manual muscle testing
	bench press/leg press
	pull-ups
	sit-ups/push-ups
	isokinetics

TABLE 7–3. Physical Examination

Height _____   Weight _____   BP _____   Pulse _____

Visual acuity   _____

CV: Pulses   _____

    Heart   _____

Abdominal   _____

Skin   _____

Genitalia   _____

Tanner   _____

Musculoskeletal

    Neck   _____

    Shoulder   _____

    Elbow   _____

    Wrist   _____

    Hand   _____

    Back   _____

    Knee   _____

    Ankle   _____

    Foot   _____

Assessment   _____

_____

_____

_____

_____

Recommendation   _____

_____

_____

_____

_____

Clearance (circle appropriate clearance)
1. No restrictions
    A. Contact/collision
    B. Limited contact/impact
    C. Noncontact
       1. Strenuous
       2. Moderately strenuous
       3. Nonstrenuous
2. Cleared after notification of coach, athletic trainer, physician
3. Clearance deferred until evaluation by a physician

Endurance	12-minute run
	1½-mile run
Power	vertical jump
	standing broad jump
Speed	40-yard dash
Sustained speed	440-yard run

Agility	Illinois agility run
Balance	Stork stand
Dynamic balance	Bass dynamic balance test
	Springfield Bram-Walking Test

It is very important that the results of the performance test are returned and explained to the coaches and athletes in a timely fashion.

CLEARANCE

Clearance can be divided into three categories:

1. Unrestricted clearance for:
   A. Contact/collision
   B. Limited contact impact
   C. Noncontact
      1. strenuous
      2. moderately strenuous
      3. nonstrenuous
2. Cleared after notification of coach, athletic trainer, team physician
3. Clearance deferred until further evaluation by physician

Clearance should be based on guidelines and the published recommendations for participation in competitive sports published by the American Academy of Pediatrics (AAP) are excellent criteria when paired with the judgment of the physician (Table 7–4). The AAP sports classification system is an accurate manner of dividing the activities for clearance (Table 7–5). These recommendations and classifications are a good guide for the physician attempting to help an athlete choose an appropriate activity.

ORTHOPEDIC SCREENING EXAMINATION FOR PARTICIPATION IN SPORTS

Many athletic activities require periodic physical examination of the participant. This information has been developed for practicing physicians who provide pediatric care as a guide to performing the orthopedic screening component of the sports preparticipation examination. The exercise should be coupled with a simple questionnaire that is easily understood by the child and his or her parent.

TABLE 7–4. Recommendations for Participation in Competitive Sports of the American Academy of Pediatrics

	Contact/ Collision	Limited Contact/Impact	Noncontact Strenuous	Noncontact Moderately Strenuous	Noncontact Nonstrenuous
Atlantoaxial instability * Swimming: no butterfly, breast stroke, or diving starts	No	No	Yes*	Yes	Yes
Acute illnesses * Needs individual assessment. e.g., contagiousness to others, risk of worsening illness	*	*	*	*	*
Cardiovascular Carditis*	No	No	No	No	No
Hypertension					
Mild	Yes *	Yes *	Yes *	Yes *	Yes *
Moderate	*	*	*	*	*
Severe	*	*	*	*	*
Congenital heart disease	†	†	†	†	†

* Needs individual assessment
† Patients with mild forms can be allowed a full range of physical activities; patients with moderate or severe forms, or who are postoperative, should be evaluated by a cardiologist before athletic participation.

	Contact/ Collision	Limited Contact/Impact	Noncontact Strenuous	Noncontact Moderately Strenuous	Noncontact Nonstrenuous
Eyes					
Absence or loss of function of one eye	*	*	*	*	*
Detached retina	†	†	†	†	†

* Availability of American Society for Testing and Materials (ASTM)-approved eye guards may allow competitor to participate in most sports, but this must be judged on an individual basis.
† Consult ophthalmologist

Condition	1	2	3	4	5
Inguinal hernia	Yes	Yes	Yes	Yes	Yes
Kidney: Absence of one	No	No	Yes	Yes	Yes
Liver: Enlarged	No	No	No	Yes	Yes
Musculoskeletal disorders	*	*	*	*	*
* Needs individual assessment					
Neurologic					
History of serious head or spine trauma, repeated concussions, or craniotomy	*	*	Yes	Yes	Yes
Convulsive disorder					
Well controlled	Yes	Yes	Yes	Yes	Yes
Poorly controlled	No	No	Yes†	Yes	Yes‡
* Needs individual assessment					
† No swimming or weight lifting					
‡ No archery or riflery					
Ovary: Absence of one	Yes	Yes	Yes	Yes	Yes
Respiratory					
Pulmonary insufficiency	*	*	*	*	Yes
Asthma	Yes	Yes	Yes	Yes	Yes
* May be allowed to compete if oxygenation remains satisfactory during a graded stress test					
Sickle cell trait	Yes	Yes	Yes	Yes	Yes
Skin: Boils, herpe, impetigo, scabies	*	*	Yes	Yes	Yes
* No gymnastics with mats, martial arts, wrestling, or contact sports until not contagious					
Spleen: Enlarged	No	No	No	Yes	Yes
Testicle: Absent or undescended	Yes*	Yes*	Yes*	Yes	Yes
* Certain sports may require protective cup					

(From American Academy of Pediatrics Committee on Sports Medicine: Recommendations for participation in competitive sports. *Pediatrics* 81:737, 1988.)

TABLE 7–5. Sports Classification System of the American Academy of Pediatrics

Contact Collision	Limited Contact Impact	Noncontact		
		Strenuous	Moderately Strenuous	Nonstrenuous
Boxing	Baseball	Aerobic dancing	Badminton	Archery
Field hockey	Basketball	Crew	Curling	Golf
Football	Bicycling	Fencing	Table tennis	Riflery
Ice hockey	Diving	Field		
Lacrosse	Field	Discus		
Martial arts	High jump	Javelin		
Rodeo	Pole vault	Shot put		
Soccer	Gymnastics	Running		
Wrestling	Horseback riding	Swimming		
	Skating	Tennis		
	Ice	Track		
	Roller	Weight lifting		
	Skiing			
	Cross-country			
	Downhill			
	Water			
	Softball			
	Squash, handball			
	Volleyball			

(From American Academy of Pediatrics Committee on Sports Medicine: Recommendations for participation in competive sports. *Pediatrics 81*:737, 1988.)

The purpose of the examination is to identify congenital or acquired musculoskeletal problems that might be adversely affected by or interfere with athletic participation. If any abnormalities are apparent from the questionnaire or the orthopedic screening examination, the physician can use this information as the basis for a specifically directed examination.

The orthopedic screening examination cannot be all things to all people—it must be a minimum standard, thus equally appropriate for the Little League baseball player, the gymnast, and the high school soccer player. The practical appeal of this examination is that it requires no special equipment, can be completed in less than 3 minutes, and can easily be a part of the preparticipation examination protocol in an office-based setting. Although not all conditions prove to be problems in all sports, once identified, the specific sports relationships can be evaluated in the directed examination.

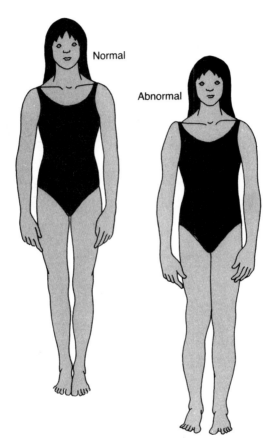

FIG. 7–1. Instructions: Stand straight with arms at sides.
Observations: Symmetry of upper and lower extremities and trunk.
Common abnormalities:
1. Enlarged acromioclavicular joint
2. Enlarged sternoclavicular joint
3. Asymmetric waist (leg length difference or scoliosis)
4. Swollen knee
5. Swollen ankle

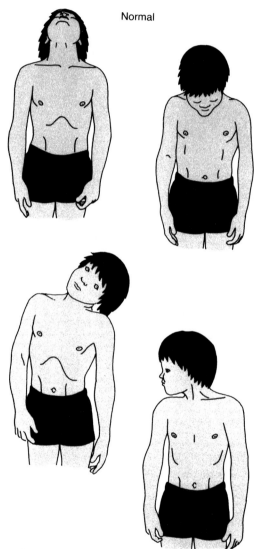

Normal

FIG. 7–2. Legend on facing page.

Abnormal

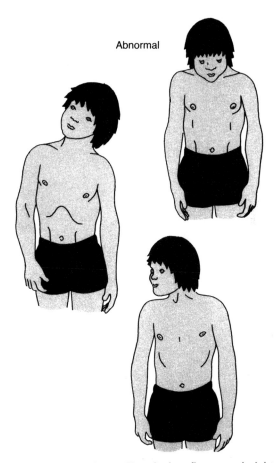

FIG. 7–2. Instructions: Look at ceiling; look at floor; touch right (left) ear to shoulder; look over right (left) shoulder.

Observations: Should be able to touch chin to chest, ears to shoulders and look equally over shoulders.

Common abnormalities (may indicate previous neck injury):

1. Loss of flexion
2. Loss of lateral bending
3. Loss of rotation

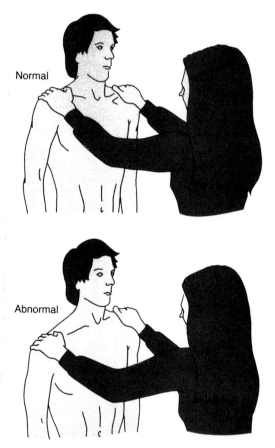

FIG. 7–3. Instructions: Shrug shoulders while examiner holds them down. Observations: Trapezius muscles appear equal; left and right sides equal strength.
Common abnormalities (may indicate neck or shoulder problem):
1. Loss of strength
2. Loss of muscle bulk

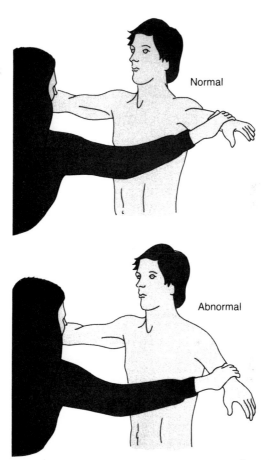

FIG. 7–4. Instructions: Hold arms out from sides horizontally and lift while examiner holds them down.
Observations: Strength should be equal and deltoid muscles should be equal in size.
Common abnormalities:
1. Loss of strength
2. Wasting of deltoid muscle

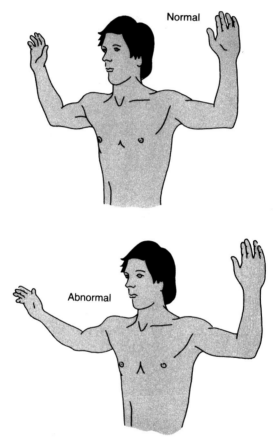

FIG. 7–5. Instructions: Hold arms out from sides with elbows bent (90°); raise hands back vertically as far as they will go.

Observations: Hands go back equally and at least to upright vertical position.

Common abnormalities (may indicate shoulder problem or old dislocation):

1. Loss of external rotation

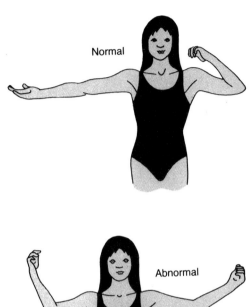

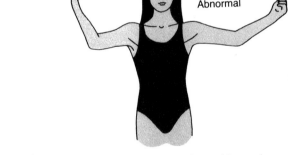

FIG. 7–6. Instructions: Hold arms out from sides, palms up; straighten elbows completely; bend completely.
Observations: Motion equal left and right.
Common abnormalities (may indicate old elbow injury, old dislocation, fracture, etc.):
1. Loss of extension
2. Loss of flexion

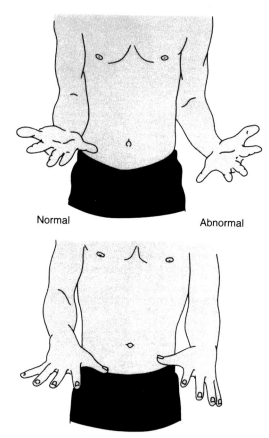

Normal   Abnormal

FIG. 7–7. Instructions: Hold arms down at sides with elbows bent (90°); supinate palms; pronate palms.
Observations: Palms should go from facing ceiling to facing floor.
Common abnormalities (may indicate old forearm, wrist, or elbow injury):
1. Lack of full supination
2. Lack of full pronation

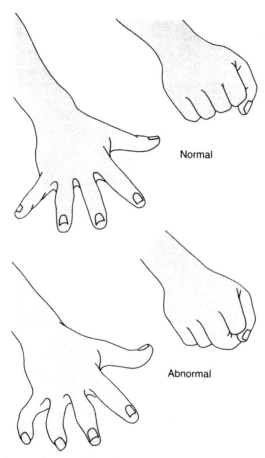

FIG. 7–8. Instructions: Make a first; open hand and spread fingers. Observations: Fist should be tight and fingers straight when spread. Common abnormalities (may indicate old finger fractures or sprains):
1. Protruding knuckle from fist
2. Swollen and/or crooked finger

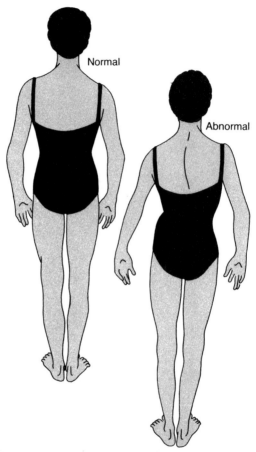

FIG. 7–9. Instructions: With back to examiner stand up straight.
Observations: Symmetry of shoulders, waist, thighs, and calves.
Common abnormalities:
1. High shoulder (scoliosis) or low shoulder (muscle loss)
2. Prominent rib cage (scoliosis)
3. High hip or asymmetrical waist (leg length difference or scoliosis)
4. Small calf or thigh (weakness from old injury)

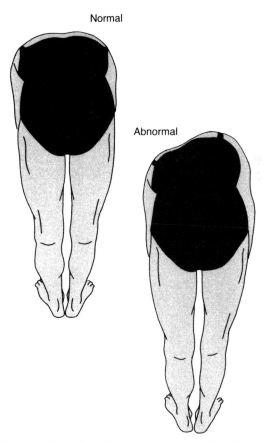

FIG. 7–10. Instructions: Bend forward slowly as to touch toes.
Observations: Bends forward straight and smoothly.
Common abnormalities:
1. Twists to side (low back pain)
2. Back asymmetrical (scoliosis)

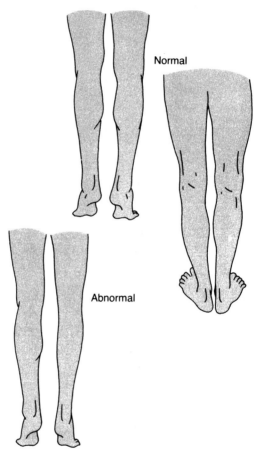

FIG. 7–11. Instructions: Stand on heels; stand on toes.
Observations: Equal elevation right and left; symmetry of calf muscles.
Common abnormalities:
1. Wasting of calf muscles (Achilles injury or old ankle injury)

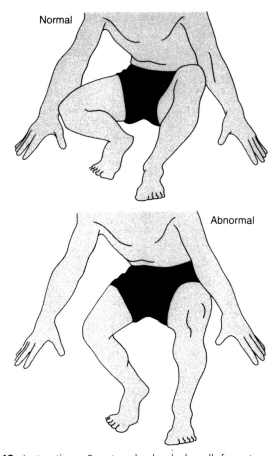

FIG. 7–12. Instructions: Squat on heels; duck walk four steps and stand up.

Observations: Maneuver is painless; heel to buttock distance equal left and right; knee flexion equal during walk; rises straight up.

Common abnormalities:

1. Inability to fully flex one knee
2. Inability to stand up without twisting or bending to one side

EXAMINATION PARAMETERS

- Appropriate for interscholastic, intramural, and extramural sports activities.
- A screening evaluation created to direct attention to problems but *not* evaluate the problems.
- Identifies the following conditions that might be adversely affected by athletic participation:
  a. Congenital problems
  b. Acquired problems

HISTORY

Questions such as the following are to be answered by the athlete and signed by *both* the athlete and the parent:
- Have you ever had an illness, condition, or injury that required you to go to the hospital, either as a patient overnight or in the emergency room or for x-rays; required an operation; caused you to see a doctor; caused you to miss a game or practice?
- Are you now or have you been under the care of a physician for any reason?
- Do you currently have any medical problems or injuries?
- Have you ever had a broken bone, joint sprain or ligament tear, muscle pull, head injury, neck injury or nerve pinch, dislocated joint, back trouble or problems?

RECOMMENDED READING

American Academy of Pediatrics Committee on Sports Medicine: Recommendations for participation in competitive sports. *Pediatrics* 81:737–739, 1988.

Lombardo JA: Preparticipation physical examination. *Primary Care Clin* 11:3–21, 1984.

McKeag DB: Preseason physical examination for the prevention of sports injuries. *Sports Med* 2:413–431, 1985.

Smith N: For the Practitioner: Orthopaedic Screening Examination for Participation in Sports. Columbus, Ohio, Ross Laboratories, 1981.

| C H A P T E R 8 |

ORGANIZATIONAL ASPECTS

James C. Puffer

The team physician plays a multifaceted role in the provision of health care to the athlete. Typically, he or she provides continuous and comprehensive medical care to the athletes for whom he or she assumes responsibility. This usually includes conduct of an appropriate preparticipation evaluation, coordination of on-site medical care during athletic competition, determination of readiness to return to play, development of appropriate procedures for injury surveillance, maintenance of accurate medication profiles, and assessment of the quality and adequacy of protective equipment. In order to provide comprehensive care in such a manner, it is critical that the team physician develop an appropriate organizational and administrative structure by which these tasks can be handled efficiently. Development of such an organizational framework will not only clearly define the expectations of each member of the sports medicine team, but more importantly, will provide a clear and concise management plan for those problems that are typically encountered or can be expected to be encountered in any situation.

SIDELINE ORGANIZATION

Perhaps no role is more important than that provided by the team physician when he or she assumes the care of athletes during athletic competition. Although the incidence of catastrophic injury is low, the potential for serious injury always exists, and it is essential that appropriate planning be undertaken to guarantee an effective and efficient response to any emergency. This requires important pre-event communication among the team physician, the certified athletic trainer (if one exists), the coaching staff, and the emergency medicine system (EMS) within the respective geographic area in which the competition will take place.

95

The development of a team approach is critical in the acute management of the injured athlete. It is important that every member of the team who will provide care for the athlete has a clear understanding of his or her responsibilities beforehand. This will require the team physician to evaluate the available resources for response to injury. If manpower for response to catastrophic injury is limited, it is the team physician's responsibility to train the coaching staff appropriately in emergency procedures that may be required at the time of an on-field emergency. This would include CPR, stabilization and movement of the athlete with suspected cervical spine injury, and the initial management of heat injury, for example. The appropriate response to on-the-field catastrophic injury needs to be practiced and rehearsed with the team that will be responsible for providing such care. These rehearsals should obviously occur prior to the beginning of the competitive season or planned event.

After identification of the team that will provide acute care to the injured athlete, the physician must plan for the appropriate transportation of the athlete to an emergency facility. Again, this requires advance planning and should be done well before the competitive season or specific event. This should include a determination of the EMS resources available to the physician, including the level of care provided by the ambulance teams, their response time to the field of competition, the equipment they carry with them, and the hospital to which they will transport the injured athlete. The hospital facility must be well equipped to handle catastrophic injury, and it is the team physician's responsibility to guarantee that such capability exists. The mechanism by which the EMS system will be notified also needs to be thought out well in advance. Will the EMS unit be available on site or must it be summoned? If it must be summoned, how will this occur, and who will be responsible for doing it? Responsibility for this task needs to be appropriately delegated in a clear and concise way, and again, this aspect of the catastrophic-care mechanism must be pretested thoroughly by rehearsal.

Finally, the team physician must develop a well-respected group of consultants to provide care to athletes on an emergency basis. Such consultants should be selected not only for their subspecialty expertise, but also for their availability and ready access in an emergency, as well as their demonstrated clinical competence in dealing with potential catastrophic injury in the athletic population.

It is the team physician's responsibility to make certain that all elements of the emergency response team are in place prior to each game or competitive event. This should include a careful checklist

TABLE 8–1. Sideline Equipment for Athletic Emergencies

1. Backboard and sandbags
2. Neck immobilizer
3. Crutches
4. Slings and splints
5. Ice, plastic bags, compression dressings
6. Appropriate emergency drugs and intravenous fluids if not readily available from the EMS unit
7. Appropriately stocked physician's bag (see reference)

approach to guarantee that identified personnel are present, the EMS system has been notified of the competition and is available for ready response if not on site, previously identified consultants are available. In addition, a careful check of sideline equipment needs to be undertaken to assess its readiness. This should include the minimum equipment outlined in Table 8–1.

In summary, precompetition organization is essential to provide rapid response to any potential injury at the competitive site. The development of a well-defined team approach to the injured athlete is critical, and the development of a well-designed organizational plan will encompass the six elements listed in Table 8–2.

PROVISION OF CONTINUOUS CARE

Optimum health care is provided to the athlete when it is continuous and comprehensive. In most university or high school settings, care is provided in a centralized training room, which should be appropriately designed and developed by both the team physician and the certified athletic trainer. In settings where re-

TABLE 8–2. Organizational Plan for Team Approach to the Injured Athlete

1. Identification of appropriately trained personnel to assist in the provision of on-site emergency medical care
2. Provision of adequate on-site emergency equipment
3. Determination of adequate emergency transportation with appropriately trained personnel on site or available on call
4. Development of appropriate communication mechanism to summon emergency transportation
5. Appropriate identification of hospital facilities with well-trained personnel
6. Identification of appropriate consultative services

sources are not available for a well-equipped, centralized training room, space should be designated in which the team physician can appropriately treat and evaluate patients in privacy, as well as maintain appropriate records.

The cornerstone of continuous and comprehensive care of the athlete is the preparticipation evaluation. This should be sports specific and should serve as the foundation for the subsequent care of the athlete. Numerous models exist for the conduct of this examination and are discussed elsewhere in this handbook.

Record keeping is equally important, and the initial database established during the preparticipation examination provides the essential element in the athlete's medical record. Subsequent evaluations should be carefully documented and maintained either in the centralized training room, the physician's office, or the previously identified sports medicine area. A frequently overlooked element of the athlete's medical record is the drug profile. Increasing attention should be paid to this important area because drug testing is now routine at many levels. Such a profile can only be obtained through a detailed and meticulous drug history documented in the athlete's medical record. This profile serves as the basis for ongoing drug education and counseling and is essential for athletes who will participate in events at which drug testing will occur.

Although individual record keeping is important, systematic, organized record keeping for the team as a whole is equally important. Such injury surveillance can be critical in helping to detect seasonal trends in the incidence of injury, can assist in modifying deleterious training techniques, and can detect inadequate equipment or less-than-optimal playing conditions. Many useful computerized injury-surveillance systems can be easily adapted to the personal computer, but for those athletics programs that do not have the resources to purchase such programs, a student trainer or student manager can be appropriately trained to maintain this information using existing database software.

A routine schedule for evaluation and examination of injured athletes needs to be established. For the team physician who works at either the professional or the collegiate level, this may occur on a daily basis; at the high school level, however, this may occur only once or twice weekly. Regardless of the frequency with which athletes are seen, a well-defined schedule should be established and communicated to coaches and athletes. An appropriate consultation panel should be developed of identified specialists or subspecialists who can provide ambulatory consultation. As mentioned previously, such consultants should be selected for their identified clinical competence as well as their specific interest in providing care for an athletic population.

INTERNATIONAL COMPETITION

For those team physicians who will have the responsibility of caring for teams that participate in international competition, it is equally important to develop an appropriate organizational schema to deal with anticipated problems. This will necessarily require the team physician to familiarize himself or herself with the local conditions and geography in which the athlete will participate. Information should be gathered from existing resources regarding endemic infectious disease, and appropriate precautions should be taken well in advance of the designated trip. This includes appropriate immunization and acquisition of health documents for travel.

In a manner described previously, the physician must assess the adequacy of the medical facilities that might be used in the host country, as well as acquaint himself or herself with the medical staff and determine their ability to handle any potential medical problem that might be encountered. Appropriate contingency plans for medical emergencies need to be developed after consulting with local authorities and assessing the availability of emergency medical transportation.

Education of the athletes is critical in preventing most of the communicable diseases contracted during foreign travel. It is appropriate that athletes be educated prior to departure with regard to specific dietary and hygienic habits. Furthermore, sleep disturbance is common when traveling across several time zones, and the team physician needs to plan appropriately for this. Education of the athletes is critical in minimizing the untoward effects of time zone shift.

Finally, drug testing is common in international competition. The team physician should review each individual athlete's drug profile with the athlete both prior to departure and on arrival, to make certain that the athlete is taking no substances or drugs that are banned. Education must be undertaken to explain the drug-testing protocol with the athletes, the importance of avoiding the use of any drugs not prescribed by the team physician, and adherence to the appropriate protocol during the drug-testing process.

SUMMARY

The role of the team physician is complex. The tasks the team physician frequently undertakes can be simplified by the development of an organizational schema that facilitates the routine care of athletes as well as their care at specific competitions, whether locally or in a distant geographical region. The team physician is a critical element in the provision of adequate health care to the athlete. Continuous and comprehensive care can be guaranteed when appropriate planning has been undertaken to ensure the ability of the team physician and other members of the sports medicine team to respond effectively to any potential problem. The development of a specific plan is determined by the setting in which the athlete competes and the availability of necessary resources.

RECOMMENDED READING

Lombardo JA: Sports medicine: a team effort. *Phys Sportsmed* 13:72–81, 1985.
Mayne BR: A team physician's bag. *Phys Sportsmed* 9:85–87, 1981.
Puffer JC: Sports medicine delivery systems for the athlete: a multisport model. *Adv Sports Med Fitness* 2:287–294, 1989.
Rice SG, Schlotfeldt JD and Foley WE: The athletic health care and training program—a comprehensive approach to the prevention and management of athletic injuries in high schools. *West J Med* 142:352–357, 1985.

ENVIRONMENTAL PHYSIOLOGY AND MEDICINE

Peter B. Raven

Four primary environments affect human athletic performance: the naturally occurring environments of heat, cold, altitude, and the environment produced as a result of urbanization—air pollution. Exercising in these environments increases the risk of injury and illness.

HEAT

Activities performed in relatively high environmental temperatures above 22° C (71.6° F) dry bulb temperature (db) can reduce exercise capacity and, depending on the humidity content of the air, can cause heat illness. When activities are performed in excessive heat (>30° C or 86° F db) or highly humidified air (rh >80%), serious heat illness or death can result if adequate medical care is not taken.

PHYSIOLOGIC RESPONSES

Heat is a byproduct of muscular activity. Even at moderate exercise intensities, the heat production is sufficient to raise the body's core temperature to lethal levels (105° +) in 15 to 30 minutes. Physiologic adaptations dissipate the excess heat and attempt to maintain a near-constant internal temperature. The excess heat is lost through radiation, convection, and conduction from the skin surface and by the evaporation of sweat in ambient conditions that are hotter than the skin.

The heat produced by the metabolic generation of energy is

brought to the surface of the skin by increasing skin blood flow. The body monitors both deep central and skin temperature through the thermoregulatory center in the hypothalamus. Based on the error signal generated in relation to the "set point" (a reference temperature in the brain similar to a thermostat's reference temperature), the hypothalamus makes circulatory adjustments. As exercise begins, blood flow increases to the active muscle to support metabolic demands and, at the same time, increases flow to the skin to dissipate the enhanced heat production. This increased flow to the muscles and skin occurs because of an increased cardiac output and redistribution of regional blood flows, i.e., reducing flow to the visceral organs via sympathetic vasoconstriction.

The body's ability to balance these competing demands can be overwhelmed by exercising in conditions of high external heat load. A high ambient temperature reduces the gradient between the air and skin, reducing effective convection and sweat evaporation. The body attempts to compensate by enhancing skin blood flow and cutaneous blood volume. This peripheral shunting of blood leads to a decline in central venous pressure, cardiac filling, and stroke volume. Heart rate must therefore increase to maintain the same cardiac output at a fixed exercise intensity. If the exercise and thermal load are sufficiently severe, heart rate reaches its maximum and cardiac output is insufficient to meet the competing demands. In these conditions heat syncope and illness may occur if specific precautions are not taken.

ACCLIMATIZATION

The ability to tolerate and exercise in the heat can be improved by repeated exposures to heat, referred to as heat acclimatization. The primary physiologic adaptations of this process include an expansion of plasma volume, increased sweat rate, and improved circulatory control. These adaptations result in a reduced core temperature and heart rate response for a given heat exposure and exercise intensity. This process is achieved most effectively by exercising moderately during repeated heat exposures, producing an elevated core temperature that is a necessary stimulus for the acclimatization process. A high level of aerobic fitness increases heat tolerance but does not replace repeated heat exposures to achieve acclimatization. No apparent difference exists in the acclimatization process between men and women.

HEAT STRESS INDEX

The assessment of the safety and effect of exercising at high temperatures necessitates quantification of the external heat load, i.e., an index of heat stress. The ordinary thermometer (dry bulb thermometer, Tdb) is not adequate because it does not take into account the ambient humidity, which has a direct bearing on the ability to evaporate sweat. The addition of the wet bulb thermometer (Twb) adds a measurement of humidity, but this instrument still omits the factor of solar radiant energy and air movement. The solar radiant energy factor can be quantitated by the additional use of a black globe thermometer (Tg). Thus, the "wet bulb globe temperature (WBGT) index" was developed. WBGT is computed as follows:

$$(\text{outdoors}) \ \text{WBGT} = 0.7 \ \text{Twb} + 0.2 \ \text{Tg} + 0.1 \ \text{Tdb}$$

$$(\text{indoors}) \ \text{WBGT} = 0.7 \ \text{Twb} + 0.3 \ \text{Tg}$$

ENDURANCE TRAINING ADJUSTMENTS

The exercise heart rate is a valid and useful indicator of the additional stress imposed by an environmental heat load. *Prolonged aerobic exercise training allows for the body heat load to increase when a high heat-stress index is present.* Training prescriptions must be adjusted downward for intensity and possibly duration to achieve the same cardiovascular load. Using target heart rates as an indicator of cardiovascular load provides a good index of the strain on the system. Very high heat-stress indices necessitate reduction of intensity/duration by a further increment to provide some safety margin. Special precautions are needed when assessing cardiac rehabilitation patients who already have narrowed tolerance limits.

HEAT ILLNESS

Heat illness (or injury) is a category of symptoms that occur as thermoregulatory mechanisms fail to cope with the competing loads of external heat load and metabolically produced heat so core temperature continues to rise. Heat illness has a spectrum of symptom severity, ranging from heat cramps and heat-induced dehydration to heat exhaustion and heat stroke.

Heat cramps are benign heat injuries, which are painful. They are typified by involuntary, painful, cramping of the muscles, usually in the calves or abdomen. They probably result from an imbalance of sodium and potassium across muscle cell membranes as a result of heavy sweating. Fluid replacement is the treatment of choice. Salting of food and a balanced diet are usually adequate to restore appropriate electrolyte levels.

Dehydration as a result of sweating accompanies and complicates other heat injuries. A 5% weight loss (3.5 kg) is common for an average-sized man in the course of a 16-km (10-mile) run in 27 to 32° C (80 to 90° F) heat. Such sweat loss must be replaced by drinking cool water or dilute electrolyte solutions. Early signs of dehydration are lethargy, anxiety, and irritability. Severe dehydration may be manifest by uncoordinated, spastic gait, faintness and altered level of consciousness. Individuals with symptoms of dehydration would be treated in the same manner as those with heat exhaustion and heat stroke.

Heat exhaustion is a potentially serious condition. It occurs in the exercise setting as a result of two events, increased "internal heat load" from physical activity and dehydration secondary to sweating. With heat exhaustion, body temperature (rectal) is elevated but is usually less than 39.5° C (103° F). Common symptoms include gooseflesh, headache, dizziness, shortness of breath, pallor, nausea, vomiting, and uncoordinated gait. Treatment is similar to that for heat stroke.

Heat stroke and heat exhaustion may be difficult to distinguish on clinical grounds. Although heat stroke casualties tend to have higher rectal temperatures (40° C (106° F) or higher), some individuals spontaneously recover from temperatures as high as 41.5° C (107° F) without sequelae. Heat stroke victims, contrary to popular belief, may sweat profusely. Symptoms of both conditions are similar, but heat stroke casualties are more likely to manifest central nervous system disturbances such as unsteady gait, disorientation, confusion, bizarre or combative behavior, and unconsciousness. Individuals who are delirious, convulsive, or comatose are more likely to have suffered heat stroke and need prompt medical attention.

Prevention

The key to the prevention of heat injuries is the avoidance of training in hot ambient conditions that place the individual at increased risk. The WBGT index integrates the primary extrinsic risk factors—absolute temperature, humidity, and solar radiant energy—into a practical indication of the relative risk for injury (Table

TABLE 9–1. WBGT Index for Outdoor Activities*

Range (°F)	Signal Flag	Activity
Below 64	None	Unlimited
64–76	Green	Alert for possible increase in index and for symptoms of heat stress
73–82	Yellow	Active exercise for unacclimatized persons should be curtailed
82–85.9	Red	Active exercise for all but the well acclimatized should be curtailed
86+	Black	All training should be stopped

*Note: Runners who are not accustomed to running in the heat must proceed with caution at any temperature.

9–1). Moderate risk exists at WBGT between 65 and 73° F, high risk between 73 and 82° F, and very high risk above 82° F.

The ACSM *Position Stand: Prevention of Thermal Injuries During Distance Running* gives further information concerning these risks levels. A summary of the recommended strategies for minimizing the risks of exercising in the heat follows:

1. Allow time for acclimatization to the heat, usually 10 to 14 days working in the heat.
2. Exercise during cooler parts of day.
3. Limit or defer exercise if WBGT is in high-risk zone red or black.
4. Plan to drink before, during, and after exercise in the heat, even during training runs (see *ACSM Guidelines*). Recommended quantities are 400 to 500 ml before and 300 ml every 20 minutes during the activity.
5. Modulate training intensity (by heart rate monitoring).
6. Monitor daily body weight closely. Acute losses are water. If losses are greater than 3% of weight, they need to be replaced by drinking (saline with additional potassium) before the next training session.
7. Salt replacement is essential. Adequate electrolyte replacement is provided by liberal salting of food and a balanced diet with adequate potassium. Use of salt tablets and exogenous potassium is generally not advised.

Treatment

Individuals who exhibit signs and symptoms of heat injury should be removed to a shaded area immediately. They should lie down with their feet elevated above the level of the heart. Excess clothing should be opened or removed. If rectal temperatures are above 39.5° C (103° F), cooling of the victims should begin immediately. Sprinkling with water and fanning to increase evaporative cooling or rubbing ice packs over major blood vessels in the armpits, groin, and neck are effective means of cooling. Cooling should proceed until rectal temperatures are 39° C (102° F). Victims should be given cool fluids to *sip* if they are conscious, but only if they are not nauseated or vomiting. If victims cannot take fluids by mouth, intravenous fluids should be administered if medical personnel are available, or they should be rapidly evacuated to the nearest hospital. All individuals who have exhibited serious disturbances of behavior or neurologic function should receive medical attention from a physician and be treated as emergency patients, especially if they fail to recover after the cessation of exercise and onset of cooling.

COLD

Performance decrements and injuries from cold exposure are reported less frequently than those from heat in the exercising adult. This difference results in part because exercise itself generates enough heat to warm the body. Nevertheless, cold weather can pose a significant threat to the exercising individual, especially cardiovascularly impaired individuals. Furthermore, cold exposure becomes a significant problem during water sports and/or survival in water.

PHYSIOLOGIC RESPONSES

Heat is lost from the body through radiation, conduction, and convection or through sweat evaporation. Although these processes are desirable and necessary when activity occurs in hot environments, they can be deleterious in cold weather. Unwanted heat loss is normally avoided by adding layers of clothing (reducing losses through radiation and convection) and keeping the skin dry. If these measures are insufficient and skin temperature falls, cutaneous vasoconstriction occurs, drawing blood away from the body surface and extremities and thereby reducing heat loss and maintaining core temperature. If the cold stress is sufficiently severe and core temperature continues to fall, shivering results in an effort to produce additional metabolic heat. Exercising in a cold environment can be helpful in most situations by producing additional heat, as with shivering. In cold-water exposure to >50° F (10° C), exercise promotes heat loss and is counterproductive in survival situations.

Humans do not have the pronounced physiologic acclimatization responses to repeated cold exposures that they do in the heat. Some evidence exists, however, that people who habitually function in cold temperatures develop the ability to burn more calories per unit of exercise than the unhabituated person and have a local vasoregulatory adaptation to protect the tissues when repeatedly exposed to the cold.

Acute cold exposure, at least to −20° C (−4° F) does not affect maximal oxygen uptake because the oxygen transport system to active muscles is not compromised. Significant cold exposure can reduce submaximal endurance performance, although the mechanism for this occurrence is not established. This reduction is not a major concern in training prescription during cold periods, and training adjustments are not necessary for the nonathlete on the basis of performance capacity.

COLD EXPOSURE INDEX

The severity of cold exposure, like that of heat, depends on air movement, humidity, and precipitation, as well as absolute temperature. Humidity is less a factor as temperatures drop below freezing. Wind velocity, however, is a major factor in the severity of cold stress by markedly increasing heat loss by radiation, convection, and evaporation. The extent of the air-velocity factor (or wind-chill effect) is shown in Table 9–2. The equivalent temperature depicted on the wind-chill chart relates to the cooling effect on exposed skin.

COLD INJURY

The cold injuries of concern during outdoor training are hypothermia and frostbite. Hypothermia is a depression in core temperature sufficient to affect body functions, usually below 35° C (95° F). Frostbite is the process of tissue water crystallization and with subsequent cell dehydration and destruction. People who suffer from Raynaud's disease (severe vasoconstriction in the cold, especially in the appendages such as the fingers and toes) are more likely than others to suffer from frostbite injury. Breathing cold air does not cause injury to the trachea and lung tissue, although it may be uncomfortable. The inhalation of very cold air by cardiac

TABLE 9–2. Wind-Chill Index

Wind Speed (mph)	Thermometer Reading (°F)										
	50	40	30	20	10	0	−10	−20	−30	−40	−50
	(Equivalent temperature (°F))										
5	48	37	27	16	6	−5	−15	−26	−36	−47	−57
10	40	28	16	4	−9	−24	−33	−46	−58	−70	−83
15	36	22	9	−5	−18	−32	−45	−58	−72	−85	−99
20	32	18	4	−10	−25	−39	−53	−67	−82	−96	−110
25	30	16	0	−15	−29	−44	−59	−74	−88	−104	−118
30	28	13	−2	−18	−33	−48	−63	−79	−94	−109	−125
35	27	11	−4	−20	−35	−51	−67	−82	−98	−113	−129
40	26	10	−6	−21	−37	−53	−69	−85	−100	−115	−132
	Minimal Risk				Increasing Risk			Great Risk			

patients can cause angina, and precautions should be taken in the rehabilitation training of these individuals.

Prevention

The primary extrinsic risk factors other than cold air temperature are wind speed, humidity or wetness, immersion in cold water, and inadequate protective clothing. Perhaps the most significant is wind, as illustrated by the wind-chill information in Table 9–2. The important intrinsic risk factors are primarily those that affect energy metabolism and/or circulation, such as fatigue, hunger, low percentage of body fat (less insulation), use of tobacco, or caffeine (vasoconstriction), and use of alcohol (vasodilation).

Most important in the prevention of cold injury during training is adequate clothing. If the wind-chill temperature is −26 to −29° C (−15 to −20° F) or lower, exposed peripheral areas such as the face, nose, ears, hands, and feet should be adequately protected with masks or scarfs, caps, mittens, and dry insulated shoes, respectively. Several layers of loose-fitting clothing should be worn under a windproof, water-repellent (not watertight) outer layer. Clothing should be kept dry from both inside (sweat) and outside (rain, mist) because water conducts cold more rapidly than air. Thus, both exercise intensity and clothing should be adjusted to maintain body heat but to prevent the accumulation of excessive amounts of sweat.

During extended training periods, the pace should be set to avoid a significant decrease toward the end and therefore loss of adequate heat production. This becomes a major problem at the end of competitive distance races in the cold. Slow runners (or skiers, etc.) need to be carefully watched. Early in the event, running, walking, or skiing into the wind may also be helpful, so the wind chill is less when the wind is behind the participant during the later phases of the activity. Additional clothing or protection from the wind may be desirable during the cool-down phase of exercise to avoid excessive cooling.

Treatment

Frostbite injuries can be serious, leading to gangrene and loss of the body part if the trauma is not recognized early and/or treated properly. The key is to leave the affected part until it can be thawed without risk of refreezing, preferably in a hospital. Injured parts can be thawed in warm water (38 to 43° C or 100 to 110° F); the temperature of the water should be measured with a thermometer.

Mild hypothermia can be managed by removing the victim to a sheltered warm location and providing dry garments and warm beverages (if the victim is alert). Moderate to severe cases should be transported gently to a hospital for rewarming. Gentle handling is crucial to avoid precipitating dangerous cardiac arrhythmias. These victims should also be kept still to avoid recirculation of cold blood from the extremities to the central circulation.

ALTITUDE

Training at high altitude is unavoidable for people who reside there. Some athletes choose to train under the conditions of reduced oxygen pressure to stimulate the training response. The reduced oxygen availability has profound effects on physical performance and can lead to illness in unacclimated individuals. This effect is highly variable and some people may be affected at altitude of less than 2424 m (8000 ft).

ACUTE PHYSIOLOGIC RESPONSES

The partial pressure of oxygen in the air decreases as barometric pressure declines with increasing altitudes above sea level. Thus, in Denver at 1600 m (5280 ft), ambient O_2 pressure declines to 132 from 159 mm Hg at sea level and is as low as 94 mm Hg at Pikes Peak, CO, 4276 m (14,110 ft). With the decline in inspired O_2 tension is a concomitant fall in arterial oxygen saturation, which triggers compensatory mechanisms in an attempt by the body to maintain oxygen transport.

On initial exposure to altitude, stimulation of pulmonary ventilation and a consequent respiratory alkalosis occur. The alkalosis, in turn, causes a leftward shift in the oxygen-hemoglobin dissociation curve, which allows oxygen to be more available to the tissue at a given inspired O_2 pressure. Additional physiologic adjustments include a temporary increase in submaximal exercise heart rate and cardiac output. The sum of these adjustments supports the transport of oxygen to the tissues despite the diminished O_2 availability.

ACCLIMATIZATION

Chronic physiologic responses as a result of altitude occur as the length of stay at altitude continues. The initial alkalosis precipitates a change in red blood cell enzymes. At the same time, red cell production increases, leading to increased hematocrit and hemoglobin volume. Prolonged high-altitude exposure leads to further adaptation at the level of the mitochondria and in exercise muscle-capillary density. These adaptive mechanisms are readily demonstrated by comparing the decreased physical performance of newly arrived lowlanders with that of persons who have lived for extended periods at altitude and who can perform heavy physical activity, such as mining or mountain climbing. The kidney responds to the alkalosis by excreting bicarbonate ion and returns blood pH to normal. This adaptation significantly reduces the blood buffering capacity for acidosis, however. Despite the significant physiologic and acclimatization responses, levels of physical performance remain decreased at altitude, even in well-acclimatized individuals.

TRAINING ADJUSTMENTS

The persistent decrement in physical performance at high altitudes should be considered in training. The magnitude of the effect of altitude on any activity is a function of its dependence on oxygen transport. Aerobic events are greatly affected, whereas anaerobic events are not. Thus, maximal oxygen uptake and submax-

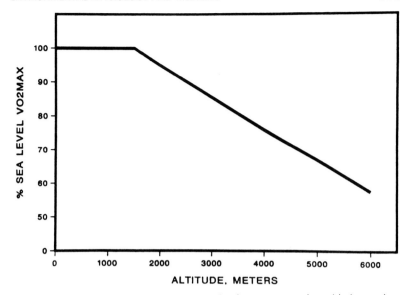

FIG. 9–1. Approximate reduction in maximal oxygen uptake with increasing altitude. (Adapted from Hartley LH: Effects of high-altitude environment on the cardiovascular system of man. *JAMA 215:*241, 1971. In American College of Sports Medicine: *Resource Manual for Guidelines for Exercise Testing and Prescription.* Philadelphia: Lea & Febiger, 1986.)

imal endurance times are decreased at altitude, whereas sprinting may be actually improved because of decreased air resistance. The decrease in maximal oxygen uptake as a function of altitude is illustrated in Figure 9–1.

HIGH-ALTITUDE ILLNESS

Pathologic conditions related to exposure to high altitude are not prominent until an elevation of about 2424 m (8000 ft). Individuals may then experience acute mountain sickness or the more severe conditions, such as high-altitude pulmonary and cerebral edema. Acute mountain sickness is a complex of symptoms that results from rapid ascent of an unacclimatized individual. Principal symptoms include severe headache, lassitude, nausea, vomiting, anorexia, indigestion, and sleep disturbances. Symptoms begin after 6 hours, peak between 24 and 48 hours, and resolve after 3 to 4 days.

High-altitude pulmonary edema is characterized by fluid accumulation in the lungs that is not associated with heart failure. Characteristic signs include increased breathing and heart rate, cyanosis,and pulmonary rales along with coughing. The condition can be confirmed radiographically, with evidence of multiple patchy infiltrates throughout the lungs. Young, active individuals seem especially susceptible to this condition. Heavy exercise and cold exposure are predisposing factors. High-altitude cerebral edema is a rare form of severe acute mountain sickness in which an individual exhibits certain abnormal neurologic signs and symptoms.

Acute mountain sickness and high-altitude pulmonary and cerebral edema result from a failure to acclimatize properly to altitude. The conditions essentially can be prevented by using a gradual ascent, thus allowing sufficient time to acclimatize. An ascent rate of no more than 303 m (1000 ft) to 606 m (2000 ft) per day at altitudes higher than 2424 m (8000 ft) is recommended. Additionally, sleep should occur at as low an altitude as possible. Acetazolamide (Diamox), a carbonic anhydrase inhibitor can be prescribed to prevent acute mountain sickness in people who cannot take time to acclimate properly.

Any pre-existing medical condition in which oxygen delivery is compromised, such as anemia or heart and lung disease, is made worse by altitude exposure. Evaluation to determine whether a person with these conditions can be exposed to altitude safely should be made by a physician.

AIR POLLUTION

Ambient air surrounding large metropolitan cities contains small quantities (in the parts-per-million (ppm) range) of gases and particulates other than its normal constituents (O_2, CO_2, N_2, inert gases, and water vapor). During times of air stagnation and temperature inversion, many air pollutants reach concentrations that produce significant detrimental effects on functional performance, morbidity, psychophysiologic performance, and subjective feelings. Among the usual atmospheric pollutants, oxidants (primarily ozone), sulfur oxides (SO_x), and nitrogen oxides (NO_x) have been suggested as possible agents of harm to the cardiovascular system; however, evidence of a direct effect is minimal. Carbon monoxide, on the other hand, interferes with cardiovascular function at remarkably low levels of exposure.

CARBON MONOXIDE

Carbon monoxide (CO) is a gas that is not easily detected by human senses, yet is readily absorbed from inspired air (when present in very low quantities) and combines with hemoglobin to interfere with tissue oxygenation. When CO is present in the ambient air (from cigarette smoking, air pollution, automobile exhaust fumes, etc.), its excretion at the lung is compromised and depends on the equilibrium pressure between blood (P_VCO) and the alveoli (P_ACO); a significant increase in blood carboxyhemoglobin (COHb) levels results.

Evidence indicates that the $\dot{V}O_{2max}$ of the healthy human is reduced linearly in relation to increased blood levels of COHb in the 5 to 35% COHb range (Fig. 9–2). The reduction in $\dot{V}O_{2max}$ was not statistically significant until levels greater than 4.3% were obtained;

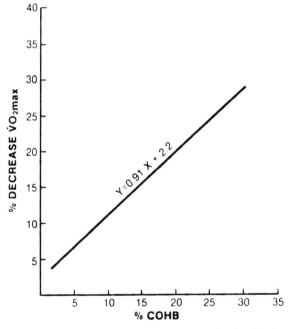

FIG. 9–2. The linear relationship between increasing levels of carboxyhemoglobin (COHb) and the decrement in maximal aerobic power ($\dot{V}O_{2max}$). r = 0.84, P < 0.05. (Reprinted with permission from Raven PB, et al. Effect of carbon monoxide and peroxyacylnitrate on man's maximal aerobic capacity. *J Appl Physiol* 36:288–293, 1974.)

however, lower levels (2.7%) have been shown to significantly decrease maximal performance time on the treadmill. COHb levels of 5% significantly increase the oxygen debt of acute work, although what portion of the debt is altered, alactacid or lactacid, was not identified. During submaximal work of short duration at $\dot{V}_{O_2}$ levels below 1.5 L/min (40 to 60% $\dot{V}_{O_{2max}}$), COHb levels of less than 15% have little effect on energy production and ventilation in the healthy person, but the submaximal heart rate is significantly increased. Hence, the efficiency of muscular exercise during CO inhalation is unaffected at levels below 15% COHb, whereas CO desaturation of hemoglobin is overcome by a hyperkinetic circulation (i.e., cardiac output is increased by an increase in heart rate alone). As work levels are increased relative to the person's maximal capacity, ventilation volume is increased by means of an increased respiratory rate. It would appear that in the healthy, noncardiovascularly compromised person, ambient CO levels resulting in COHb levels below 15% do not alter functional ability to do low levels of work (35 to 60% $\dot{V}_{O_{2max}}$). Because of the physiologic requirements during aerobic training, however, the inroads into the cardiopulmonary reserves incurred by CO loading will prove detrimental to elite performance and most certainly will affect the person exercising with compromised cardiovascular reserves.

PHOTOCHEMICAL OXIDANTS

Any person who has had the unpleasant experience of exercising in high ambient levels of oxidants (ozone constitutes 90% of photochemical oxidants) is subjectively convinced that his or her ability to function is significantly reduced. Many complaints of eye irritation (burning sensation and scratchy feelings on the eyeball, with significant conjunctivitis), pain sensations below the sternum, chest tightness, dyspnea, and cough with a feeling of nausea sometimes strong enough to produce wretching or the "dry heaves" have been reported.

OZONE

The primary targets of ozone action appear to be the lungs and respiratory tract. If exposure to low levels of ozone (0.1 to 0.5 ppm) occurs for long periods of time (days and weeks), significant changes in lung function parameters, suggestive of structural changes, occur even at rest. Decrements in capacity and expiratory flow rates have been observed during acute exposures, indicating increased airway resistance caused by the bronchoconstriction effect of ozone. The primary findings of studies carried out with subjects at rest and O_3 concentrations of <0.30 ppm were that this type of exposure had minimal, if any, impact on lung function. In contrast to these few studies on resting subjects, numerous investigations have been reported using exercising subjects exposed to ozone levels up to 0.30 ppm. One particularly interesting observation was that subjects who exercised during 0.3-ppm ozone exposure exhibited markedly greater responses and significantly greater decrements in lung function than resting subjects. Significantly, when athletes have been asked to perform maximally at levels of ozone <0.2 ppm, a large proportion were unable to complete performance events because of subjective symptoms.

In summary, pronounced responses have been shown in heavily exercising subjects (who consequently breathe more), whereas little response has been seen in lightly exercising individuals. As would be expected, short exposures have elicited smaller functional changes than longer exposures. Thus, athletes competing in events lasting from 30 minutes to 2 or more hours while exposed to 0.10 to 0.30 ppm O_3 could experience alteration in lung function with potential consequences for ventilatory and endurance performance.

PEROXYACETYLNITRATE AND NITROGEN OXIDES

The few investigations concerning humans and other oxidant pollutants [peroxyacetylnitrate (PAN) and oxides of nitrogen (NO_x)] suggest a mechanism of action similar to that of ozone. Sufficient data are not available to describe the levels above which performance will be affected. A level of 0.24 ppm PAN, however, appears to be a critical threshold at which human pulmonary and exercise performances are decreased.

Even less is known about the exercise-related effects of another oxidant, nitrogen dioxide (NO_2). Concentrations of 0.62 ± 0.12 ppm NO_2 were evaluated after 2 hours of exposure at 40% $\dot{V}O_{2max}$, with no significant alterations in cardiorespiratory function. Hence, it appears that in the case of photochemical pollutants (ozone, PAN, and NO_2), cardiovascular impairment has not been demonstrated. It has been reported, however, that oxidant-like pollutants cross the alveolar membrane and interact with blood components, increasing both red blood cell fragility and specific enzyme activities. In addition, some indications of central nervous system functional decrements have been reported.

SULFUR OXIDES

Sulfur dioxide (SO_2) is generally regarded as an upper-airway and bronchial irritant. Exposure to different levels of SO_2 while at rest produces strikingly similar responses; airway resistance increases rapidly, reaching a maximum at 4 to 10 minutes of exposure. Subsequently, a decrease in resistance occurs with continued exposure, regardless of SO_2 concentrations. The probable cause of the increased resistance is reflex bronchospasm initiated by irritation of the bronchial receptors in the smooth muscle. Investigation suggests that SO_2 stimulates the subepithelial receptors in the larynx, trachea, and bronchi and, via the vagus nerve, causes increased tension in the tracheobronchial tree.

Few experiments have been done on maximal working capacity and submaximal work performance during SO_2 exposures. It is certain, however, that ambient levels of SO_2 above 1.0 ppm cause significant discomfort and prove detrimental to performance. When

TABLE 9–3. Possible Adverse Health Effects of Air Pollutants Greater Than Federal Alert Levels

Pollutant	Averaging Time (hr)	Primary NAAQS*	Symptoms
CO	8	9 ppm	Impaired exercise tolerance in persons with cardiovascular disease.
	1	35 ppm	Decreased physical performance in normal adults.
SO_2	24	0.14 ppm	Increased hospital admissions for respiratory illness in elderly patients with related illness.
TSP*	24	250 pg/m³	Aggravation of chronic lung disease and asthma.
			Aggravation of cardiorespiratory disease symptoms in elderly patients with heart or chronic lung disease.
			Increased cough, chest discomfort, and restricted activity.
Ox*	1	0.08 ppm	Aggravation of chronic lung disease and asthma. Irritation of the respiratory tract in healthy adults.
			Decreased visual acuity; eye irritation.
			Decreased cardiopulmonary reserve in healthy subjects.

* TSP refers to total suspended particulates and Ox refers to oxidants where O_3 usually represents 90% of the total oxidant. NAAQS refers to the National Ambient Air Quality Standards.

inhaled in combination with dry cold air, SO_2 induces bronchoconstriction at even lower concentrations (0.25 ppm), and cold exacerbates the effect of a higher concentration; however, a fairly broad range of sensitivity to SO_2 exists in asthmatics, with the least sensitive asthmatics no more sensitive than the most sensitive normal subjects.

The major concern with SO_2 is that it affects asthmatic individuals at concentrations lower than 1 ppm. At concentrations as low at 0.50 ppm SO_2, exercising asthmatics may experience marked changes in airway resistance. Two reports have demonstrated at least 100% increases in airway resistance in asthmatics after only 5 minutes of exercise with SO_2 concentrations in the range of 0.5 ppm. With repeated exposures within the same day, however, the responses become much less severe.

Another factor, formerly of concern with exposure to SO_2 in conjunction with ozone, was the possibility that the pulmonary function response to the combination of SO_2 plus O_3 would be worse than the sum of their individual effects. In conclusion, SO_2 probably causes problems with athletic performance in asthmatics, but at current ambient levels, it is unlikely to be of concern to the performer with otherwise normal lungs. Furthermore, the SO_2-induced bronchoconstriction can be inhibited by the prior administration of cromolyn sodium (disodium cromoglycate).

Obviously, persons whose cardiopulmonary system is impaired and who wish to perform exercise in the outdoors should be cautioned against heavy exercise on days of high pollution indices.

Table 9–3 summarizes the air quality standards and possible health effects.

C H A P T E R   1 0

MEDICAL-LEGAL ISSUES

David L. Herbert and William G. Herbert

For physicians and some other health-care providers, the provision of professional services attendant to an individual's participation in sport or exercise activity encompasses the practice of sports medicine. Despite the clear existence of this practice area and the provision of service by both licensed and nonlicensed personnel, attempts at definitional reference for the term "sports medicine" have not been universally accepted to date. Those practicing in this provider area include physicians, chiropractors, podiatrists, psychologists, nutritionists, therapists, trainers, and a host of other nonlicensed personnel, even though the term "medicine" is utilized in most definitional references. For physician practitioners, there is no American Medical Association (AMA) or American Board of Medical Specialties (ABMS) recognition of a specialized practice area for sports medicine; however, currently three sports medicine specialty certifications are in existence and are available for some practitioners who wish to obtain recognition of their specialized competencies. These are provided by the American Osteopathic Association of Sports Medicine (AOASM), the American Academy of Sports Physicians (AASP), and the American Academy of Podiatric Sports Medicine (APSM). Those who practice nonphysician-performed sports medicine services are generally, if at all, governed by a variety of state regulatory enactments. Most of these regulatory enactments are nonspecific to sports medicine services, but some do provide certain regulation for a few of the professionals engaged in some sports medicine activities. Statutory authority exists in fewer than half the states for licensure and/or regulation of athletic trainers, most of whom provide "front-line" first aid and rehabilitative services to athletes, which services might be loosely described as "sports medicine." Certification, as opposed to licensure, is available for trainers principally through two organizations, the American Athletic Trainers Association and Certification Board, Inc.,

(AATA) and the National Athletic Trainers Association, Inc. (NATA).

State laws governing the practice of medicine and allied health care generally provide that only licensed physicians have the legal authority to evaluate, diagnose, and treat individuals for the purposes of relieving pain, reducing physical impairment, and restoring health . . . whether such activities are sports related or not. Despite such enactments and their statutory companions, which provide criminal penalties for the violation of unauthorized-practice-of-medicine laws, many nonphysicians are providing services independent of licensed practitioners and even independent of any state licensing authority. In other situations, where a "team approach" is used to provide care under the broad or direct authority of a physician, a clear delineation for the provision of sports medicine services does not exist through any state statutory scheme. As a result of the lack of clear statutory authorization for these services, and the diverse involvement of many allied practitioners in the provision of care to athletes, some services are clearly being provided that would not meet accepted standards of practice and may even increase the rate or severity of injuries to exercise or sports participants or may delay, prevent, or compound appropriate treatment or rehabilitation of injury. When one adds to this a variety of competing interests and viewpoints from those participating in sport or exercise activities—athletes, parents, coaches, trainers, therapists, physicians, fans, and others—it is no wonder that a variety of legal and ethical concerns often arise in the treatment and provision of health-care services to athletes. These competing interests lead to legal questions related to a variety of concepts including negligence and malpractice, informed consent, counseling, contract/constitutional/privacy rights, and a host of other considerations related to preparticipation: physicals, reentry to play/exclusion from play determinations, privileged communication and privacy, drug or other substance abuse testing or counseling activities, the provision of prescriptive medications, counseling, and other similar concerns.

All these practice concerns carry with them certain risks of litigation based on a variety of potential claims. Both licensed and unlicensed providers are at risk. With the dramatic growth in sport and exercise participation by millions of Americans and the billion-dollar enterprise involved with this growth has been a concomitant increase in the related legal problems. The litigation epidemic that has affected all provider areas has begun to engulf sports medicine providers and others involved in the provision of sport and exercise-related health care.

The delivery of service and the risk of claim and suit against practitioners arising from sports medicine activities can be minimized by an increased understanding and utilization of the applicable standard of practice, the adoption of a low-risk approach to the delivery of care, the maintenance of qualified and appropriately licensed personnel at "state of the art" levels, and the appropriate documentation of the timely delivery of care in accordance with relevant standards of practice.

Standards of practice, guidelines, position statements, and similar written pronouncements issued by many organizations may have application to sports medicine provider activities or programs. These standards define the elements of care that a particular association deems minimally or optimally acceptable for a particular service or program. These standards are not uniform in their professional perspective, detail, or comprehensiveness. The contents of these documents are not limited to the development of practice guidelines that may be cited in legal proceedings and used to judge provider acts or omissions. They are used as a framework for determining, in the course of resolving issues of negligence and malpractice, questions centering on whether a particular provider or program acted safely and effectively in the rendering of service in accordance with the applicable and appropriate standard of practice. Thus, it becomes critical for each practitioner to know, understand, and apply in their service all those standards that, when considered collectively, are likely to define the minimum expectation for care that "peers" would judge to be appropriate. Obviously, this is not easy to do given the diversity of professions in the field and the various standards of practice in existence when compared against state regulatory and licensure requirements.

Regardless of the origin of applicable standards of care, these benchmarks of expected practice should govern the application of one's knowledge and skills in the provision of professional service. Written protocols should be prepared to prescribe how these services will be applied for all major areas of care in which exercise/sports clients may be considered vulnerable to untoward outcomes. Thus, the creation of an operating guide for an individual sports medicine practice or administrative center and documenting that such is based on accepted standards are first steps in defining the appropriate provision of patient care and in minimizing legal risk and exposure to those providing that care.

Given this broad and basic discussion related to the legal concerns associated with sports medicine practices, the delivery of sports medicine services can result in specific legal concerns that should be briefly examined. A short review of each such practice area would seem to be appropriate—especially in making practitioners aware of potential problems that may deserve more thorough study and examination, for which various sources of information are available for reference.

PREPARTICIPATION/REENTRY TO PLAY EXAMINATIONS AND DECISIONS

Preparticipation physicals and reentry to play examinations, processes, and decisions have been the subject of frequent litigation. Physicians and other sports medicine providers have been named in such litigation as a result of alleged negligence in allowing athletes to participate or recommence play where it was claimed that those athletes should not have been allowed to do so. Other suits have also been brought against practitioners where decisions have been made to exclude individuals from participation under circumstances where athletes wanted to participate despite obvious personal risks (Note 1). Although most of these latter cases usually result in court affirmance of reasonable practitioners' decisions to exclude athletes from play, the litigation arising from practitioners' decisions to allow play have not been so uniform. Such cases have involved a variety of claims beyond mere negligence, including negligent/fraudulent concealment of medical information (Note 2), negligent failure to monitor an athlete's condition during competition thereby improperly allowing the athlete to play despite undue fatigue (Note 3), negligent mismatch of athletes leading to injury (Note 4), and recent allegations of negligence and other wrongful conduct related to alleged coach-practitioner conspiracy to withhold appropriate treatment in claimed violation of the appropriate standard of care (Note 5).

Judicial development in these areas, as well as the ongoing promulgation of practice standards, will continue to affect practices for years to come. Sports medicine practitioners will necessarily need to keep abreast of judicial and professional developments in this and other areas to protect their own practices adequately.

INFORMED CONSENT/PROVISION OF INFORMATION TO ATHLETES

Informed consent is a process by which relevant information on a given medical procedure is provided to patients—including athletes—followed by an affirmative decision by the patient to undergo a particular procedure or treatment. Much litigation has arisen over the years related to this particular topic. Much of this litigation in the traditional sports medicine setting has centered on claims that information was withheld—either negligently or intentionally—from athletes on the true nature of their conditions, thereby preventing the informed choices that every patient has the right to make (see, for example, Note 2). Clearly, the competing interests of athletes, physicians, coaches, fans, and others all bring different perspectives and pressures to bear on this matter; however, physicians and other practitioners have the obligation to put such interests aside and deal with athletes and their interests, as opposed to anyone else's interests or views.

The information-disclosure part of the informed-consent process is subject to frequent judicial review. Most of this litigation has centered on alleged failures to make sufficient disclosure on which the patient could make an informed decision (Note 6). The law is clearly moving toward the requirement of broader and more complete disclosure of risks and benefits attendant on particular procedures, including those that may only be possible rather than probable or even part of what might be considered a traditional risk. Given this trend, practitioners may wish to review their disclosure procedures with their legal advisors to ensure adherence to the current state of the law.

DRUG TESTING/COUNSELING

Drug and substance abuse among the entire population has resulted in recent years in a variety of legislative, judicial, and professional reactions. Many of these reactions have been directed at the detection, prosecution, or exclusion from play of athletes found to be engaged in substance abuse. Sports medicine providers are often asked to become involved in substance abuse testing or counseling programs developed for sports programs. Whereas practitioners have a rightful place in consulting activities and in the development of testing protocols and procedures, involvement in programs that would violate the confidentiality of the physician-patient relationship would seem to be clearly inappropriate. Physicians supplying sports medicine services to athletes should not be involved in the selection of athletes for testing, in testing, or in otherwise communicating medical information or testing results on that patient. Any such activity might well be deemed to be violative of the physician's duties towards his or her athlete/patient and should be avoided.

DISPENSING PRESCRIPTION MEDICATIONS TO ATHLETES

The provision of medications to athletes by nonphysician sports medicine practitioners raises a number of concerns related to the authority of both the physician and the dispensing allied health-care practitioner. The provision of medication by those who are not legally authorized to do so by state legislative enactments or similar federal legislation, however, can result in criminal charges and prosecution, as well as civil lawsuits by athletes if harm results from the activities (Note 7).

Although physicians may be able to utilize standing orders for dispensing medications in their absence under established and defined circumstances, care must be taken to ensure that medications are provided only by those who are qualified to carry out the standing orders and sometimes only pursuant to state authorizing legislation.

UNAUTHORIZED PRACTICE OF MEDICINE

Because of the nature of modern sports medicine programs, a number of licensed and nonlicensed practitioners are engaged in the provision of services to athletes. Whereas some practitioners may be authorized to provide specific services, e.g., therapists delivering therapy or rehabilitative service, many are not so authorized. The authority for the provision of such activity is defined by state law. Often statutes also delineate the unauthorized practice of health care as well.

The unauthorized practice of medicine has been defined as "the diagnosis of an individual's symptoms to determine with what disease or illness he is afflicted, and then to determine on the basis of that diagnosis what remedy or treatment should be given or prescribed to treat that disease and/or relieve the symptoms" (Note 8).

Whereas athletic trainers are licensed in some states, and other licensed providers such as therapists, nurses, podiatrists, chiropractors, and physician assistants all provide service to athletes, many others are not so licensed. Some of these practitioners may not be properly authorized to provide certain services to athlete patients under particular circumstances. Where a practice is determined to be beyond a particular statute authorizing the delivery of services or where the provision of care rendered by a nonlicensed practitioner has been determined to be reserved for licensed practitioners only, two separate and distinct legal concerns may arise: (1) a judicial finding resulting in an elevation of the standard of care required of the practitioner to that expected of a physician (a standard that a nonlicensed provider cannot possibly meet, almost always resulting in a finding of negligence and concomitant liability); and (2) exposure of the nonlicensed practitioner to the criminal charge of the unauthorized practice of medicine, usually a misdemeanor punishable by fine and/or imprisonment for up to 1 year.

RELEASES, WAIVERS, ASSUMPTIONS OF THE RISK

Many sports programs at different levels of competition utilize written documents commonly referred to as releases, waivers, or assumptions of risk. Some practitioners in sports medicine settings utilize these forms to offset potential liability for untoward events arising during participation, treatment, or rehabilitation. Such documents are sometimes used where athletes wish to participate despite contrary medical or coaching advice, frequently where they have secured a second opinion from outside the program supporting their decision to play. Although these documents are not foolproof, and putting aside the need to address and maintain control over such decisions by program personnel as opposed to outside practitioners, the use of these documents in certain circumstances should be considered and reviewed by program counsel. In some states, however, the use of such documents is against public policy, rendering them of no worth to a program.

ADHERENCE TO THE STANDARD OF CARE

The health-care profession as a whole has made significant movement toward the development and promulgation of written practice standards or guidelines for utilization by those rendering care. In fact, the movement toward these written practice guidelines was deemed to be the top medical story of 1988 by the American Medical Association (Note 9).

In the sports medicine area, some groups, including the American College of Sports Medicine (ACSM), are involved in the development and promulgation of standards that affect sports medicine practices. The development of such written standards in the years ahead will certainly continue and will more accurately define the duty of care owed by practitioners to their athlete patients. Adherence to such standards will undoubtedly become of major importance to practitioners in years to come and may be one risk-management response to the litigation epidemic that has engulfed so many practitioners in so many diverse practice areas.

SUMMARY

A variety of legal concerns face those engaged in sports medicine practices. A basic and ongoing knowledge of these legal concerns can greatly assist practitioners in planning their activities and in delivering care in accordance with the applicable standard of practice.

NOTES

1. See, for example, *Sitmoer v. Half Hallow Hills Central School District, et al.*, 520 N.Y.S. 2d 37 (A.D.2 Dept. 1987).
2. *Krueger v. Bert Bell N.F.L. Players Retirement Plan*, 234 Cal. Rptr. 579 (Cal. App. 1 1987), *analyzed in* Herbert: Proof of fraudulent concealment of medical information requires finding in favor of professional football player. *Sports, Parks, Recreation Law Reporter* 1:23–25, 1987, *and in* Negligent fraudulent concealment of medical information claims. *Sports Med Standards Malpractice Reporter* 1:40–43, 1989.
3. *Benitez v. New York City Board of Education*, 530 N.Y.S.2d 825 (A.D.1 Dept. 1988) *analyzed in* Herbert: Reentry to play decisions: new legal concerns. *Sports Med Standards Malpractice Reporter* 1:58–60, 1989, *reversed in* 73 N.Y.S.2d 650 (1989)) *reversal analyzed in*, Update on responsibility for injuries due to fatigue and mismatch—No responsibility says New York Court of Appeals in *Benitez v. New York City Board of Education*, 73 N.Y.S.2d 650 (1989). *Sports Med Malpractice Reporter* 1:79–80, 1989.
4. *Tepper v. City of New Rochelle School District*, 531 N.Y.S.2d (A.D.2 Dept. 1988) *analyzed in* Herbert: Coach and administrator responsibility for mismatches and injuries due to fatigue—An examination of recent trends. *Sports, Parks Recreation Law Reporter* 2:33–38 1988.
5. Recent lawsuit filed by the Estate of College Basketball Star Hank Gathers against Loyola Marymount University, among others, *Gathers v. Loyola Marymount University, et al.*, Los Angeles Superior Court, Case No. C759027.
6. See *Hedgecorth v. United States*, 618 F.Supp. 627 (E.D.Mo. 1985) *analyzed in* Herbert: Informed consent and new disclosure responsibilities for exercise stress testing: The case of *Hedgecorth v. United States*. *Exercise Standards Malpractice Reporter* 1:30–32, 1987.
7. See Herbert: Dispensing prescription medications to athletes: Pitfalls and potential problems. *Sports Med Standards Malpractice Reporter* 1:67–73, 1989.
8. Herbert and Herbert: *Legal Aspects of Preventive and Rehabilitative Exercise Programs*, 2nd ed. Canton, OH: Professional Reports Corporation, 1989.
9. See Year end review: Medicine by the book. *Am Med News* 1:28, 1989.

RECOMMENDED READING

BOOKS

Herbert DL and Herbert WG: *Legal Aspects of Sports Medicine Programs*. Canton, OH: Professional Reports Corporation, 1990.

Herbert DL and Herbert WG: *Legal Aspects of Preventive and Rehabilitative Exercise Programs*, 2nd Ed. Canton, OH: Professional Reports Corporation, 1989.

NEWSLETTERS

The Exercise Standards and Malpractice Reporter. Canton, OH: Professional Reports Corporation.

The Sports Medicine Standards and Malpractice Reporter. Canton, OH: Professional Reports Corporation.

The Sports, Parks and Recreation Law Reporter. Canton, OH: Professional Reports Corporation.

BRACING, SPLINTING, AND TAPING TECHNIQUES

Bruce E. Baker

Bracing, splinting, and taping techniques are commonly prescribed by the team physician for injured athletes. These techniques can be used in various stages of treatment and subsequent rehabilitation. Preventive techniques are also available and can reduce the potential for injury to certain joints while the athlete participates in running and jumping activities. Strains and sprains of the upper and lower extremities are the most common reasons to use such techniques and devices. Joints treatable by these techniques include fingers, thumbs, wrists, elbows, and shoulders in the upper extremity. Lower extremity joints include the great toe, ankle, and knee.

LOWER EXTREMITY

Sprains of the metatarsophalangeal joint of the great toe occur commonly in running and jumping sports, particularly on artificial surfaces. Discomfort and ligamentous laxity can be assisted by taping techniques that reduce the range of motion at the metatarsophalangeal joint and provide collateral stabilization (Fig. 11–1). Additionally, a firm-soled shoe can reduce the range of motion and assist the athlete in his or her effort to return to a functional state.

The most common injury associated with the ankle joint during competitive athletics is an inversion sprain of the ankle. The calcaneofibular and the anterior talofibular ligaments are commonly sprained in varying degrees. Following the application of ice after the initial injury, consideration can be given to bracing the ankle with commercially available ankle corsets with metal stays that limit range of motion and rest the injured ligaments. A type of stirrup

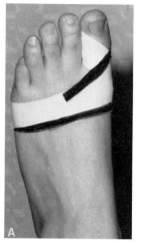 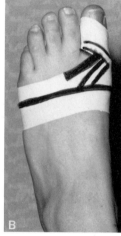 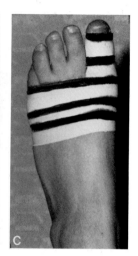

Fig. 11–1. Great toe. Materials used include tape adherent and 1-inch adhesive tape. The knee is in extension and the foot is off the table. After placing the tape adherent over the toe and forefoot, an anchor strip around the forefoot is used (*A*). Additional figure-of-eight strips are then placed, as in *B*. The taping is completed with overlapping strips applied initially on the two and then extending proximally over the distal forefoot (*C*).

called an air splint can also be used during the initial phase of treatment and during the rehabilitative phase when the patient is increasing his or her activity pattern (Fig. 11–2). Following the restitution of normal function in the ankle and prior to returning to competitive activity, three types of support can be used. These include ankle corsets with or without metal stays (Fig. 11–3),ankle wrapping with cotton muslin, and taping with adhesive tape (Fig. 11–4).

These techniques can also be used prophylactically in situations where concern exists about the potential for injury in a competitive athlete.

Instability problems about the knee most commonly relate to the patella, the medial collateral ligament, and the anterior cruciate ligament. Immediate treatment following an acute injury is best provided by a knee immobilizer (Fig. 11–5). This allows modification of the splint in the course of initial treatment and knee immobilization limiting the potential for further injury and reduces discomfort associated with the injury. The potential for recurrent subluxation or dislocation of the patella can be reduced by the use of a patellar stabilization brace following rehabilitation (Fig. 11–6). This

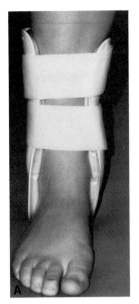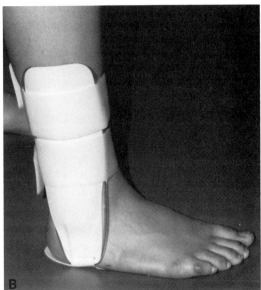

Fig. 11–2. *A* and *B*, Commercial air splint used for postinjury medial and lateral support.

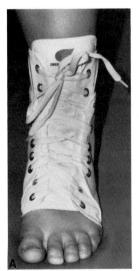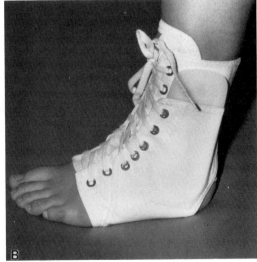

Fig. 11–3. *A* and *B*, Laced ankle corset with medial and lateral struts that can be used for prophylactic purposes or for medial and lateral support after injury.

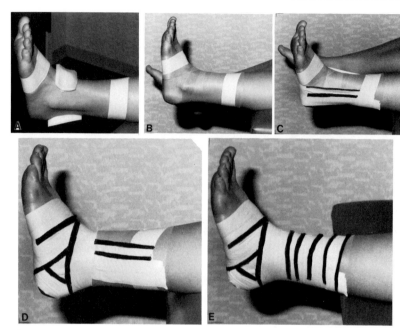

Fig. 11–4. Ankle. Materials required include heel and dorsal pads with lubrication, tape adherent, underwrap, and 1½-inch adhesive tape. The athlete sits with the knee extended and the distal half of the lower leg beyond the edge of the table. The foot is in a neutral position. *A,* Heel and dorsal pads may be applied, as may underwrap. *B,* Two anchor strips are applied with 1½-inch adhesive tape, one below the gastrocnemius and the second at the distal arch. *C,* The next step is to apply stirrup strips under the foot and heel. This produces eversion of the foot. Heel locks can then be applied in both directions, as indicated in *D.* Following this, figure-of-eight strips with force to cause slight eversion is done. Following this, circular strips of tape are placed around the leg, foot, and ankle in an overlapping fashion, as indicated in *E.*

device is most commonly manufactured as a knee sleeve with an opening for the patella, with padding and strapping around the distal thigh and proximal tibia for static stabilization of the patella.

The most common type of knee sprain occurs with a valgus external rotation stress with or without a lateral impact load. Injury can occur to the superficial and deep portions of the medial collateral ligament, as well as the menisci, the anterior cruciate ligament, and the posterior cruciate ligament. The situation may dictate surgical repair. Some medial collateral ligament injuries without complete

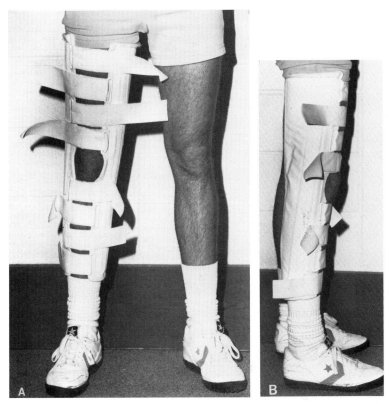

Fig. 11–5. *A* and *B,* Commercial knee immobilizer used for postinjury stabilization of the knee.

disruption and without anterior cruciate ligament injury can be
treated with bracing or taping, however. A rehabilitation knee brace
is defined as a device used following surgery or knee injuries treated
nonoperatively that allows limited range of motion controlled by the
physician (Fig. 11–7). This device is not compatible with a functional
state following completion of rehabilitation, but can be of great assistance in protecting the injured ligaments or in postoperative situations while allowing limited range of motion during the early
rehabilitation phase.

Prophylactic braces have been advertised as having the capacity
to limit the potential for injury to the knee by the so called clipping
mechanism secondary to lateral contact to the knee. There is significant controversy about the efficacy of these types of braces. Cur-

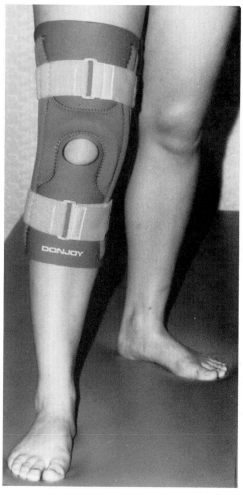

Fig. 11–6. Commercially available patellar stabilization brace with Velcro straps above and below the patella and a U-shaped stabilizing component surrounding the patella.

rently, the position statement of the American Academy of Orthopedic Surgeons and the Medical Society of the State of New York is that these types of braces cannot be definitively shown to produce a protective effect and, therefore, cannot be recommended for prophylactic use.

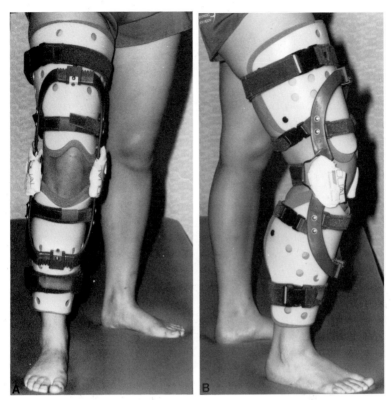

Fig. 11–7. *A* and *B,* Commercially available rehabilitation brace with hinges that can be adjusted for limited mobilization of the knee following injury or surgical procedure.

Functional braces, such as the one shown in Figure 11–8, most commonly consist of rigid double uprights with hinges, rigid crossing struts, and some form of soft tissue containment. They have a capacity to limit abduction stresses. Controversy exists currently as to the capacity of functional braces to control anteroposterior translation of the tibia on the femur, as would be seen with an anterior cruciate ligament injury. These braces can be constructed with extension stops that have the potential for controlling hyperextension mechanisms that can occur during competition. The most common types are form fitted following a casting of the patient's knee and fabrication by the manufacturer. These can be particularly useful in

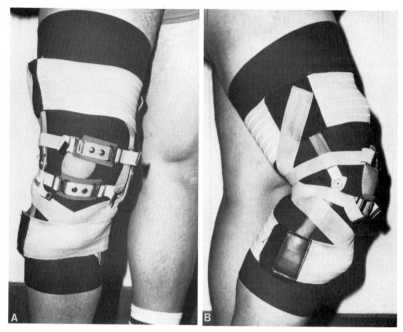

Fig. 11–8. *A* and *B*, Functional brace with hinged medial and lateral uprights with rigid crossing struts and significant soft tissue containment above and below the knee.

situations of injury to the medial collateral ligament where resistance to recurrent stress to the medial aspect of the knee is desired.

Neoprene nylon-lined knee sleeves can be beneficial to the individual with inflammatory problems, such as patellar tendinitis or symptoms secondary to previous patellar instability. Knee instability is not improved; however, the insulation frequently makes the patient subjectively more comfortable and can be used in situations where the static stability is intact.

Taping techniques can be used in situations where the knee does not demonstrate gross instability (Fig. 11–9). Taping can be particularly useful in situations of first-degree injury to the medial collateral ligament without gross instability. This may allow advancement to a functional state in situations where the knee is not grossly unstable.

Achilles tendon injuries can be helped during the stages of rehabilitation and subsequent return to activity with taping techniques outlined in Figure 11–10.

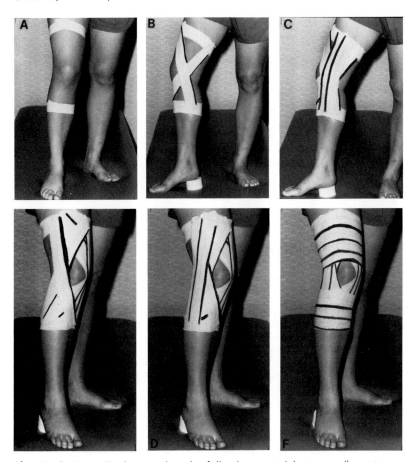

Fig. 11–9. Knee. Taping requires the following materials: tape adherent, underwrap, 1½-inch adhesive tape, and 3-inch elastic tape. The patient stands with the heel of his foot elevated on an object of approximately 1½ inches in height. The knee should be in a position of approximately 20° of flexion. *A,* Tape adherent and underwrap are applied initially with anchor strips of 1½-inch, adhesive tape placed at the midthigh and midcalf. *B,* Two-inch elastic tape is then applied in a crossing fashion over the knee joint with crossing in the midportion of the joint. *C,* Additional vertical strips of elastic tape can then be applied. Crossing strips of tape (*D*) can then be applied to the lateral aspect of the knee with vertical strips (*E*) applied subsequently. *F,* Circular anchor strips are then applied to the calf and thigh regions and are reinforced with adhesive tape.

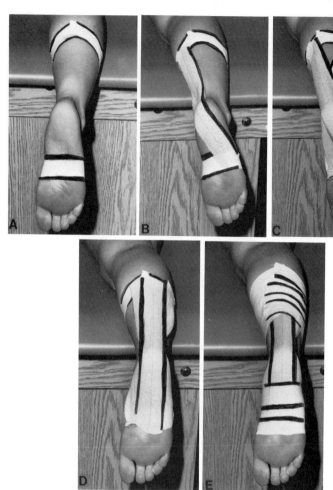

Fig. 11–10. Achilles tendon. Taping requires tape adherent, heel pad, 2- or 3-inch elastic tape, and 1½-inch adhesive tape. The patient lies in the prone position with the leg extending over the end of the table. *A*, Anchor strips are applied over the metatarsal region and the midcalf with 1½-inch adhesive tape. *B* and *C*, Crossing strips of 2-inch elastic tape are then applied extending to the anchor strips. *D*, A longitudinal strip is then placed over the gastrocnemius, Achilles tendon, and plantar surface of the foot, extending from one anchor to another. *E*, Circular anchor strips of adhesive tape are then applied over the foot and calf regions to anchor the vertically applied tape.

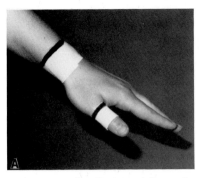
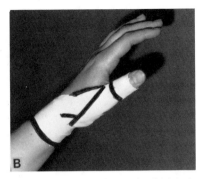

Fig. 11–11. Thumb. Materials required include tape adherent and 1-inch adhesive tape. The thumb is placed in a neutral position. *A,* Initial circular anchor adhesive tape is placed at the base of the distal phalanx of the thumb and around the wrist. Crossing strips extending from the distal anchor strip to the wrist anchor strip are then placed. *B,* Longitudinal reinforcement strips can then be applied with reinforcement of the taping completed in a figure-of-eight fashion.

UPPER EXTREMITY

Injuries to the interphalangeal joints and metacarpophalangeal joints of the fingers are probably the most common upper extremity injury. Sprains of these joints can be protected by buddy taping. This involves taping the injured digit to the adjacent finger allowing motion at the interphalangeal joints and metacarpophal-

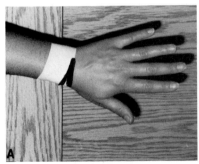
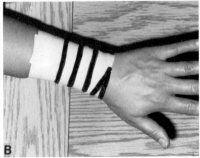

Fig. 11–12. Wrist. Materials required include 1½-inch adhesive tape and tape adherent. The patient holds the affected wrist in a neutral position with the fingers flat. *A,* A strip is placed at the base of the wrist with a circular configuration. *B,* Additional strips overlapping the preceding one are continued for approximately four applications.

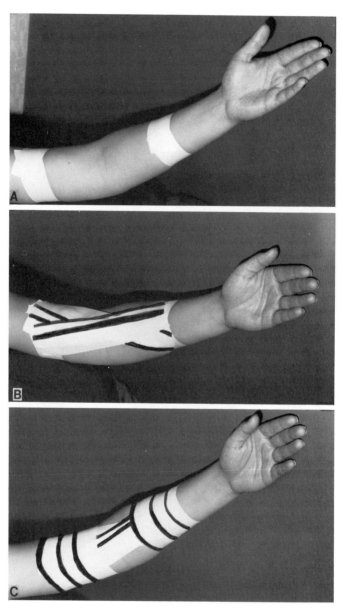

Fig. 11–13. Elbow. Materials required include 1½-inch adhesive tape, tape adherent, and 2-inch elastic tape. *A,* The patient maintains the elbow flexed while strips are applied around the midupper arm and midforearm. *B,* Crossing strips of elastic tape are then applied over the antecubital fossa from one anchoring strip to another. *C,* Circular strips of adhesive tape are then placed above and below the elbow to anchor the elastic tape.

angeal joints with splinting. This can be done in situations where there is no gross instability of the joint. Injuries to the thumb, particularly the metacarpophalangeal joint, can be disabling for people who play skill positions in sports. Taping to protect structures such as the ulnar collateral ligament of the metacarpophalangeal joint of the thumb, in many cases, will allow a functional return to activity (Fig. 11–11).

Injuries to the wrist that do not involve fracture or dislocation can initially be treated with a splint over the volar aspect of the forearm and hand. Following completion of treatment and rehabilitation, the wrist can be taped for increased stabilization (Fig. 11–12). In situations where limited wrist motion is required, a modified volar splint can be applied for additional stabilization.

Soft tissue injuries to the elbow include dislocation, as well as sprain and strain (Fig. 11–13). The use of a sling and posterior splint following the initial injury allows stabilization and reduction of pain. Following completion of rehabilitation, taping techniques to limit

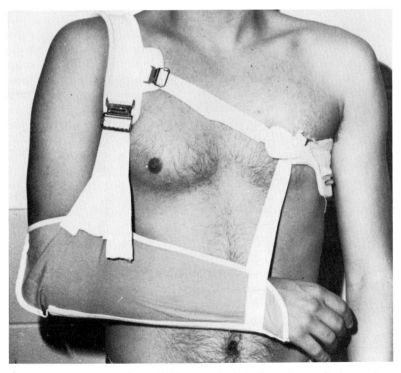

Fig. 11–14. Commercially available acromioclavicular splint applied to reduce the distal clavicle at the acromioclavicular joint.

hyperextension can reduce the potential for recurrent injury to the elbow, particularly following dislocation.

Injuries to the shoulder most commonly seen include acromioclavicular sprains, with acromioclavicular separation the most severe. Dislocation or subluxation of the glenohumeral joint is another common injury to the shoulder. Following reduction and immobilization with a sling, range of motion and rehabilitation can be started for dislocation. Situations where limitation of abduction and external rotation can be controlled, such as recurrent subluxation or dislocation, may be limited by the use of taping that reduces abduction and external rotation.

Initial treatment of third-degree acromioclavicular sprains or separations in the common vernacular include reduction of the distal clavicle and application of a Kenny-Howard splint (Fig. 11–14). This can be used as a form of treatment if surgery is not indicated. Some commercially available splints can be used in the treatment phase prior to the institution of rehabilitation.

SUMMARY

Bracing, splinting, and taping techniques are commonly prescribed by the team physician for athletes following injury. These can be used in various stages of treatment and subsequent rehabilitation. Preventive techniques are also available and can reduce the potential for injury to certain joints while an athlete participates in running and jumping activities.

ACKNOWLEDGMENTS

The author is grateful to Reatha Baker, Suzanne Sesnie-Orth, A.T.C., and Steven Parker.

COMPETITION PHASE

C H A P T E R   1   2

LIFE-THREATENING EMERGENCIES

Jack E. Young and Robert C. Cantu

Catastrophic injuries in sports medicine are rare, usually fewer than 1/100,000 reported injuries. High school injuries produce the highest incidence and contact sports the highest rate. Any sport may involve emergencies, however. Evaluation of the cause of catastrophies followed by appropriate measures can prevent some injuries. Preparation can lead toward better management of emergencies. As a rule, trainers should have Basic Life Support (BLS) experience and at least one team physician Advanced Cardiac Life Support (ACLS) experience. Periodically, drills should be conducted to assess the availability of necessary medical equipment and supplies and to determine the proper routes for mobilization of the local emergency medicine system (EMS).

Athletic emergencies are managed in the same manner as any type of emergency. Initial assessment establishes the level of consciousness: "How are you? Are you OK?" This is followed by the ABCs of emergency care.

*A*irway management with cervical spine stabilization: Establish the patency of the airway and foreign body removal. Suction is essential to establish patency and visualization of the vocal cords. Without EMS, suction can be obtained in the field with a mechanical Ambu minipump and a tonsilar (Yankauer) suction tip. The chin lift and jaw thrust are utilized to open the airway, and an oropharyngeal airway is used to maintain patency.

*B*reathing by observation and feel: If necessary, initiate mouth-to-mouth or preferably mouth-to-pocket-mask ventilation. When available, follow with bag-valve-to-mask resuscitation, and endotracheal intubation if necessary. Again, suction is often mandatory for proper tube placement. Laryngoscopes contained in most commercial emergency kits should be replaced by larger battery-operated scopes with a large (Macintosh) blade. Cricothyroidotomy may be required in massive facial trauma.

Circulation: Estimate systolic BP by palpating a pulse: radial (>80 mm Hg), femoral (>70 mm Hg), or carotid (>60 mm Hg). Apply direct pressure to control open bleeding. Use of the pneumatic antishock garment (PASG) is controversial but indicated for pelvic and lower-extremity fractures. Shock is treated with oxygen, and fluid replacement with 16-gauge IV apparatus and balanced salt solution. ECG monitoring will reveal rhythm disturbances that can be treated by following the ACLS algorithm guidelines. In addition to CPR, the following is initial treatment for the corresponding dysrhythmia: ventricular fibrillation (VF)—if pulseless, immediate defibrillation with a progression from 200 to 360 joules p.r.n.; asystole—epinephrine, 1:10,000, 0.5 to 1.0 mg IV bolus; electromechanical dissociation—same as asystole and consider underlying causes; stable ventricular tachycardia (VT)—lidocaine, 1 mg/kg IV; unstable VT—cardioversion with a progression from 50 to 360 joules p.r.n.; bradycardia with symptoms, hypotension, or ventricular ectopy—atropine, 0.5 to 1.0 mg IV; ventricular ectopy (when suppression is indicated)—lidocaine, 1 mg/kg IV and consider underlying causes; stable paroxysmal supraventricular tachycardia (PSVT)—verapamil, 5 mg IV; unstable PSVT—cardioversion as in unstable VT.

Disability: conduct a rapid neurologic evaluation. This also establishes a baseline in tracking the patient's course. Follow the AVPU system: Alertness, Vocal stimuli response, Painful stimuli response, and Unresponsiveness.

SUDDEN DEATH

In athletes younger than ages 30 to 35 the most common causes of sudden death include: hypertrophic cardiomyopathy (idiopathic concentric left ventricular hypertrophy, aortic rupture associated with Marfan's syndrome, congenital coronary anomalies, and atherosclerotic coronary artery disease (CAD). The presumed mechanisms of death in most of these conditions involve fatal dysrhythmias, the terminal event being ventricular fibrillation.

In athletes over the ages of 30 to 35, CAD is the primary cause. Congenital anomalies may also be causes.

Cocaine abuse may produce aortic dissection, ventricular tachycardia, pulmonary edema, or coronary artery spasm leading to sudden death with or without CAD. Cocaine toxicity is treated with IV propranolol 1 mg q5min to 0.1 ml/kg. Seizures are titrated with diazepam and dysrhythmias according to the proper ACLS algorithm. Over-the-counter sympathomimetic agents can create similar life-threatening emergencies. Steroid abuse has been associated with premature CAD. Approximately half of young athletes at risk of sudden death can be identified by medical history and physical examination. Family history should focus on sudden death; personal history on syncope, palpitations, and exertional chest pain. Physical examination should emphasize the characteristic outflow tract murmur of hypertrophic cardiomyopathy (murmur increases with Valsalva maneuver, standing, tachycardia, and amyl nitrate), marfanoid features (tall, upper-to-lower body segment ratio of <0.9, hyperextensibility, lens dislocations, or striae), and evidence of congestive heart failure. Massive cardiac testing is neither cost effective nor medicolegally feasible.

THORACIC AND PULMONARY EMERGENCIES

Blunt trauma may be caused by contact sports, falling on objects such as a football, weights falling on an athlete, horse rolling, or vehicles involved in sports. Penetrating injuries can result from equipment associated with any sport. Both can produce life-threatening emergencies that are identified and managed in the primary survey.

Tension pneumothorax ("one-way valve" air leak) causes collapse of the ipsilateral lung and is usually caused by blunt trauma. Signs include dyspnea, tracheal deviation, decreased breath sounds on the affected side, and jugular venous distension. Treatment is immediate decompression with a large-bore needle in the second intercostal space.

An open pneumothorax (sucking chest wound) is usually caused by penetrating trauma. Initial management is with a sterile occlusive dressing.

Massive hemothorax occurs after blunt or penetrating trauma and is usually associated with shock. The affected side has decreased breath sounds and is dull to percussion. Initial treatment is with fluid resuscitation.

Flail chest results from multiple rib fractures within the same or serial ribs resulting in paradoxic movement of the chest wall. External immobilization is no longer considered effective treatment. The underlying pathologic process involves lung parenchyma; thus, initial treatment consists of adequate ventilation, oxygenation, and fluid resuscitation.

Cardiac tamponade usually results from penetrating injury. Beck's triad forms the classic signs: increased venous pressure (JVD), decreased arterial pressure (BP), and decreased heart sounds. Failure of ACLS resuscitative efforts after any trauma should produce a high index of suspicion for tamponade, which then requires pericardiocentesis and is best performed via the subxyphoid route.

A variety of chest injuries may be diagnosed during the secondary survey, including: pulmonary or myocardial contusion; uncomplicated pneumothorax or hemothorax; fractured ribs; or pulmonary embolism. The last has been postulated in athletes who practice blood doping, become dehydrated, and develop deep-vein thrombophlebitis. Presentation, in order of frequency, includes: tachypnea, chest pain, dyspnea, and apprehension. All the foregoing require hospital evaluation and, pending their seriousness, hospitalization.

Anaphylaxis with acute bronchospasm can occur in individuals allergic to airborne pollens, grass pollens inoculated through skin abrasions, or stings and bites from Hymenoptera insects (bees, wasps, or ants). Administer epinephrine 1:1000, 0.3 to 0.5 ml subcutaneously followed by diphenhydramine 25 to 50 mg IM, and fluid resuscitation p.r.n. Steroids minimize delayed symptoms, and secondary infection at the site should be considered. All allergic individuals should be instructed in the use of insect sting kits.

ABDOMINAL EMERGENCIES

Primary survey: Initial management of abdominal trauma is usually associated with shock secondary to rupture of a solid organ, pelvic fracture, or laceration of a major vessel. The ABCs with fluid resuscitation are necessary for stabilization prior to transport. Pelvic fractures may lead to exsanguinating hemorrhage, and the PASG is indicated. Impaled objects in any trauma should be left in place with careful stabilization until definitive care can be rendered because removal may result in uncontrollable hemorrhage.

Secondary survey: Most abdominal emergencies are identified during the secondary survey. Thoracic trauma may be associated with injuries to the spleen, stomach, liver, or diaphragm. Direct blows to the upper abdomen may cause rupture and hemorrhage of the liver or spleen. Direct contact without proper padding, falls in various sports, and horse kicking can lead to lethal abdominal injuries. With conservative management of ruptured spleen, splenectomy is not needed in greater than half the cases.

Retroperitoneal injuries to the kidney, ureter, pancreas, or duodenum usually develop more slowly and require a high index of suspicion. Intramural duodenal hematoma results from deceleration and jarring and may be associated with football, cycling, and equestrian sport. Direct blows can also produce this injury. The proposed mechanism is shearing of the blood vessels between the submucosa and muscularis at the transitional zone of the duodenum.

HEAD INJURIES

The central nervous system, consisting of the brain and the spinal cord, is unique in that nerve cells are incapable of regeneration. Injury to these structures takes on a singular importance because cells that die are forever lost, incapable of regrowth, transplantation, or replacement with artificial hardware. Although virtually every major joint (ankle, knee, hip, elbow, shoulder) and most of the body's organs are capable of replacement, the central nervous system housed in the skull and spine is the sole organ where this is not possible.

With these sobering facts in mind, the clinical evaluation of the head- or spine-injured athlete takes on a singular importance. The clinical assessment must be expeditious, precise, and forever bearing in mind the hippocratic prohibition: "First, do no harm."

Whenever the injury involves a loss of consciousness, several important simultaneous observations and assumptions must be made. Assume that the patient has a fractured neck and carry out the examination with this in mind. First, determine whether the patient has an adequate airway; then conduct a rapid baseline medical and neurologic examination. This should include blood pressure, pulse, respiratory rate, state of consciousness (alert, stupor, semicomatose, comatose), pupillary size and reactivity, extremity movement spontaneously and in response to painful stimulation, and deep-tendon and Babinski reflexes.

The leading cause of death from athletic head injury is intracranial hemorrhage. The examining trainer or physician must be alert to four types of hemorrhage in every instance of head injury. Because all four types of intracranial hemorrhage may be fatal, rapid, accurate initial assessment, as well as appropriate follow-up, is mandatory after an athletic head injury.

An epi- or extradural hematoma is usually the most rapidly progressive intracranial hematoma. It is frequently associated with a fracture of the temporal bone and results from a tear in one of the arteries supplying the covering (dura) of the brain. The hematoma accumulates inside the skull but outside the covering of the brain. Arising from a torn artery, it may progress rapidly and may reach a fatal size in 30 to 60 minutes. Although this does not always occur, the athlete may have a lucid interval; that is, the athlete initially may regain consciousness after the head trauma and before starting to experience increasing headache and progressive deterioration in the level of consciousness as the clot accumulates and the intracranial pressure increases. This lesion, if present, will almost always declare itself within an hour or two of the time of injury. Usually, the brain substance is free of direct injury; thus, if the clot is promptly removed surgically, full recovery is to be expected. Because this lesion is rapidly and universally fatal if missed, all athletes receiving a head injury must be very closely and frequently observed during the ensuing several hours, preferably the next 24 hours. This observation should be done at a facility where full neurosurgical services are immediately available.

A subdural hematoma, a second type of intracranial hemorrhage, occurs between the brain surface and the dura. It is thus located under the dura and directly on the brain. It often results from a torn vein running from the surface of the brain to the dura. It may also result from a torn venous sinus or even a small artery on the surface of the brain. With this injury, there is often associated injury to the brain tissue. If a subdural hematoma necessitates surgery in the first 24 hours, the mortality is high not because of the clot itself, but because of the associated brain damage. With a subdural hematoma that progresses rapidly, the athlete usually does not regain consciousness, and immediate neurosurgical evaluation is obvious. Occasionally, the brain itself will not be injured, and a subdural hematoma may develop slowly over a period of days to weeks. This chronic subdural hematoma, although often associated with headache, may initially cause a variety of very mild, almost imperceptible mental, motor, or sensory signs and symptoms. Because its recognition and removal will lead to full recovery, it must always be suspected in an athlete who has previously sustained a head injury and who, days or weeks later, is not quite right. A computed tomographic (CT) scan of the head will definitively show such a lesion.

An intracerebral hematoma is the third type of intracranial hemorrhage seen after head trauma. In this instance, the bleeding is into the brain substance itself, usually from a torn artery. It may also result from the rupture of a congenital vascular lesion such as an aneurysm or arteriovenous malformation. Intracerebral hematomas are not usually associated with a lucid interval and may be rapidly progressive. Death occasionally occurs before the injured athlete can be moved to a hospital. Because of the intense reaction such a tragic event precipitates among fellow athletes, family, students, and even the community at large, and because of the inevitable rumors that follow, it is imperative to obtain a complete autopsy in such an event to clarify fully the causative factors. Often the autopsy will reveal a congenital lesion that may indicate that the cause of death was other than presumed and was ultimately unavoidable. Only by such full, factual elucidation will inappropriate feelings of guilt in fellow athletes, friends, and family be assuaged.

A fourth type of intracranial hemorrhage is subarachnoid, confined to the surface of the brain. Following head trauma, such bleeding is the result of disruption of the tiny surface brain vessels and is analogous to a bruise. As with the intracerebral hematoma, brain swelling often occurs, and such a hemorrhage can also result from a ruptured cerebral aneurysm or arteriovenous malformation. Because bleeding is superficial, surgery is not usually required unless a congenital vascular anomaly is present.

Such a contusion of the brain usually causes headache and, not infrequently, an associated neurologic deficit, depending on the area of the brain. The irritative properties of the blood may also precipitate a seizure. If a seizure occurs in a head-injured athlete, it is important to log-roll the patient onto his or her side. Any blood or saliva will thus roll out of the mouth or nose, and the tongue cannot fall back, obstructing the airway. If one has a padded tongue depressor or oral airway, it can be inserted between the teeth. Under no circumstances should one insert one's fingers into the mouth of an athlete who is having a seizure because a traumatic amputation can easily result from such an unwise maneuver. Usually, such a traumatic seizure will last only a minute or two. The athlete will then relax, and transportation to the nearest medical facility can be effected.

CERVICAL SPINE INJURIES

The same traumatic lesions that affect the brain may also occur to the cervical spinal cord, that is, concussion, contusion, and the various types of hemorrhage. The major concern with a cervical spine injury is the possibility of an unstable fracture that may produce quadriplegia. At the time of injury, there is no way to determine the presence of an unstable fracture until appropriate x-rays are taken. There is also no way of determining a fully recoverable from a permanent case of quadriplegia. If the patient is fully conscious, a cervical fracture or cervical cord injury is usually accompanied by rigid cervical muscle spasm and pain that immediately alerts the athlete and physician to the presence of such an injury. The unconscious athlete, who is unable to state that the neck hurts and whose neck muscles are not in protective spasm, is susceptible to potential cord severence if one does not always think of the possibility of an unstable cervical spine fracture. With an unconscious or obviously neck-injured athlete, it is imperative that no neck manipulation be carried out on the field. Definitive treatment must await appropriate x-rays at a medical facility, and all the precautions discussed previously must be taken.

RECOMMENDED READING

Cantu RC: Head and neck injuries in the young athlete. In *Sports Injuries In The Young Athlete*. Edited by LJ Micheli. Philadelphia: W.B. Saunders, 1988.

Cantu RC: Head injury in sports. In *Advances In Sports Medicine and Fitness*. Vol. 2. Edited by WA Grana and JA Lombardo. Chicago, Year Book Medical Publishers, 1988.

TRANSPORTATION/IMMOBILIZATION

Robert C. Cantu

The initial examination is crucial to subsequent evaluation and treatment. If the patient shows improvement within a few minutes, then subsequent transportation and diagnostic evaluation can proceed in a routine manner. If, however, deterioration, especially in the state of consciousness, is seen, then transportation and subsequent treatment must be immediate. Every unconscious athlete should be transported on a fracture board. The head should be secured in a neutral position with sandbags, a four-poster collar, or a traction device if available.

If the unconscious athlete is wearing a helmet and has a good airway, do not remove the helmet, because this may precipitate quadriplegia if an unstable cervical fracture is present. If breathing is obstructed, the face mask should be removed to gain access to the mouth. The oral pharynx should be searched for a foreign body and an oral airway inserted. Only if the airway is questionable should the helmet be removed, and then never forcibly and always with the neck in a neutral (neither flexed nor extended) position. The helmet can be used for cervical traction. The chin strap serves as the halter and the ear holes and/or immediately adjacent edge of the helmet as a site for attachment of neutral traction. While the unconscious athlete is being moved onto the spine board, the ear holes of the helmet also may serve as a convenient site for inserting one's index finger to effect gentle neutral cervical traction. Only after appropriate cervical spine x-rays have excluded a cervical spine fracture, malalignment, or instability can the helmet be safely removed from the unconscious athlete.

In the event that a fracture board is not readily available to transport the unconscious athlete from the site of injury, a decision must be made whether to wait for the ambulance to arrive with its stretcher or to transport the athlete using the locked-arm technique. Although one might generally favor waiting for the ambulance, it is true that if an adequate number of players or spectators are present, by locking hands to the elbows of individuals standing opposite each other, a secure surface for transporting an injured athlete a short distance is provided. When transporting an unconscious athlete in this manner, one person applies neutral traction to the helmet or otherwise secures the head in a neutral position.

RECOMMENDED READING

Cantu RC: Head and neck injuries in the young athlete. In *Sports Injuries in the Young Athlete*. Edited by LJ Micheli. Philadelphia: W.B. Saunders, 1988.

Cantu RC: Head injury in sports. In *Advances In Sports Medicine and Fitness*. Vol. 2. Edited by WA Grana and JA Lombardo. Chicago: Year Book Medical Publishers, 1988.

| C H A P T E R   1   4 |

LIMB-THREATENING EMERGENCIES

Preston M. Wolin

Although it may be unusual, the sports medicine physician
can be confronted with an injury that represents a limb-threatening emergency. In that situation, proper disposition is critical. For
the purposes of this discussion, limb-threatening emergency is defined as one in which the extremity as a whole or its proper function
is placed at risk. As with all emergencies, prompt initiation of treatment is critical. Careful planning can minimize problems. Every
event should have a prearranged plan for emergency transport of
the injured athlete utilizing standard protocols.

ENVIRONMENTAL CONDITIONS

Two special environmental conditions can produce limb-
threatening emergencies. The first of these is cold. A detailed
description of cold injuries is beyond the scope of this chapter; however, frostnip and frostbite can occur in the sports medicine setting.
Prevention is crucial. The athlete/team must be advised of the predisposing factors to cold injuries. These include: inadequate insulation of all potentially exposed areas; decreased peripheral circulation due to tight clothing (especially footwear) and/or arterial
disease; fatigue; and the use of alcohol, tobacco, and other drugs.
A mild cold injury (frostnip) is characterized by skin changes, a
frosted appearance, and numbness. The symptoms are reversible
by warming. Frostbite is the freezing of soft tissue. The longer the
exposure, the larger the area of necrosis. The extremity swells and
reddens as the patient complains of numbness. The body part then
becomes white with a yellow-blue waxiness. Skin is initially firm
but can become hard. Emergency treatment is required to avoid
further injury and to save borderline tissue. Overlying clothing or

equipment should be removed. The extremity should be rapidly rewarmed by immersion in water heated to 104 to 108° F (40 to 42° C). Antibiotic ointment and fluffy dressings should be applied thereafter. The extremity should not be used after rewarming because repeat exposure to cold can cause even greater harm. Emergency transport for definitive care should be arranged as soon as possible.

The second environmental condition predisposing to limb-threatening situations is gas gangrene. The infection is characterized by fulminating myonecrosis. In the sports medicine setting, Clostridium perfringens can occur with an open fracture or dislocation. This may be especially true where animals are present such as in equestrian events or rodeo. Initial symptoms may be few, but the onset can occur between 12 and 72 hours after injury, depending on the extent of contamination. The patient may present with localized pain, swelling, or crepitus (indicative of gas production). A thin, brownish discharge may be noted along with an unpleasant odor and bronze skin color. Systemically the patient may have fever, tachycardia, hypotension, and eventual coma.

Prevention of gas gangrene is by debridement of all nonviable tissue. If any question exists, the wound should be left open. Penicillin or more broad-spectrum antibiotics are appropriate. Once frank infection develops, emergency debridement is required to salvage the limb. High doses of antibiotics need to be administered. Hyperbaric oxygen, if available, may also be useful. If this treatment is insufficient, amputation may be required as a lifesaving procedure.

GENERAL CONSIDERATIONS

Although many individual limb-at-risk situations exist, several general principles are common. The most obvious emergency is that caused by trauma to part of an extremity in continuity with a vital structure, e.g., a nerve or artery. Every extremity injury must be initially evaluated with a complete neurovascular examination. The presence/absence of pulses, normal capillary refill, and skin color should be noted. Sensation and motor examination specific to the relevant nerve must also be documented. If swelling limits the examination, that too should be noted. To prevent further injury the injured extremity should be splinted and the *prearranged* method of emergency transport completed. Definitive reduction of the fracture and/or dislocation must be accomplished as soon as possible.

A nerve can be contused (ulnar nerve—medial collateral epicondyle fracture), compressed (radial nerve—distal humerus fracture), or disrupted (peroneal nerve—lateral knee ligament injury). Prompt reduction of a fracture and/or dislocation can avoid further insult to a compressed nerve. An artery can be lacerated as a result of a fracture (tracheal artery—humeral shaft fracture), its intima can be disrupted (popliteal artery—dislocation), or it can be contused resulting in thrombus formation. Although pulselessness often is an indicator of arterial insufficiency, it may not always be present. Distal collateral circulation may provide enough flow to generate a pulse. Hypoesthesia or paresthesia in a stocking-glove distribution, cyanosis, and pain disproportionate to the injury should alert the examiner to the diagnosis. Emergency angiography may be needed. Arterial repair/reconstruction has the best result if performed promptly within 6 to 8 hours of the injury.

Another general class of emergencies is the compartment syndrome. The pathophysiologic features of this condition result when impeded blood flow causes capillary leakage, thus increasing compartment pressure in a closed compartment. Common causes include decreased-arterial-flow vascular injury or diminished venous return caused by constricting bandages. Contusion or exercise can also result in muscle swelling that precipitates a compartment syndrome. Compression injuries to muscles and nerves within the compartment can result. The diagnosis must be suspected when pain is out of proportion to the initial injury. On examination the compartment is tense. There is pain to passive motion of the digits activated by the involved muscles (i.e., passive finger extension to check volar forearm involvement). Pulselessness and sensory-motor changes are late sequelae. *If these signs are present the time for effective intervention may well have passed.* If the injury is left untreated, the breakdown products of muscle are released resulting in systemic acidosis and possible renal tubular damage.

Once a compartment syndrome is suspected, all constricting bandages should be removed or casts at least bivalved with underlying padding released. The extremity should be placed level to the heart. Elevation may increase compartment pressure. If symptoms do not resolve promptly, intracompartmental pressure readings should be obtained. Some disagreement exists regarding indication for surgery. The current recommendation is for fasciotomy when intracompartmental pressure exceeds 30 mm Hg and positive clinical findings exist. To avoid permanent damage, fasciotomy should be completed promptly. Muscle shows functional changes within 2 to 4 hours of ischemia, and irreversible functional loss begins at 4 to 12 hours.

REGIONAL CONSIDERATIONS

Although many extremity injuries can be potentially limb threatening, several of the more common ones are mentioned here.

Shoulder. Anterior shoulder dislocations do occur about the brachial plexus, but they rarely endanger the entire limb. Care must be exercised in attempting relocation of an anterior dislocation, however, especially in a patient over 50 years of age. There are reports of injury to the subclavian vessels with attempted reduction when the dislocation has been present for more than several hours. Gentle reduction should be attempted only after complete relaxation. Complete pre- and postreduction neurovascular examinations must be documented.

Humerus. Brachial artery lacerations have been reported following humerus fractures. The key to treatment is recognition. If the patient with a suspected humerus fracture (pain, tenderness, and ecchymosis, with or without deformity about the humerus) presents with pallor, pulselessness, and diffuse paresthesias, the diagnosis of arterial injury must be entertained and appropriate studies completed. Compartment syndrome should also be considered.

Elbow and Forearm. Volkmann's ischemic contracture of the forearm muscles was originally described as a complication of supracondylar humerus fracture; moreover, volar forearm compartment syndrome can also occur following elbow dislocation, both-bone forearm fracture, or contusion. Prevention by removal of constricting bandages and recognition by clinical examination and compartment pressure readings can save the limb.

Thigh. Fractures of the femur can result in femoral artery lacerations, whereas thigh contusions have been reported to result in compartment syndromes. Both should be suspected in any case where pain exceeds what would normally be expected for the injury.

Knee. The incidence of vascular damage following traumatic knee dislocation (tibiofemoral, not patellofemoral) is reported to be between 20 and 38%. Combined neurovascular involvement is 50 to 54%. The attitude of the joint on first presentation often belies the severity of the injury to the popliteal artery. The presence of pulses does not rule out vascular involvement, which can include laceration, intimal damage, or thrombus formation. *Therefore, all knee dislocations should be considered a limb-threatening emergency until proved otherwise.* Reduction should be accomplished gently. Care should be taken in initial evaluation to avoid hyperextension of greater than 15° or excess varus opening to test lateral ligament integrity. Both maneuvers can stretch the peroneal nerve. Complete neurovascular status should be documented. All patients with knee dislocations should undergo arteriography as soon as possible after injury. The study should always precede ligament repair/reconstruction. Amputation is the only alternative if ischemic changes are of sufficient magnitude.

    Leg. Fractures of the tibia and fibula can be complicated by injuries to the anterior tibial artery. If this occurs proximally, blood can be shunted from the posterior tibial to the peroneal and from there to the dorsalis pedis artery. Thus both pulses may be intact in the presence of signs of ischemia. An emergency arteriogram is indicated. If either pulse is absent before reduction (and is present on the contralateral limb) and does not return thereafter, vascular investigation is warranted.

    Compartment syndrome can complicate fractures or contusions of the leg. Although the anterior compartment (containing the anterior tibial and toe extensor muscles) is most commonly affected, the lateral (peroneals), superficial posterior (gastrocnemius and soleus) and deep posterior (posterior tibial and toe flexors) compartments can also be involved. Severe pain referable to the compartment and pain on passive lengthening of the affected muscle (i.e., passive extension to test the posterior compartment) should alert the examiner to the diagnosis.

    One special circumstance should be mentioned: acute exertional compartment syndrome of the leg. Most often this condition resolves after ceasing the precipitating activity, such as running. If symptoms persist, however, emergency treatment as outlined previously should be instituted.

    Ankle and Foot. Arterial injury is a well-known complication of severe midfoot injury such as a Lisfranc (tarsometatarsal) dislocation. The accompanying swelling can result in a compartment syndrome of the foot. An inversion ankle injury has been reported to cause a dorsalis pedis pseudoaneurysm. Because of the relatively closed space, a foot compartment syndrome can result. Pseudoaneurysm of the peroneal artery after inversion ankle injury has also been reported. Any of these problems may represent a limb-threatening emergency.

This review is not meant to be exhaustive. It is provided as a guide to the sports medicine physician who may encounter these unusual problems. Early recognition and definitive treatment can clearly be of immense significance to the athlete.

RECOMMENDED READING

Axe MJ: Limb threatening injuries in sport in emergency treatment of the injured athlete. *Clin Sports Med 8;* 1989.

Epps CH Jr: *Complications In Orthopedic Surgery,* 2nd Ed. Vols. 1 and 2. Philadelphia: J.B. Lippincott, 1986.

Fritz RL and Perrin DH: Prevention and treatment in emergency treatment of the injured athlete. *Clin Sports Med 8;* 1989.

Kym MR and Worsing RA Jr: Compartment syndrome in the foot after an inversion injury to the ankle—a case report. *J Bone Joint Surg 72H:*138–139, 1990.

Maguire DW, Huffer JM, Ahlstrand RA and Crummy AE Jr: Traumatic aneurysm of perforating peroneal artery: arterial bleeding—cause of severe pain following inversion, plantar flexion, ankle sprains. *J Bone Joint Surg 54A:*409–412, 1972.

Mubarek SJ: Compartment syndrome. In *Operative Orthopedics.* Edited by MW Chapman. Philadelphia: J.B. Lippincott, 1988, pp. 179–196.

Rockwood CA and Green DP: *Fractures in Adults.* Vols. 1 and 2. Philadelphia: J.B. Lippincott, 1984.

Rockwood CA, Wilkins KE and King RE: *Fractures in Children.* Vol. 3. Philadelphia: J.B. Lippincott, 1984.

Walls RM and Rosen P: Traumatic dislocation of the knee. *J Emerg Med 1:*527–531, 1984.

FIRST AID OF INJURIES IN SPORTS

Jack Harvey

Participation in sports carries with it certain risks, many of which have been defined in the sports medicine literature. Effective care of athletes requires the team physician to become familiar with the type and frequency of injuries in specific sports. A thorough knowledge of this information allows the team physician to be prepared to intervene to prevent these risks, as well as to deal with specific injuries as they occur. Familiarity with the sport makes the team physician a more trusted and valuable member of the team.

Injury rates vary not only among sports, but also as the intensity of the sport changes. For instance, football and wrestling both carry injury rates of 80 to 85% and have the potential for serious injury including paralysis or death. A sport such as gymnastics may on the surface seem less risky, with an injury rate of about 30% in recreational gymnastics, but a rate of 80% in competitive gymnastics has been reported. Therefore, coverage of athletic events should vary according to the risk. A collegiate football game requires doctors, trainers, and an ambulance in attendance, whereas a track meet may only require a coach trained in first aid and ready access to a telephone to summon aid. Injury rates also change as the intensity of training increases. Frequency, intensity, and time (FIT) of training increase the injury rate for overuse injuries. Today the young teenage athlete runs 6 to 8 miles/day, swims 5000 to 7000 yards/day, trains 4 hours/day in the gym, or rides the bike 250 to 350 miles/week. This increased FIT produces more injuries as well as more advanced overuse injures that do not respond to simple conservative treatment plans (rest, ice, and aspirin). Now team physicians are faced with the decision of using more potent anti-inflammatory agents, physical therapy techniques, injections, and surgery for these budding champions.

First aid of athletic injuries begins with preparation of a kit and a system of communication and backup. The kit needs to be rela-

159

tively complete for coverage of events in remote areas or international travel. For coverage of a local event, however, an effective communication system to summon a doctor or ambulance is more important than an elaborate medical kit. In fact, on the field or sidelines very little is used except the physician's five senses and common sense. A stethoscope, light, and pin are the most frequently used diagnostic equipment. Ice bags, elastic wraps, and tape make up the bulk of the sideline therapeutic equipment.

Situational awareness, clinical judgment, and experience greatly enhance the effectiveness of the team physician. Situational awareness is the ability to synthesize all the relevant information on type and severity of injury, age of player, and game situation while analyzing the risk : benefit ratio of allowing the player to return to play.

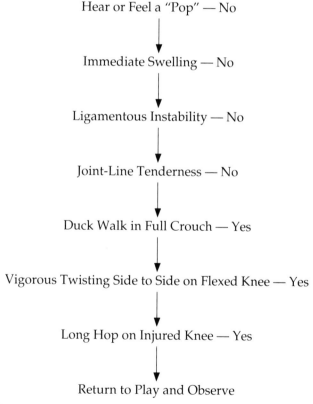

FIG. 15–1. Sideline knee screening examination.

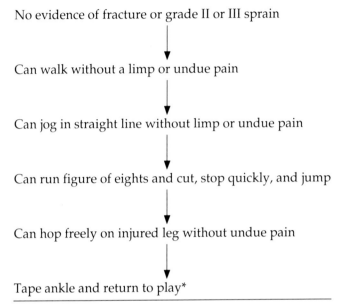

No evidence of fracture or grade II or III sprain

↓

Can walk without a limp or undue pain

↓

Can jog in straight line without limp or undue pain

↓

Can run figure of eights and cut, stop quickly, and jump

↓

Can hop freely on injured leg without undue pain

↓

Tape ankle and return to play*

---

*Observe athlete closely during remainder of game and remove from play if athlete's performance deteriorates or is hampered by pain or limp.

FIG. 15–2. Sideline ankle sprain screening examination.

Clinical judgment is of paramount importance. Because sideline medicine often is devoid of diagnostic equipment and medical backup, the physician must rely on his or her clinical skills to make judgments about diagnosis, treatment, and return to play. Experience in the sport is a tremendous asset because the more one knows about a certain sport, the better equipped the physician is to know what injuries to expect, how to treat them, and the risks of return to play in that particular sport. The additional input of a trainer in providing taping, bracing, and a series of functional drills to demonstrate the fieldworthiness of the injured player is also an asset. In general, "the younger the player the more conservative the decision, the younger the doctor the more conservative the decision" is a good rule to follow. Prior to allowing the player to return to the game, a physician needs to exclude serious injury by physical examination and to demonstrate adequate functional ability of the athlete (Figs. 15–1, 15–2). On returning to play an athlete must be watched carefully. If not performing up to par (i.e., limping, avoiding cutting) he should be removed from the game.

Players with musculoskeletal trauma who are not allowed to return to play should be treated by immobilization of the injured extremity, ice packs, and an elastic wrap. The ice needs to be placed over no more than one layer of the wrap and kept in place for 20 to 30 minutes. This is followed by removal of the ice and replacement of the elastic wrap. Icing should be performed as much as is reasonably practical in the 24- to 36-hour postinjury period. The injured limb should also be kept elevated above the level of the heart as much as practical. Neurovascular checks should be repeated as often as appropriate for the injury. Early application of the RICE (rest, ice, compression, and elevation) principle markedly reduces the period of disability and speeds rehabilitation.

Field treatment of the injured player begins with the trainer and/or physician initially assessing the severity of the injury from the sidelines. Actually seeing the injury occur may help in establishing the diagnosis because the doctor is aware of the mechanism of injury. Any life-threatening injury (i.e., a player that does not move once he is down) should bypass the tradition of the trainer or coach first seeing the player then summoning the doctor onto the field. In these instances all members of the health-care team need to arrive rapidly at the scene. Communication via pre-established hand signals or radio is used to request a stretcher, CPR equipment, or an ambulance. Emergency procedures need to be well rehearsed by all members of the team.

On reaching the athlete, one performs an initial on-field triage while calming the athlete. Often this may be the athlete's first experience with a significant injury. Initially the athlete may be almost hysterical even with a minor injury. After the initial on-the-field triage, the athlete should be transported to the sidelines using husky teammates or a stretcher. A more thorough examination or series of examinations can then be performed prior to making a decision about the disposition of the injured player. Do not hesitate to remove protective gear (except the helmet in the case of suspected head or spinal injury) or transport the athlete to a warm private training room to obtain an adequate examination.

INJURY RECOGNITION AND EVALUATION: UPPER EXTREMITY

Lyle J. Micheli and Angela D. Smith

SHOULDER

Injuries to the shoulder can affect one or more of its three joints: the glenohumeral joint, the scapulothoracic joint, and the acromioclavicular joint. A blow to the shoulder may also cause injury to the sternoclavicular joint. Even if only one portion is injured initially, the other portions of the shoulder may become symptomatic because of secondary changes, such as muscle atrophy.

As with any other musculoskeletal injury, the physician needs to determine whether the problem was caused by an acute injury. The athlete may have been involved in activities that predisposed the joint to injury, such as the overhand maneuvers of pitching, serving, or swimming. The history should also include questions about possible injury to the neck because cervical spine injuries may cause pain in the shoulder region.

The physical examination of the shoulder begins with inspection of both the right and left shoulder girdles of the athlete, with the muscles relaxed and contracted. This provides important information regarding atrophy of specific muscle groups. The bones to be palpated include the glenoid rim, the humeral head, the clavicle, and the acromion. Specific soft tissue structures are all examined, including the sternoclavicular joint, the acromioclavicular joint, and the anterior and posterior capsules of the glenohumeral joint. The subacromial bursa and the bicipital tendon in its groove on the anterior surface of the humeral head should also be checked for tenderness.

The range of motion of the injured shoulder should then be compared to the range of motion of the uninjured side. Pitchers and racket sports players frequently have excessive external rotation of the dominant shoulder, with decreased internal rotation compared to the opposite side. The total range of rotation of the dominant shoulder should be at least equal to the nondominant side and may be slightly increased. While the range of motion of the shoulder is being tested, other specific tests can be performed. For the apprehension test, an athlete who has recurrent subluxation or dislocation of the shoulder will experience apprehension when the abducted shoulder is externally rotated. The impingement sign is elicited by moving the athlete's arm passively, taking the internally rotated shoulder forward into 90° of flexion, and then adducting the arm across the athlete's body. This causes pain when impingement is present. Some athletes, such as swimmers and pitchers, may have symptoms that are consistent with both subluxation and impingement.

The athlete's shoulder should then be tested for stability. With the athlete sitting in a relaxed position, the examiner attempts to subluxate the humeral head anteriorly or posteriorly within the glenoid fossa. Inferior instability can be demonstrated by a positive sulcus sign, obtained by pulling both the relaxed arms distally. If a depression is noted in the lateral portion of the shoulder, signifying that the upper portion of the glenoid becomes empty when the humeral head is pulled downwards, there is inferior instability. The physician can also check the athlete for anterior and posterior instability in the abducted position with the athlete lying supine, the shoulder at the edge of the table, and the shoulder abducted to 90°. With the scapula stabilized, the humeral head can then be forced anteriorly or posteriorly.

Fractures of the shoulder may involve the humeral head, proximal humerus, glenoid, or acromion. More proximally, the clavicle may fracture, or the acromioclavicular joint may separate. The diagnosis of a fracture or separation is often made from the physical examination. The exact location of a proximal humerus or glenoid fracture usually requires radiographs for determination, however, magnetic resonance imaging or computed tomographic scans may also be useful when a smaller lesion of the humeral head or glenoid is suspected.

Neurovascular structures may be damaged by any of these injuries. The brachial plexus lies immediately adjacent to the anterior and inferior shoulder structures. Injury to the shoulder may be accompanied by contusion or disruption of the plexus. One of the more common nerve injuries accompanying shoulder injuries is neurapraxia of the axillary nerve. If an athlete has sustained a shoulder dislocation, the sensation over the proximal lateral shoulder should be examined to ascertain the status of the axillary nerve.

Several cases of vascular injury about the shoulder have been reported. Often these were not noted initially, but came to the attention of a physician later, when pain or swelling of the entire upper limb became a problem. These late sequelae of shoulder injury are probably related to intimal tears of either arterial or venous vessels, followed by occlusion of the vessel.

Treatment of most acute shoulder injuries involves rest, using a sling or a sling and swathe. Some fractures of the humerus may require open reduction and internal fixation. When fractures of the glenoid cause recurrent instability of the shoulder, the fracture fragment may need to be replaced, either arthroscopically or by open reduction. Treatment of the acromioclavicular joint separation depends on the degree of the separation. For a grade 1A to C separation (notable for only tenderness over the joint, but not accompanied by radiographic changes), a simple sling and limitation of activities until pain free are usually sufficient. Grade 2 injuries are generally treated the same way. A Grade 3 injury signifies complete separation of all the acromioclavicular ligaments. Some physicians believe that this should be treated more aggressively, either by use of a confining brace or by surgery. Most orthopedists now do not treat these so aggressively unless the athlete is an elite throwing athlete. Even in that group, treatment is somewhat controversial.

Acute injuries of the soft tissues about the shoulder may involve the rotator cuff muscles, the bicipital tendon, or contusion of one of the muscles about the shoulder. In a very young person, rotator cuff tears and biceps tendons ruptures are extremely rare. In the older person, they are more common, but often muscle strengthening alone (rather than anatomic restoration) is sufficient to sustain the level of function of an older person. The initial role of the team physician is to diagnose the soft tissue injury appropriately. Once the diagnosis is firm, then appropriate therapy can begin, consisting primarily of ice, strengthening and flexibility exercises, and relative rest. In the event of a severe muscle contusion, therapy must proceed more gradually because overaggressive stretching and strengthening exercises may lead to myositis ossificans. The goals for an athlete with a soft tissue injury about the shoulder are to restore the full motion of the shoulder, including rotation and abduction, and to strengthen the entire shoulder girdle, including the stabilizers of the shoulder.

Most overuse injuries of the shoulder result from repetitive stresses of the soft tissues. Biceps tendinitis is generally a problem of the older athlete. Recurrent subluxation of the shoulder and impingement syndrome occur in both adolescents and older athletes. The most important treatment for overuse shoulder injuries is an appropriate strengthening program for the shoulder girdle muscles, generally beginning with exercises that allow the shoulder to remain in an adducted position.

ELBOW

In an acute elbow injury, as in all acute injuries, a careful history should be obtained. The mechanism of injury should be defined. Any neurologic abnormality, even temporary, should be identified.

The examination of the elbow requires thorough knowledge of the anatomy of the region. Often the diagnosis is made from the physical examination, by location of the area of maximal tenderness. This is especially true in very young children, whose radiographs may be difficult to interpret. The function of distal neurovascular structures should also be examined.

Radiographs may need to include oblique views as well as the usual anteroposterior and lateral views. In children, comparison views of the unaffected elbow may be very useful. If a posterior fat pad sign is seen, then significant injury should be suspected, even if no bony injury is immediately obvious on initial interpretation of the radiograph.

The specific location of fractures about the elbow is related to the age of the athlete. As the multiple ossification centers of the elbow develop, the fracture patterns change. For example, very young children almost never sustain epicondylar fractures, but rather suffer either condylar or supracondylar fractures of the distal humerus. Olecranon fractures occur infrequently in children, but are much more frequently seen in adolescents and adults. Fractures of the radial head and neck may occur at any age.

True dislocations of the elbow are usually obvious on initial physical examination very soon after the injury occurs. Swelling occurs rapidly in this injury, however, and the true diagnosis may be difficult to appreciate visually. When an elbow is dislocated, it is rarely appropriate to reduce the dislocation on the field, because fractures of either the distal humerus or the proximal radius or ulna may accompany the dislocation. If the circulation to the distal portion of the extremity is severely disrupted because of the dislocation, however, the physician may consider immediate reduction. In general, it is best to transport the athlete to an appropriate facility for radiographs, and then allow reduction of the elbow when the athlete is relaxed under sedation.

Sprains of the elbow ligaments are diagnosed by physical examination and by the lack of any fractures on radiographs. Athletes

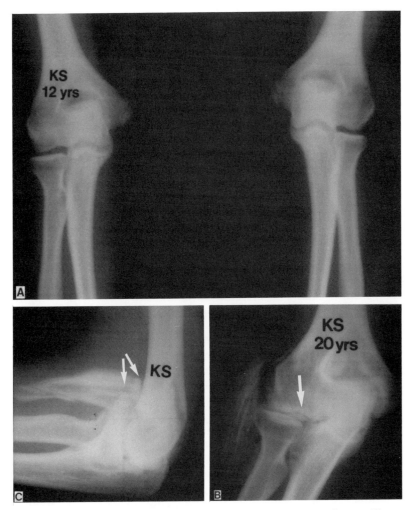

FIG. 16–1. *A*, This competitive swimmer's bouts of recurrent elbow stiffness responded to rest and physical therapy at age 12; radiographs were normal. *B* and *C*, at age 20, radiographs showed osteochondritis of the capitellum (arrow, *B*) and intra-articular loose bodies (arrows, *C*).

with elbow sprains may require brief periods of immobilization, either in a splint or a sling. As usual, the rehabilitation is extremely important.

Medial and lateral epicondylitis occurs among athletes whose elbows sustain repetitive rotary and angular stresses. The "tennis elbow" usually responds to rest, ice, and nonsteroidal anti-inflammatory agents. A below-elbow circumferential strap may be useful. "Little League elbow" is usually osteochondritis dissecans of the capitellum of the distal humerus. This overuse injury can lead to permanent disability if the child attempts to continue playing with a painful elbow. Figure 16–1 shows radiographs of a swimmer with elbow stiffness and subsequent osteochondritis.

WRIST AND HAND INJURIES

Fractures are the most common sports injuries to the wrist and hand in child and adolescent athletes. Among older athletes, however, overuse injuries occur more frequently. Fractures of the distal radius and ulna, as well as of the carpal and hand bones, should be splinted and then referred for orthopedic care. Sprains of the wrist occur less often; many injuries that are initially thought to be sprains are actually fractures or even dislocations. Any sport that requires frequent snapping motions of the wrist, particularly combined with rotation, may cause an overuse injury.

One of the most frequently missed wrist fractures is that of the scaphoid, or carpal navicular. These fractures are diagnosed by tenderness to palpation of the anatomic snuffbox between the extensor tendons of the thumb, just distal to the radius. Any athlete who has tenderness in this area should be treated as if the scaphoid is fractured, even if the fracture does not appear on the initial radiographs (Fig 16–2). Repeat films 10 to 14 days later may show the fracture line as bone resorption progresses. Appropriate immobilization for this fracture is a thumb spica. Another fracture frequently missed on routine plain radiographs is fracture of the hook of the hamate bone, on the ulnar side of the hand, just distal to the wrist crease. This injury is generally caused by repetitive microtrauma, such as golfing or batting. Rather than immobilizing the wrist in an attempt to heal this fracture, the usual recommendation is to excise the hook of the persistently painful fractured hamate.

Other overuse injuries related to repetitive impact include Kienböck's syndrome and stress fractures of the growth plates. Kienböck's syndrome (avascular necrosis of the lunate) may lead to collapse of the wrist. In a skeletally immature athlete such as an adolescent gymnast (Fig. 16–3), wrist pain may be caused by epiphysiolysis, or Salter I stress fracture, of the distal radius or ulna. The problem of epiphysiolysis is frequently difficult to solve even with splinting and rest and may end in growth arrest.

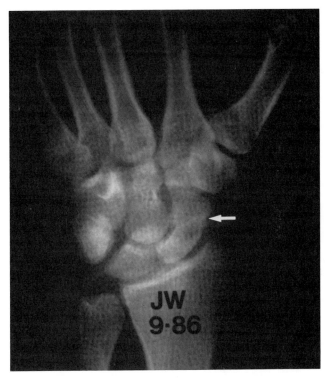

FIG. 16–2. A scaphoid fracture was suspected despite normal initial radiographs. The athlete removed his cast, however, to play basketball. He returned to his orthopedist 3 weeks later because of continued pain. Radiographs obtained in the new cast showed that the fracture had become displaced, and the athlete was referred for surgical treatment.

Athletes who must repetitively flex and extend their wrists and fingers through a large range of motion risk tendinitis. Numerous tendons traverse the wrist through narrow tunnels, and the great excursion of these tendons increases the likelihood of inflammation from overuse. Tenosynovitis and ganglion cysts of the wrist tend to occur in similar locations. With greater overuse of the wrist, the swelling related to both increases. Initial treatment for both conditions is relative rest, ice, and perhaps splinting. The injection of corticosteroid, followed by splinting, may be considered in certain cases. However, treatment for persistent tenosynovitis is surgical release of the constricting tendon sheath, where the persistently

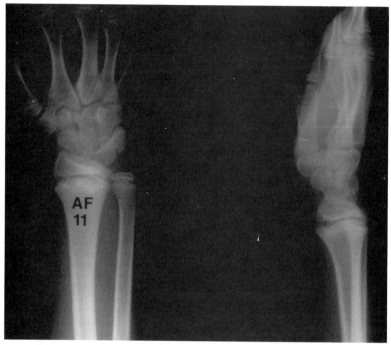

FIG. 16–3. A prepubertal gymnast with chronic wrist pain had widened, abnormal growth plates of the distal radius and ulna. Athletes who continue to overstress such an injured growth plate may permanently destroy the growth potential of the plate.

symptomatic ganglion cyst requires complete excision of the cyst for relief. It is clear from this discussion that anyone who treats wrist injuries needs an excellent knowledge of the anatomy of the region and of the types of injuries that are likely to occur.

Metacarpal fractures such as boxers' fractures are sustained fairly frequently by athletes who do not seek any medical attention for the hand injury. If the angulation is excessive, the resulting malunion can cause future disability. Therefore, orthopedic referral is recommended for a metacarpal fracture unless the fracture is nondisplaced and the team physician feels comfortable treating it with an appropriate splint. Similarly, finger fractures that appear to be minimally displaced and innocuous may undergo shortening and rotation, healing with an unacceptably deformed result. Therefore, significant injuries to the digits should be referred for care by appropriate fracture specialists. Treatment of volar plate injuries requires familiarity with digital anatomy, so the injured structures can be identified. Isolated volar plate injuries are usually treated by splinting the injured proximal interphalangeal joint in flexion. Once the tenderness and swelling have decreased, the digit is buddy taped to adjacent digits. In children and adolescents, special care must be taken for the finger tip crush injury, such as that resulting from a blow with a stick. In these types of injuries, the growth plate may be injured; often the nail bed is also violated, leading to permanent deformity of the nail unless the nail bed is repaired and the fracture is maintained in good position.

Overuse injuries of the digits are relatively rare. Occasionally fencers develop overuse strains of the intermetacarpal ligaments or of the sagittal bands that stabilize the extensor tendon at the level of the metacarpophalangeal joint. Inflammation of the ulnar digital nerve of the thumb occurs among bowlers.

RECOMMENDED READING

Dehaven KE: Throwing injuries of the elbow in athletes. *Orthop Clin North Am* 4:801–808, 1973.

DiStefano V: Functional anatomy and biomechanics of the shoulder joint. *Athletic Training* 12:141–144, 1977.

Emans JB: Upper extremity injuries in sports. In *Pediatric and Adolescent Sports Medicine*. Edited by LJ Micheli. Boston: Little, Brown, 1984, pp. 49–79.

Kalenak A, et al.: Athletic injuries of the hand. *Am Fam Physician* 14:136, 1976.

INJURY RECOGNITION AND EVALUATION: LOWER EXTREMITY

Lyle J. Micheli and Angela D. Smith

INJURIES TO THE PELVIS

The child's pelvis consists of membranous bones, connected through growth plates. Near puberty, the secondary ossification centers of the iliac crests, iliac spines, and ischial tuberosities appear. From the time of the secondary ossification centers' appearance until the time of final fusion with the underlying pelvic bones, the young athlete is at risk of sustaining either overuse or acute injuries to these structures. The secondary ossification centers are traction apophyses; large muscles tend to pull the secondary ossification center away from the underlying bone, through the weaker apophyseal growth plate.

An acute avulsion injury, usually of the anterior superior iliac spine, anterior inferior iliac spine, or ischial tuberosity, often is preceded by a period of time when the athlete notices a dull ache in the region. Pre-existing inflammation at the apophyseal region is probably associated with weakening of the growth plate itself. Chronic apophysitis may be relieved by increasing the flexibility of the muscles that attach to the apophysis, and by using ice application and nonsteroidal anti-inflammatory agents (NSAIDs). Some cases persist for years, however, until fusion of the growth plate is complete. The athlete who has significant chronic pain at the site of a pelvic apophysis should be cautioned against activities such as sudden sprints and high jumps. The rapid, forceful muscle contractions required for such maneuvers are frequently implicated in the actual avulsion of chronically painful apophyses (Fig. 17–1). If avulsion does occur, it is almost never necessary to return the avulsed portion to its anatomic position. Rest, ice, and nonweight bearing are the usual initial treatments. A thorough rehabilitation program is required before the athlete returns to full activity.

Adult athletes rarely develop injuries of the bony pelvis. Pubic

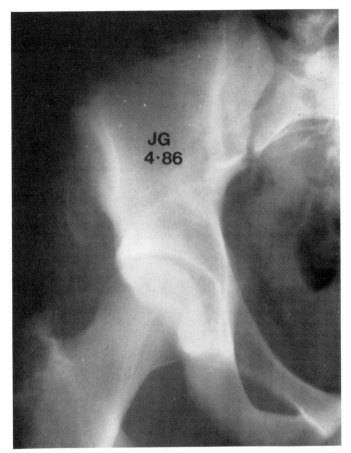

FIG. 17–1. Avulsion fracture of the anterior superior iliac spine occurred as this adolescent boy began to sprint.

ramus stress fractures have been reported in female runners, however, and stress reactions in the same area occasionally occur among elite soccer players.

INJURIES TO THE HIP

The hip joint is unique in several ways. Normally, the spherical femoral head fits into a deep bony socket, which is further deepened by a thick, fibrous rim. A true suction fit is obtained, so dislocation of the hip joint requires a great amount of force. Despite the bony and ligamentous restraints of the hip joint, it has a large range of motion.

Because the range of hip joint motion is constrained primarily by the muscles that cross it, injuries to these muscles can occur. The muscles that are strained frequently are the adductor muscles; others include the rectus femoris anteriorly and the hamstrings posteriorly. When an athlete strains any of the muscles about the hip, initial treatment consists of rest of the injured muscle, local ice application, and possibly NSAIDs. Rehabilitation of the injured muscle must be carried out carefully, without performing exercises that cause significant discomfort, to avoid the development of myositis ossificans. Early in the rehabilitation program, the team physician should recommend strengthening exercises for the uninjured muscles about the hip. These muscles must be prepared to help compensate for the injured muscle by taking on extra loads as the athlete begins to return to activity. Otherwise, an athlete frequently strains additional muscles adjacent to the muscle that was originally injured.

Tight muscles can cause two other injuries at the level of the proximal femur. In the skeletally immature athlete, a tight iliopsoas muscle may lead to avulsion of the secondary ossification center of the lesser trochanter. On the lateral side of the proximal femur, a tight tensor fasciae latae muscle (causing a tight iliotibial band) may cause bursitis at the greater trochanter. Treatment of both these injuries is symptomatic, consisting of rest and possibly systemic anti-inflammatory therapy. Occasionally, it is useful to inject the greater trochanteric bursa with corticosteroid when the inflammation is severe.

Many female athletes notice a "clunk" in the anterior hip with flexion and extension. This sometimes becomes a painful problem for ballet dancers. The most frequent cause of the sound and of the pain is the iliopsoas tendon snapping past a bony prominence in the anterior hip region. Many athletes simply need reassurance that the sound does not represent a serious abnormality that is likely to cause them problems. In ballet dancers and gymnasts, however, tendinitis or bursitis may develop. These patients are treated initially with anti-inflammatory therapy and physical therapy, and these conditions usually resolve without invasive treatment.

Injuries to the skeletal structures of the hip tend to be serious. Dislocation of the hip joint must be treated as an emergency. The longer the hip remains dislocated, the more likely avascular necrosis of the femoral head is to develop, resulting in severe degenerative joint disease at an early age. Reduction of a dislocated hip generally requires either sedation or anesthesia. Hip dislocation may be associated with fractures of the femoral head or femoral neck, so generally it is best to obtain radiographs before attempting reduction maneuvers.

Fractures may occur at several locations along the proximal femur. Stress fractures of the proximal femur generally are located in the femoral neck region. If radiographs of the hip show a fracture line that completely traverses the femoral neck, then internal fixation with hardware is indicated. If the plain x-rays show an incomplete fracture line with no displacement, and a radionuclide bone scan indicates stress reaction rather than a complete stress fracture, however, then rest may be indicated instead, possibly including a period of nonweight-bearing time on crutches.

In childhood and adolescence, two other pathologic entities must be considered when the athlete complains of either hip, groin, anteromedial thigh, or even knee pain. Legg-Calvé-Perthes disease (avascular necrosis of the femoral head) occurs most often in children between the ages of 6 and 10 years. These children should be referred for orthopedic care, which may consist of physical therapy, bracing, or surgery. A slipped capital femoral epiphysis is generally found in older children, most commonly between 11 and 14 years of age. Most of the affected children are obese, but approximately 10% of the affected children are slender. Slipped capital femoral epiphysis may present as chronic pain or may follow an acute event. As is seen with other growth plate injuries, an acute event may be superimposed on chronic pain. The treatment for this problem is usually surgical fixation of the slipped capital femoral epiphysis.

Hip, groin, and thigh pain may also be caused by a number of less-common disorders. An osteoid osteoma in the trochanteric region may be difficult to diagnose. A tip-off to this diagnosis is pain that is worse at night and is relieved by aspirin. Other neoplasms in this area are very rare. Infectious arthritis of the hip does not occur frequently in adulthood or adolescence, but may occur in young children. This must be differentiated from transient synovitis. Transient synovitis often follows a viral illness, the affected hip has minimal limitation of range of motion, and log rolling of the hip does not cause significant discomfort. It improves rapidly over a few days and generally resolves completely within 2 to 3 weeks. On the other hand, septic arthritis of the hip is a surgical emergency. An infected hip causes much more pain with any attempted motion of the hip and is generally accompanied by abnormal laboratory tests, such as white blood cell count and sedimentation rate. Finally, hip pain may be caused by hereditary syndromic or metabolic problems, or by a hereditary spondylarthropathy such as ankylosing spondylitis.

INJURIES TO THE THIGH

Probably the most frequent injury to the thigh is a contusion. Contusions may be very deep, very broad, and may lead to the accumulation of a large hematoma. First aid for a thigh contusion includes the application of ice and compressive wrap as soon as possible to prevent the hematoma formation. Physical therapy must proceed gradually and carefully to prevent the development of myositis ossificans. Strains of the quadriceps and hamstring muscles also occur with regularity. Their initial treatment and rehabilitation differ little from the treatment of thigh muscle contusion.

Acute fractures of the femoral shaft are relatively rare in athletics because so much force is required. If the patient has a pathologic lesion such as cyst in the femoral shaft, however, then the bone may break with minimal trauma. Stress fractures of the femoral shaft have also been reported. Following appropriate treatment of a femoral shaft fracture, it generally takes 6 to 12 months for the athlete to return to his or her former level of activity.

INJURIES ABOUT THE KNEE

The knee is a hinge joint, but with approximately 15° of rotation through the joint between the femur and tibia. The patella glides on the anterior and distal surfaces of the femur, depending on the degree of flexion of the knee. The patella functions to increase the amount of force that the quadriceps can apply to extend the knee. The four major ligaments and the two meniscal cartilages stabilize the tibiofemoral joint. The medial and lateral collateral ligaments provide stability against varus/valgus forces, and the cruciate ligaments restrain anterior and posterior translation and rotation. The menisci distribute the joint reaction force more equally throughout the joint and also increase the stability of the knee in both translation and rotation.

Injuries to the knee may involve any structure of the knee. The mechanism of injury provides many clues about the structures that might be injured. The injured area is frequently painful, usually accompanied by swelling or ecchymosis. A presumptive diagnosis can usually be made from the history and physical examination alone. This diagnosis may be confirmed by plain radiographs (which may also disclose unsuspected neoplasms or developmental anomalies), magnetic resonance imaging examination, or direct visual inspection by arthroscopy. Arthrograms are used much more rarely in the knee. Ultrasound examination may play a role in the diagnosis of a mass in the knee.

LIGAMENT INJURIES

Knee sprains are graded according to the standard systems for other sprains. In a grade 1 sprain, tenderness is felt over the ligament, but the ligament maintains its normal length. A ligament that has sustained a grade 2 sprain is still in continuity, but it has been stretched. In a grade 3 sprain, the ligament has completely ruptured, and there is no continuity of the fibers. In general, an athlete with a grade 1 or grade 2 sprain of a single knee ligament is able to walk off the field with minimal or no assistance. The swelling is moderate, and the swelling progresses slowly over many hours. The athlete with a grade 3 knee ligament tear frequently is unable to walk in the minutes following the injury. Swelling occurs quite rapidly, within 1 to 2 hours. A complete dislocation or an acute subluxation of the patella may present similarly, with the athlete unable to bear weight and the rapid occurrence of swelling.

Following inspection of the knee, the physical examination begins with the structures thought to be uninjured, based on the mechanism of injury and the sites of pain. The medial and lateral collateral ligaments are palpated along their entire length. If the injured athlete is not skeletally mature, then the palpation should continue along the distal femoral and proximal tibial growth plates to rule out fracture. The joint lines are also palpated to detect concurrent injury to the menisci. The medial and lateral patellar retinacula are also palpated to rule out acute patellar subluxation or dislocation.

Following palpation, stress tests of the ligaments are performed. Patellar mobility is checked to determine instability or apprehension. To test the collateral ligaments, valgus and varus stresses are applied with the knee in full extension and then in 30° of flexion. If varus or valgus instability is noted with the knee in full extension, then the posterior capsule is probably also disrupted. The status of the anterior cruciate ligament may be studied by many physical tests. One of the most sensitive is the Lachman test. In this test, the knee is flexed approximately 20°, and the examiner attempts to subluxate the tibia anteriorly on the femur. The amount of translation of the injured knee is compared with that of the uninjured knee. This is the least painful of the anterior cruciate ligament tests in an acutely injured knee.

Another frequently used anterior cruciate ligament stability test is the anterior drawer test. The injured knee is flexed to 90°, the ipsilateral foot is stabilized, and the examiner again attempts to translate the tibia anteriorly on the femur. The test is repeated with the tibia rotated medially and laterally on the femur. A test of the anterior cruciate ligament that usually indicates the likelihood of marked instability that will debilitate the athlete is the pivot shift test. For this test, the examiner holds the injured knee in full extension and applies medial rotation to the tibia and a gentle valgus stress to the proximal tibia. In this position, if the anterior cruciate ligament is deficient, the tibia will subluxate anteriorly on the distal femur. As these forces are maintained gently, and the knee is flexed slightly by the examiner, the tibiofemoral joint can be seen to jump slightly as it relocates.

Treatment of most isolated grade 1 or grade 2 ligament injuries is by protected mobilization. When the stability of the knee can be controlled effectively by an external device such as a brace, then the injured ligament heals more rapidly and more completely with motion through a protected arc than with complete immobilization in a cast. Special considerations must be made for the apparent grade 2 injury of the anterior cruciate ligament. If the structures that provide additional restraint to anterior translation of the tibia on the femur are intact, then a complete tear of the anterior cruciate ligament may seem to be only a grade 2 injury on physical examination. The injury is likely to be more severe than grade 2 if the mechanism of injury is suggestive, if the athlete heard a "pop," if the onset of swelling was rapid, and if there is a history (in a chronically injured knee) of giving way with pivoting. In these situations, an apparent grade 2 injury of the anterior cruciate ligament may require magnetic resonance imaging or arthroscopic examination for correct diagnosis.

Grade 3 collateral ligament injuries may require a brief period of immobilization followed by protected motion. Most surgeons now recommend nonoperative treatment for the isolated grade 3 medial collateral ligament injury, but some recommend operative treatment for the lateral collateral ligament injury, because a grade 3 lateral collateral ligament injury rarely occurs in isolation. Among athletes, most grade 3 anterior cruciate ligament tears should be reconstructed. Special considerations may need to be made, however, for the older athlete who does not wish to continue to play at his or her current level, or for the very young child athlete. For isolated grade 3 posterior cruciate ligament tears, nonoperative treatment is currently recommended by most orthopedic surgeons. If chronic instability becomes a problem, however, then reconstruction may be indicated. When two or more ligaments are injured, or when a meniscus or other secondary stabilizer is also injured, then surgical treatment may be required.

TORN MENISCUS

The medial and lateral menisci may be torn as isolated injuries, or they may be torn in conjunction with other injury to the knee. Meniscal injuries may result from twisting injuries, particularly when the knee is hyperflexed, or when the twisting injury sprains a ligament as well (Fig 17–2). When the tear is in a relatively avascular region of the meniscus, then swelling may be negligible and may occur over several days. Acute tears in the vascular region of the meniscus frequently lead to the rapid accumulation of a bloody effusion, however.

Torn menisci are generally diagnosed by tenderness to palpation, positive McMurray's test, imaging studies, or arthroscopy. Most of the meniscal stress tests involve moving the injured knee through

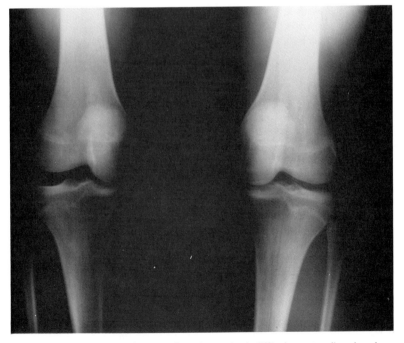

FIG. 17–2. This figure skater, who always had difficulty extending her knee fully, sustained a minor twisting injury to her flexed knee that caused severe pain and an effusion. These weight-bearing radiographs show a widened lateral compartment cartilage space and broad lateral tibial spine, indicative of a discoid lateral meniscus.

a range of motion while some rotation is placed on the tibiofemoral joint. This causes torn portions of the meniscus to be displaced into the joint or to be pinched between the tibia and femur.

Some very small tears may heal with nonoperative treatment. If the athlete wishes to continue sports with full participation, however, the size of the tear should be delineated by magnetic resonance imaging or arthroscopic examination. Larger meniscal tears may require surgical repair, or resection if they are nonrepairable.

Osteochondral fractures of the knee may occur with an acute dislocation of the patella. In a lateral patellar dislocation, the osteochondral fragment may arise from either the crest of the patella or from the lateral femoral condyle. Palpation of the articular surfaces of the femoral condyles occasionally reveals an area of tenderness. This may be also be indicative of osteochondritis dissecans of the lateral or medial femoral condyle. Acute fractures of osteochondral fragments should be repaired back to their underlying bed if possible, and excised if not.

In a young person, typically less than 20 years of age, a tibial eminence fracture may mimic an anterior cruciate ligament sprain. These fractures frequently occur from a hyperextension injury while the athlete is bicycling. The osteochondral fragment is usually elevated anteriorly with a posterior hinge, but it may become completely displaced. When the fragment is not completely displaced, closed reduction in extension is often successful. If the anterior horn of the medial meniscus is entrapped in the fracture, then arthroscopic or open reduction may be necessary. Completely displaced fractures almost always require fixation.

Intra-articular fractures of the distal femur or the proximal tibia, or growth plate fractures of these regions, need to be treated in such a way that anatomic reduction is obtained. This often requires surgical therapy.

OVERUSE INJURIES OF THE KNEE

Most overuse injuries of the knee involve the extensor mechanism of the knee: the quadriceps muscles, quadriceps tendon, patella, patellar tendon, and tibial tubercle. Overuse injuries of the knee are often associated with rotational or angular malalignments of the lower extremity (Fig. 17–3). Like other overuse injuries, they may be caused by a change in activity level, equipment, or training intensity. Sometimes overuse injuries follow inadequately rehabilitated acute injuries. They may be related to growth spurts in children and adolescents because of muscle flexibility deficits.

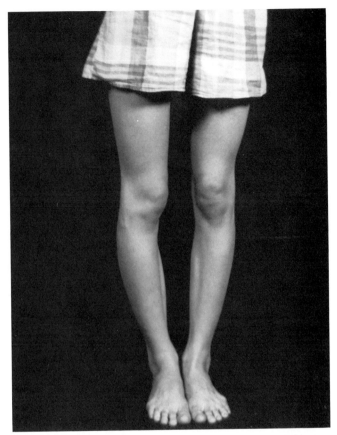

FIG. 17–3. Rotational and angular malalignment in an adolescent girl.

Among athletes of all ages, patellofemoral dysfunction is probably the most commonly noted overuse injury. It is frequently related to either malalignment, congenital malformation, or muscular imbalance. The symptoms are pain around and beneath the kneecap, occasionally radiating to the posterior aspect of the knee. The pain is made worse by climbing or descending stairs, by increasing activity, or by sitting for a long period of time with the knees flexed (movie theater sign). There may be occasional slight swelling.

Physical examination generally elicits tenderness about the patellofemoral joint, either the medial or lateral retinaculum or the patellofemoral joint itself. The crest of the patella can be used as an extension of the examiner's fingers to palpate the surfaces of the femoral sulcus for irregularity. Usually, atrophy of the quadriceps is noted, and the hamstrings are frequently tight.

Almost all cases of patellofemoral pain syndrome can be resolved by having the athlete perform straight leg raising exercises, or knee extensions only through the last few degrees of extension. (That is, in an arc of motion from 20° of flexion to 0° of flexion.) If the hamstrings or quadriceps are too inflexible, then stretching exercises are also done.

More distal along the extensor mechanism, traction problems may occur at either the inferior pole of the patella or at the tibial tubercle, or tendinitis of the patellar tendon itself may be present. Often these problems are seen in athletes who are jumpers. They are also found in athletes who have inflexible quadriceps muscles. Treatment includes rest and ice when symptomatic. If the quadriceps or hamstrings are tight, they should be stretched. Almost all athletes with pain in this region require strengthening exercises for the quadriceps, because those muscles atrophy in the presence of knee pain. Occasionally, inflammatory disorders of the patellar tendon and its attachments are recalcitrant to treatment. In these cases, NSAIDs and prolonged rest may be necessary. A few jumping athletes are forced to retire from a competitive level because of refractory patellar tendinitis.

Osteochondritis dissecans of the distal femoral condyles is often regarded as an overuse injury. It may well be developmental in nature, or it may be related to a single episode of acute macrotrauma. The osteochondral fragment that is separated from the underlying bone is often tender. This tenderness is best located when the athlete's knee is flexed approximately 90°. The radiograph that best shows the fragment is usually the tunnel view. Treatment must be individualized according to symptoms. If the osteochondritis dissecans is simply a serendipitous finding on a radiograph, then usually no treatment is necessary. If the athlete experiences recurrent effusions and pain, however, then limitation of activity, immobilization, or even surgical treatment may even be required.

Iliotibial band friction syndrome causes pain on the lateral aspect of the knee, as the tight iliotibial band slips back and forth against the prominent lateral femoral condyle. Athletes with bowlegs are more likely to develop this condition. Sometimes the anatomic malalignments can be improved by orthotic devices in the shoes. Stretching of the tensor fasciae latae muscle relieves the pressure. On the medial side of the knee, the pes anserinus bursa may become inflamed. The distal attachment of the medial hamstrings overlies this bursa, and it may become irritated. If ice and oral antiinflammatory medications are unsuccessful in relieving the pain of this bursitis, then the injection of a small amount of corticosteroid into the bursa itself usually brings rapid relief.

INJURIES TO THE LEG

Acute fractures of the tibia and fibula need to be referred for appropriate treatment. Stress fractures occur frequently among athletes, however, and these may be appropriately treated by the primary-care team physician. A stress fracture is usually caused by a rapid increase in activity level, intensity, or training time. It may also be associated with changes in technique or equipment. Occasionally, pre-existing tendinitis in the region eventually develops a stress reaction or a stress fracture. Once a stress fracture becomes established, there is usually point tenderness over the bone itself. The tenderness may be reproduced by three-point bending of the bone, without any pressure over the painful area itself. Radionuclide bone scans show a focal area of increased uptake of the isotope. Plain radiographs may show periosteal new bone formation or the presence of one or more fracture lines. When the findings are those of a stress reaction (meaning that the area of increased uptake on the bone scan is slightly diffuse, the area of increased uptake does not completely cross the bone, or plain radiographs show only periosteal reaction rather than a complete fracture line), then the athlete frequently can continue with competitive activities. The athlete should not perform any activities that make the pain worse, however. The level of activity needs to be changed so the rate of the healing process can exceed the rate of the injury process. For many athletes, that just means avoiding certain specific moves or skills. If the fracture line is complete, then it may be inappropriate for the athlete to continue full activities. At times, it is necessary to immobilize the fracture in a cast.

Two other conditions of the lower leg should be differentiated from stress fracture. These include tendinitis and compartment syndrome. Tendinitis may occur on the medial or lateral side of the leg. When it occurs on the medial side, it is sometimes considered part of the spectrum of posteromedial tibial stress syndrome. Pain along the medial border of the tibia and the posterior tibial tendon often responds rapidly to a program of strengthening the posterior tibial tendon. If the calf muscles are inflexible, then they should be stretched appropriately. Orthotic shoe inserts may be indicated. Pain over the peroneal muscles and musculotendinous junctions is less common. If the pain is mainly distal, then the diagnosis of tendinitis must be differentiated from that of subluxating peroneal tendons.

Compartment syndromes can occur in any of the compartments of the lower leg. These disorders most often affect the anterior compartment, but some athletes have problems with the deep posterior compartment. Athletes who seem to be the most prone to develop compartment syndromes are those who have significantly hypertrophied muscles, because their muscle tissue is more likely to be compressed by the overlying fascial envelope as the muscle increases in size during exercise. Rest, ice, and stretching may be useful for some patients with anterior compartment syndrome. Some athletes find relief with orthotics in their footwear; however, many athletes find it necessary to limit activity or to undergo fasciotomy to relieve symptoms.

Achilles tendinitis may cause posterior leg pain. When the tendon is inflamed in its tendinous portion, there is often also inflammation at the musculotendinous junction. Frequently an athlete reports a searing pain that shoots up the posterior aspect of the leg. This can usually be differentiated from posterior tibial nerve pain, because the athlete with Achilles tendinitis feels as if the pain begins distally and then shoots proximally. The usual anti-inflammatory measures and stretching generally solve the problem. Until the athlete has been able to relieve the inflammation by those measures, however, a lift in the shoe (or wearing of high heels), will help to relieve symptoms.

RECOMMENDED READING

Clancy WG: Runners' injuries. Part II: Evaluation and treatment of specific injuries. *Am J Sports Med* 8:287–289, 1980.

Desai ST, Patel MR, Micheli LJ, Silver JW, and Lidge RT: Osteochondritis dissecans of the patella. *J Bone Joint Surg* 69B:320–325, 1987.

Hunter LY and Funk FJ Jr (eds.): *Rehabilitation of the Injured Knee*. St. Louis, C. V. Mosby, 1984.

Micheli LJ: Injuries to the hip and pelvis. In *The Pediatric Athlete*. Edited by JA Sullivan and WA Grana. Park Ridge, IL: American Academy of Orthopaedic Surgeons, 1990, pp. 167–172.

Micheli LJ: Lower-extremity overuse injuries: overuse injuries in the recreational adult. In *The Exercising Adult*, 2nd Ed. Edited by RC Cantu. New York: Macmillan, 1987, pp. 275–285.

Micheli LJ: Lower extremity overuse injuries. *Acta Med Scand (Suppl.)* 711:171–177, 1986.

Nicholas JA (ed.): *Lower Extremity Injuries*. St. Louis: C. V. Mosby, 1985.

C H A P T E R   1 8

INJURY RECOGNITION AND EVALUATION: FOOT AND ANKLE

Elliott B. Hershman

The foot and ankle area are common locations for athletic injuries. They sustain a variety of traumatic events that necessitate immediate intervention to allow early and safe return to sports participation. Accurate diagnosis is imperative so appropriate treatment can be administered in the immediate postinjury period.

When evaluating an athlete with a foot or ankle problem, ascertain the mechanism of injury. For acute injuries, the athlete should describe the position and movement of the injured foot and ankle. The possibility of previous similar injuries should be explored. If the problem is chronic, then details regarding inciting activity, changes in activity level, and previous injuries must be elucidated. Any variation in training techniques or equipment should be documented. Early treatment of an overuse injury such as peroneal tendinitis is quite different from the initial treatment of an acute injury such as peroneal tendon dislocation.

The complete physical examination of the region includes observation of gait, lower extremity alignment, skin integrity, tender areas, neurovascular function, range of motion, joint stability, and motor strength. The examination must be tailored to the suspected type and severity of injury. If appropriate, watch the athlete walk both in athletic shoes and barefoot. Static weight-bearing evaluation should include analysis of the heel-to-leg alignment, integrity of the longitudinal arch, and forefoot alignment. Nonweight-bearing observation of the forefoot-midfoot-hindfoot alignment is important in the assessment of acute injuries such as tarsometatarsal injury. Subtalar dislocations and ankle fractures can usually be identified clinically by the positions of the foot and ankle structures.

The foot and ankle should be carefully palpated to locate areas of tenderness. Any ecchymosis or other skin lesion should be documented. Calluses or corns are also noted. Localized swelling, if present, aids in diagnosis. Neurovascular integrity must be documented so any changes following injury can be easily identified. The speed of capillary refill and the presence or absence of pulses are determined. Gentle range of motion evaluation can be performed if appropriate. The limits of ankle dorsiflexion/plantar flexion, subtalar inversion/eversion, forefoot abduction/adduction, and toe dorsiflexion/plantar flexion are measured. The integrity of the anterior and lateral ankle ligaments can be evaluated by the anterior drawer test. The heel is gently brought forward as the tibia is stabilized, and the degree of anterior motion is compared to the opposite side. The calcaneofibular ligament is tested by holding the ankle in neutral position and inverting the heel. Deltoid ligament stability may be determined by eversion of the heel.

The motor function is assessed by having the patient demonstrate all active movements of the foot and ankle. This includes plantar flexion and dorsiflexion of the ankle, inversion and eversion of the heel, and supination and pronation of the forefoot. Active toe motion is also evaluated. If indicated, strength should be assessed against resistance. If a maneuver causes pain, then the specific region of the pain should be noted.

In the setting of an acute injury, the athlete is treated with the basic first aid principles of RICE: rest, ice, compression, and elevation. Rest is started on the playing field—the acutely injured athlete should not bear weight on the injured extremity. Ice is applied to the area of injury for a 20-minute period, with an ice bag or in an ice water bath. For acute injuries, application of an ice bag may be preferred because the limb can also be elevated and compressed. Ice treatment can be continued intermittently with sufficient periods of warming between ice treatments to prevent frostbite or other cold injury. One rule of thumb is 20 minutes on and 40 minutes off, repeating as tolerated.

Compression is important in ankle and foot injuries. This can be combined with immobilization (rest) by judicious use of a variety of materials. A Jones compression bandage can be applied by wrapping cotton wadding (Webril) sequentially from distal to proximal around the injured foot and ankle. Elastic (Ace) wrap or adhesive elastic material (Coban) is then applied over the cotton material. If available, an inflatable splint, designed for use on the foot and ankle, can also be applied. These air splints should be avoided, however, if significant deformity or circulatory compromise exists. If necessary, plaster of Paris can also be used to immobilize the injured region, by adding a posterior splint or coaptation splint to the bulky compression dressing. This type of compression/immobilization is particularly useful in more severe injuries and is generally safer than an air splint.

Because the foot and ankle are the most dependent portions of the musculoskeletal system, elevation is critical in acute injuries to prevent further swelling and tissue trauma. The foot and ankle should be placed at a position at the level of, or above, the heart to facilitate venous return and reduce dependent edema.

Once first-aid treatment has been rendered, further diagnostic studies can be performed. Radiographs of the foot and ankle are indicated in most instances of athletic injury, and standard views (ankle—AP, lateral, mortise; foot—AP, lateral, oblique) should be obtained. Specialized views such as Harris heel views, sesamoid views, stress radiographs, and tomography can be useful in evaluating a wide variety of ankle and foot disorders, but their indications are for further evaluation of the injury following initial assessment.

Most ankle sprains can be treated by early protected mobilization, as long as care is taken to control edema. Athletes with ankle fractures should be referred for orthopedic care. Most acute metatarsal fractures are displaced little and are often treated simply with a hard-soled shoe. The Jones fracture of the proximal shaft of the fifth metatarsal (diaphyseal-metaphyseal junction) is notorious for nonunion, however. It is usually best treated by immobilizing the athlete in a below-knee cast, nonweight-bearing, for at least 6 weeks. Most toe fractures require minimal immobilization. In the skeletally immature athlete, however, a distal phalanx fracture is often accompanied by a nail bed injury, classifying it as an open fracture. Such fractures require appropriate emergency irrigation, nail bed repair, fracture reduction, and antibiotic therapy.

Early intervention and disposition of foot and ankle injuries can reduce morbidity and allow faster recovery from athletic injuries, so prompt attention to the injured ankle and foot is mandatory.

RECOMMENDED READING

Fetto JF: Anatomy and physical examination of the foot and ankle. In *The Lower Extremity and Spine in Sports Medicine*. Edited by JA Nicholas and EB Hershman. St. Louis, C. V. Mosby, 1986.

Lindenfeld TN: The differentiation and treatment of ankle sprains. *Orthopedics* 11:203, 1988.

McMaster WC: A literary review of ice therapy on injuries. *Am J Sports Med* 5:124, 1977.

Roy S and Irvin R: *Sports Medicine*. Englewood Cliffs, NJ: Prentice-Hall, 1981.

Vegso JJ: Nonoperative management of ankle injuries. In *Current Therapy in Sports Medicine*. Edited by J Torg, RP Welsh and RJ Shephard. Toronto: B. C. Decker, 1990.

POSTCOMPETITION PHASE

C H A P T E R   1 9

REHABILITATION

Stanley A. Herring and W. Ben Kibler

Participation in sports continues to grow both as organized team sports and as individual participation. Comcomitant with an increase in sporting activity is an increase in injury. Approximately 18 million Americans suffered sports-related injuries in 1988. Not surprisingly, collision sports have high injury rates. Over 100% of 5-year college football players sustain injuries significant enough to miss practice or play. Noncontact sports are not shielded from regular injury, however; 60 to 70% of runners, 40 to 50% of swimmers, and as many as 80 to 90% of serious triathletes report injuries at some point in their career. Not only is the incidence of injury high in almost all sports, but also frequently recurrent injury to the same body part or limb is reported very soon after return to activity. Flexibility, strength, biomechanical alignment, and other parameters have all been assessed as predictors of injury; however, the most consistent predictor of new injury is the history of a previous injury.

Most athletes sustain injury, and once injured they may very well be hurt again.

The remarkable frequency of injury in sports and the information that previous problems portend recurrent injury emphasize the essential role of rehabilitation. Proper rehabilitation may break the injury/reinjury cycle, particularly if a complete program addressing return to function, not just relief of symptoms, is instituted.

After an injury occurs and the tissue undergoes repair, symptoms abate. During this recovery process, however, changes in strength, flexibility, proprioception, endurance, and other factors occur. To decrease the chance of reinjury, rehabilitation must extend beyond relief of pain. The functional deficits that have developed must be corrected. Complete rehabilitation addresses return to function, not just relief of symptoms. The goals of such a rehabilitation plan can be stated as:

1. Establishment of an accurate diagnosis.
2. Minimalization of deleterious local effects of the acute injury.

191

3. Allowance for proper healing.
4. Maintenance of other components of athletic fitness.
5. Return to normal athletic function.

ESTABLISHMENT OF AN ACCURATE DIAGNOSIS

A precise diagnosis is essential in order to select and initiate a complete rehabilitation program. The anatomic injury and accompanying functional deficits must be identified. The diagnosis of "runner's knee" fails to provide anatomic localization (patello-femoral joint? meniscus? iliotibial band? pes bursa? etc.) or functional information (muscle inflexibility, strength deficits, strength imbalances, biomechanical malalignments, etc.). A vague diagnosis leads to a general rehabilitation plan often oriented toward symptomatic relief. If the injury is not accurately and completely diagnosed, rehabilitation will be incomplete.

MINIMALIZATION OF DELETERIOUS LOCAL EFFECTS OF THE ACUTE INJURY

Certainly rest is initially indicated after some injuries. Protracted immobilization and lack of weight bearing have deleterious effects on the injured structure and surrounding tissue, however. Biochemical and microscopic changes occur in cartilage and subchondral bone within days of immobilization, and these changes may be permanent by 8 weeks. The same type of changes occur in the bone-ligament complex. After 8 weeks of immobilization, up to 1 year is required to regain approximately 90% of the normal strength and stiffness of these structures. After 6 weeks of complete rest the joint capsule stiffens to a point where the torque necessary for movement increases up to 10 times normal. The muscle may lose as much as 20% of its strength per week of immobilization. Relative rest is appropriately employed in the initial stages of rehabilitation, but steps must be taken to avoid unnecessary deterioration of the injured and surrounding local structures. Relative rest can occur while still adhering to the next goal of rehabilitation, allowance for proper healing.

ALLOWANCE FOR PROPER HEALING

Appropriate controlled early motion will help to avoid the foregoing side effects of immobilization. In addition, recovery from injury may be promoted. The formation of adhesions between the healing tissues and adjacent structures may be decreased and proprioception better maintained with early motion. Early tensile loading stimulates collagen fiber growth and realignment, aiding recovery from injury. Physical modalities help allow for proper healing. Therapeutic cold acutely limits inflammation via its vasoconstrictive effect. It also is beneficial to decrease pain and spasm. The addition of compression and elevation to cold modality increases efficacy. Therapeutic electricity may also decrease pain, spasm, and swelling and can be helpful acutely after injury. Therapeutic heat, superficial or deep, should be utilized in cases of subacute or chronic injury. Physical modalities do not constitute a complete rehabilitation program. Many claims particularly concerning new applications of electrical and laser modalities are testimonial. A thorough understanding of the biophysics of physical modalities and utilization of these modalities by trained personnel help to ensure maximum benefit. Along with early motion and physical modalities medication helps to allow for proper healing. Nonsteroidal anti-inflammatory drugs (NSAIDs) limit the inflammatory response via their antiprostaglandin effect. They are also pain relievers. NSAIDs may have a role, particularly during the acute phase of injury, but the potential for side effects must be remembered. Oral corticosteroid use has been reported by some for acute musculoskeletal injury. Although this medication is a potent anti-inflammatory agent, few helpful data on efficacy are available and significant side effects can occur.

MAINTENANCE OF OTHER COMPONENTS OF ATHLETIC FITNESS

While measures are implemented to treat the local area of injuries, substitute exercises should be prescribed to maintain cardiovascular fitness and general body strength. The athlete can decrease total rehabilitation time by retaining general fitness during a period of recovery from an injury.

RETURN TO NORMAL ATHLETIC FUNCTION

Substitute activities for general fitness are essential during injury rehabilitation, but more specific fitness is needed before return to play. The athlete must be able to demonstrate sports-specific skills including proper aerobic and strength parameters for these skills before full rehabilitation has occurred.

Early intervention is paramount in injury rehabilitation to avoid the local and systemic effects of deconditioning. This intervention is most effective if closely monitored. Proper supervision ensures compliance, proper execution, and correct timing of rehabilitation measures. Athletic participation places significant demands on the musculoskeletal and cardiovascular systems, and rehabilitation to a proper level of performance requires input from trained personnel. This also allows for education of the player, coach, family, and others as to the severity of the injury and the necessity for complete treatment. Early intervention, close supervision, and education increase the chance that all the goals of rehabilitation will be met. This allows the player to obtain all the necessary criteria for return to play. These criteria are a reflection of the goals of rehabilitation and can be stated as:

1. Painless full range of motion.
2. Equivalent strength/power and flexibility of the injured/uninjured body part.
3. General body conditioning for strength and cardiovascular fitness.
4. Sports-specific skills.
5. Appropriate protective equipment.

These criteria can serve as a checklist for a rehabilitation program. If they are achieved, then a thorough function-based rehabilitation plan has been completed. The athlete can return to play with, one hopes, a decreased chance of reinjury and an increased opportunity for maximum performance.

RECOMMENDED READING

Cahill JG and Griffith EH: Effect of preseason conditioning on the incidence of severity of high school football knee injuries. *Am J Sports Med* 6:180, 1978.

Canale ST, Cantler ED Jr, et al.: A chronicle of injuries of an American intercollegiate football team. *Am J Sports Med* 9: 384, 1981.

Dahl S: Nonsteroidal anti-inflammatory agents: chemical pharmacology/adverse effects/usage guidelines. In *Therapeutic Controversies in the Rheumatologic Diseases.* Edited by R Williams and S Dahl. Orlando: Grune and Stratton, 1987.

Garrick JG and Regua RK: Injuries in high school sports. *Pediatrics* 61:465, 1978.

Herring SA: Rehabilitation of muscle injuries. *Med Sci Sports Exerc* 22:453, 1990.

Kellett J: Acute soft tissue injuries—a review of the literature. *Med Sci Sports Exerc* 18:489, 1986.

Kibler WB: Concepts in Exercise Rehabilitation of Athletic Injury. In *Sports Induced Inflammation.* Edited by W Ledbetter, J Buckwalter, and S Gordon. Park Ridge, IL: American Academy of Orthopedic Surgeons, 1990.

Leach RE: The prevention and rehabilitation of soft tissue injuries. *Int J Sports Med* 3:18–20, 1982.

Lehmann JF (ed.): *Therapeutic Heat and Cold*, 3rd Ed. Baltimore: Williams & Wilkins, 1982.

Lysens R, Steverlynck A, et al.: The predictability of sports injuries. *Sports Med 1*:6, 1984.

Paulos LE, Payne FC and Rosenberg TD: Rehabilitation after antrior cruciate ligament surgery. In *The Anterior Cruciate Deficient Knee.* Edited by D Jackson and D Drew. St. Louis: C. V. Mosby, 1987.

Pollock ML, Gettman LR, et al.: Effects of frequency and duration of training on attrition and incidence of injury. *Med Sci Sports 9*:31–36, 1977.

Prentice WE: *Therapeutic Modalities in Sports Medicine.* St. Louis: Times Mirror/Mosby College, 1986.

Renstrom P and Johnson RJ: Overuse injuries in sports. *Sports Med 2*:316–333, 1985.

Robey R and Blyth C: Athletic injuries: applications of epidemiologic methods. *JAMA 217*:184, 1971.

Roy S and Irvin R: *Sports Medicine: Prevention, Evaluation, Management and Rehabilitation.* Englewood Cliffs, NJ: Prentice-Hall, 1983.

Rutherford OM: Muscular coordination and strength training: implications for injury rehabilitation. *Sports Med 5*:196–202, 1988.

Scott SG: Current concepts in the rehabilitation of the injured athlete. *Mayo Clin Proc 59*:83–90, 1984.

Zarins B: Soft tissue injury and repair—biomechanical aspects. *Int J Sports Med (Suppl) 3*:9, 1982.

CRITERIA FOR RETURN TO COMPETITION AFTER MUSCULOSKELETAL INJURY

Douglas B. McKeag

The decision surrounding whether an athlete should return to play is the most important made by a community sports medicine network. The team physician heading that network must have the *final* decision on all return-to-play concerns. This question is so important because its answer sets the tone for how *all* injuries will be handled and how respected the entire network will become within the entire community. In the current medical-legal climate such decisions can have far-reaching ramifications. It is wise, then, to consider the entire process *proactively* and clearly indicate to all involved exactly what the process will be in determining the answer to the question, "Should the athlete return to play?"

Criteria for return to participation are also fundamental because they are truly a matter of sports mortality and morbidity. Every year several hundred athletes (recreational as well as competitive) die while participating in sports activities. Some die suddenly and unexpectedly, having had no reason (or at least inclination) to see a physician prior to their unfortunate demise. Some die after ignoring medical advice not to compete. Regrettably, some die after clearance has been obtained from medical personnel and team physicians, assuring them that all was well. Finally, some die after suffering traumatic or medical emergencies for which treatment was absent or insufficient. One hopes that most needless sports-related deaths have decreased as the sophistication of exercise screening techniques has increased.

Such screening represents a major *area of preventive impact* for any population of athletes in a sports medicine network system (Fig. 20–1). Injury and morbidity data clearly demonstrate a specific profile of injuries for a specific sport. With such information the team physician as head of the community sports medicine network should

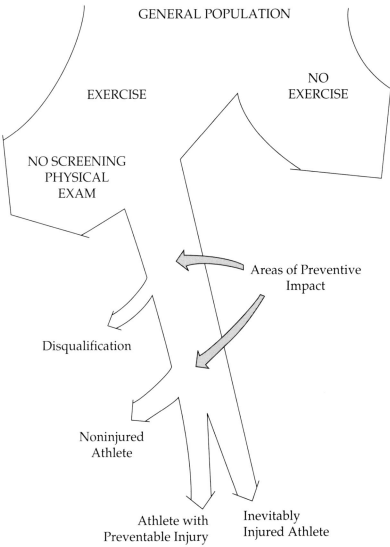

FIG. 20–1. Preventive sports schema in the community.

be able to prepare all personnel appropriately and to determine protocols for treating most of the common sports injuries encountered with that specific sport in that community. It is absolutely imperative that the team physician have a good understanding of the epidemiologic frequency of injury within the community sports system.

Consideration of sports medicine morbidity data is affected by many factors. First, the number of individuals participating in sports has grown steadily across the general population as well as within specific population groups. Children, always involved in sports, are now much more involved in *formal* sports programs. Sports opportunities for women have expanded well past traditional high school activities. Exercise has provided a potent rehabilitative technique and has increased the quality of life for the elderly and the handicapped. Many activities are currently available. In general, return-to-play guidelines have been discussed, but never regulated by any governing body. For the team physician, such subsequent inconsistency can be confusing and frustrating.

The community sports medicine schema also reveals a second area of preventive impact (Fig. 20–1). This area addresses conditions surrounding sports participation itself:

1. Environmental injuries (e.g., heat injury, playing conditions).
2. Training and conditioning techniques (e.g., inappropriate stretching, overconditioning).
3. Biomechanics (e.g., poor execution, improper coaching).
4. Equipment (e.g., poorly fitting or defective equipment).
5. Rules (e.g., spearing; nonuse of batting helmets).

Another way to prevent sports injuries is to adhere to return to competition principles regardless of where those principles need to be evoked. Studies inform us that 65 to 75% of all sports-related injuries occur in *practice* (Garnich, 1977). A well-organized, integrated system in which return-to-competition principles are practiced even in the absence of the team physician is a desired goal. Importantly, it represents the maturation of a sports medicine community network as well as the guiding philosophy behind that network. This guiding philosophy should reflect the values of the community and the physician. These values need to be communicated *before the fact* to all members of the network (colleagues, trainers, athletes), as well as to interested, involved parties (parents, coaches, administrators).

BASIC PRINCIPLES

The basic principles of "return to participation" relative to all situations, regardless of sport or level of competition, are relatively simple (McKeag, 1984). One must first look at the principal responsibility of the team physician as it relates to the coverage of the sports medicine network. *Before competition* the principal goal of the team physician is *injury prevention. During competition* the primary responsibility is *triage* of the acutely injured athlete. *After competition,* proper and appropriate rehabilitation is a prime concern.

BEFORE COMPETITION

Guidelines for return to play at this juncture are really guidelines for *beginning to play.* The following guidelines reflect the need for appropriate and thorough screening of potential athletes or returning athletes:

1. Cardiovascular and musculoskeletal health should be assessed and determined appropriate to withstand the rigors of the contemplated activity.
2. All pre-existing defects and conditions predisposing to injury should be uncovered and corrected where possible.
3. Level of competition should be appropriate to the level of physical and psychological maturation.

DURING COMPETITION

Reiterated here for the sake of emphasis, the primary responsibility of the team physician during competition is triage of the acutely injured athlete. The team physician must realize that return of an athlete to competition will subject that individual to the *same* forces that initially caused the injury. Guidelines for return to play during competition are as follows:

1. A definite diagnosis has been made.
2. The injury will not worsen with continued play.
3. The injury will allow the athlete to compete fairly and not render the athlete incapable of protecting him or herself.
4. The injury or its treatment will not increase risk to other athletes.

Within the context of these guidelines, other factors can and do come into play, affecting "sideline" philosophy concerning return to play. It should be given that any team physician allow an athlete every reasonable chance to resume play. Evaluation of acute athletic injuries on site should result in neither excessively conservative nor dangerously liberal conclusions. The athlete deserves a fair, unbiased medical decision concerning his or her opportunity to con-

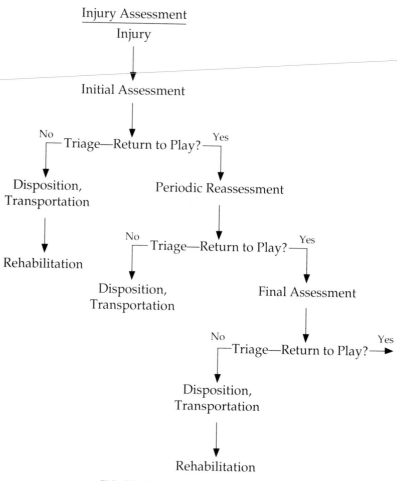

FIG. 20–2. Injury assessment pathway.

tinue playing. The team physician who can successfully and consistently follow the foregoing philosophy will find such decision-making rewarding and will be respected by both coach and athlete, for each will realize that the physician has done everything possible to allow the participant a chance to play. The team physician should have previous knowledge of the individual. Then, factors such as age, ability, situation, and knowledge of the patient's motivation can be factored in. The clinical expertise and experience of the team physician are other important factors. The ability to recognize early signs of sports-induced injury can only help when rendering decisions concerning return to play.

Clinical examination findings on the field will similarly affect the ultimate return-to-play decision. Immediate initial assessment, when possible, is extremely helpful. A quick evaluation will uncover signs and symptoms in the athlete prior to the onset of secondary reactions (e.g., pain, swelling, inflammation, decreased range of motion, guarding) that inhibit diagnosis. The concept of serial assessment should be applied during the course of competition. Injuries can and do evolve and change. It is important to consider a stepwise assessment of the injury. If the capacity of the athlete to return to competition is not clear, repeated assessments should be made (Fig. 20–2). Any injury that is in the process of evolution and in which signs and symptoms are changing should be watched; the athlete should be removed from play and not left alone. If the final decision on participation following injury is to allow return to play and the same injury recurs, then the athlete should be removed from play for the remainder of the contest. Subsequently, if the decision is to disqualify participation, periodic assessments should be continued and initial treatment begun.

Regarding disqualification from participation, some criteria have been outlined. What guidelines can be used when determining contest disqualification? To help the team physician, the following is a list of situations generally precluding further participation (Garnick, 1977):

1. Obvious swelling, with the possible exception of the digits.
2. Limited passive or active range of motion (compared to opposite side) unless artificially limited by a brace.
3. Significant pain within the normal range of motion.
4. Decreased strength through the normal range of motion.
5. Obvious uncontrolled significant bleeding.
6. Any injury the examiner cannot diagnose or properly manage.
7. Obvious loss of normal functions (e.g., sight, ability to move extremity).
8. Any injury that requires the athlete to have assistance getting off the field, mat or court.
9. Anytime an athlete says he or she is injured and cannot participate (regardless of what the examiner thinks of the injury).

Both the short- and long-term well-being of the athlete must always take precedence over the needs of the individual, team, coach, parents, and fans.

AFTER COMPETITION

Return-to-play principles for the completely rehabilitated athlete involve the following three general rules:

1. Full function of the injured/ill area/part has been restored.
2. For neurologic and musculoskeletal injuries, neuromuscular performance is not compromised.
3. The athlete is psychologically ready to return.

SIMPLE RETURN-TO-PLAY CRITERIA: FOR SPECIFIC INJURED AREAS

SHOULDER

May return to play if the athlete has:
1. Minimal pain.
2. Full range of motion.
3. Good resistance to involved muscle groups.
4. No deformity.
5. Normal neurovascular examination.

ELBOW

Return to play if the athlete has:
1. Minimal pain.
2. No deformity.
3. Stable joint.
4. Painless resistance to involved muscle groups.
5. Normal neurovascular examination.

WRIST

May return to play if the athlete has:
1. No pain over anatomic snuff box.
2. Good resistance to involved muscle groups.
3. Normal neurovascular examination.

FINGER AND THUMB

May return to play if:
1. Joints are stable.
2. Pain is minimal.
3. The initial injury is protected and splinted.
4. The athlete is able to function.

QUADRICEPS

The athlete with a quadriceps contusion may return to play if he or she has:
1. Symmetrically full range of motion of quadriceps.
2. Minimum tenderness to palpation.
3. Minimum pain with range of motion against resistance.
4. Functional progression (see knee).

HAMSTRING

The athlete with a hamstring strain may return to play if he or she has:
1. Symmetric flexibility of hamstrings.
2. Minimal tenderness to palpation.
3. Minimal pain on range of motion against resistance.
4. Functional progression (see knee).

KNEE

No return to play is allowed if the athlete has effusion, ligament instability, or a positive apprehension test. The athlete may return to play if the foregoing are not present, and if he or she is capable of functional progression as follows:
1. Hop on one foot.
2. Duck walk.
3. Run and cut at half speed, then full speed to right and left.
4. Run backward.
5. Run functional figure-of-eights.

If able to complete functional progression without problem or pain, then the athlete may return to play.

ANKLE

No return to play is allowed if moderate bony tenderness or any new instability is noted. The athlete may return to play if functional progression is passed as follows:

1. Run forward.
2. Run backward.
3. Hop.
4. Run and cut.
5. Run figure-of-eights at full speed without limp.

SUMMARY

Please realize that the team physician should always use all available information (e.g., previous knowledge of the patient, an initial examination done by appropriate personnel immediately after injury, etc.) to render a decision. Dogma has little place when dealing with the disposition of an injured athlete.

RECOMMENDED READING

Garrick JG: Sports medicine. *Pediatric Clin North Am* 24:737–747, 1977.
McKeag DB: On-site care of the injured youth. In *Practice in Pediatrics.* Edited by VC Kelley. Philadelphia: Harper & Row, 1984, pp. 4–9.

CRITERIA FOR RETURN TO COMPETITION AFTER HEAD OR CERVICAL SPINE INJURY

Robert C. Cantu

The head and spine are unique in that their contents are incapable of regeneration. The brain and spinal cord cannot regrow lost cells, as can the other organs of the body, and thus injury to these structures takes on a singular importance. Many parts of the body are today capable of being replaced, either by artificial hardware or transplanted parts. The list is long, with virtually every major joint (ankle, knee, hip, elbow, shoulder) and most organs capable of replacement. The head and spine are not included because their contents cannot be transplanted. The most complex and vital area of the body, the central nervous system housed in the skull and spine, is capable of recovery from injury to cells, but once a cell or cells have died, no replacement is possible.

RETURN-TO-PLAY CRITERIA AFTER A HEAD INJURY

Table 21–1 describes the classification of concussion by severity.

Grade 1. Following a first mild concussion, if the athlete has no symptoms at rest or exertion, return to the game may be permissible after a period of observation on the bench. Usually, though, and in every instance when symptoms are present, removal from the game is mandatory. All symptoms (e.g., headache, dizziness, impaired orientation, concentration, or memory) must have disappeared, first at rest and then during exertion (e.g., running wind sprints) before return to competition is considered.

A second mild concussion mandates removal from competition

205

TABLE 21–1. Severity of Concussion

Grade	Feature	Duration of Feature
Grade 1 (mild)	PTA	<30 minutes
	LOC	None
Grade 2 (moderate)	PTA	>30 minutes, <24 hours
	LOC	<5 minutes
Grade 3 (severe)	PTA	>24 hours
	LOC	>5 minutes

PTA, Post-traumatic amnesia; LOC, loss of consciousness.

for at least 2 weeks. Return is allowed only if the athlete is asymptomatic during rest and exertion for at least 1 week.

It is recommended that three grade 1 concussions terminate a player's season and that the athlete not engage in another contact sport for at least 3 months, and then only if asymptomatic at rest and exertion.

> **Grade 2.** Return to competition after a first moderate concussion may be as soon as 1 week after the athlete is asymptomatic at rest and exertion. Return to contact or play should be deferred for at least 1 month after a second grade 2 concussion, and termination of the season should be considered. Terminating the season for that player is mandated by three grade 2 concussions, as would any abnormality on computed tomographic or magnetic resonance scans consistent with brain contusion or other injury.

TABLE 21–2. Guidelines for Return after Concussion

	First Concussion	Second Concussion	Third Concussion
Grade 1 (mild)	May return to play if asymptomatic* for 1 week	Return to play in 2 weeks if asymptomatic at that time for 1 week	Terminate season; may return to play next season if asymptomatic
Grade 2 (moderate)	Return to play after asymptomatic for 1 week	Minimum of 1 month; may return to play then if asymptomatic for 1 week; consider terminating season	Terminate season; may return to play next season if asymptomatic
Grade 3 (severe)	Minimum of 1 month; may then return to play if asymptomatic for 1 week	Terminate season; may return to play next season if asymptomatic	

*Asymptomatic means no headache, dizziness, or impaired orientation, concentration, or memory during rest or exertion.

TABLE 21–3. **Number and Severity of Concussions in Single Season That Preclude Future Participation That Season**

Grade 1	Grade 2	Grade 3
3	2 or 3	1 or 2

Grade 3. One month is the minimal period the athlete should be held from contact after a first severe concussion. Return to play after 1 month is allowed only if the athlete is asymptomatic at rest and exertion for at least 1 week. If the athlete is asymptomatic, conditioning drills may be resumed prior to 1 month. A season is terminated by two grade 3 concussions but may be considered after a first. The above are summarized in Tables 21–2 and 21–3. Other conditions that contraindicate return to competition after a head injury are listed in Table 21–4.

RETURN-TO-PLAY CRITERIA AFTER CERVICAL SPINE INJURY

When an athlete is unconscious, assume that he or she has a neck injury in addition to a head injury. Maintain the airway, breathing, and circulation. Treat as a serious, life-threatening injury and follow the procedures as outlined in Chapters 12 and 13.

If the athlete is conscious, return to competition after a neck injury should not be permitted until the athlete is asymptomatic. Specifically the athlete must be free of all neck tenderness and spasm, neck and arm pain, numbness, paresthesias, and weakness not only at rest, but at full range of motion with and without axial compression.

Rockett has described further criteria used at Harvard University. Each athlete is measured to determine the maximum weight he or

TABLE 21–4. **Conditions That Contraindicate Contact Sports Competition After Head Injury**

Symptomatic neurologic or pain-producing abnormalities about the foramen magnum
Permanent central neurologic sequelae from head injury (e.g., organic dementia, homonymous hemianopsia)
Spontaneous subarachnoid hemorrhage from any cause
Presence of postconcussion syndrome

she can pull with the neck in flexion, extension, and to each side. This becomes the athlete's neck profile. Athletes with neck injuries are not allowed to return to competition until they are asymptomatic and can perform to the level of their neck profiles.

RECOMMENDED READING

Cantu RC: Guidelines for return to contact sports after a cerebral concussion. *Phys Sports Med* 14:75–83, 1986.

Cantu RC: Head and neck injuries in the young athlete. In *Sports Injuries in the Young Athlete*. Edited by LJ Micheli. Philadelphia: WB Saunders, 1988.

Cantu RC: Head injury in sports. In *Advances in Sports Medicine and Fitness*. Edited by WA Grana and JA Lombardo. Chicago: Year Book Medical Publishers, 1988.

Rockett FX: Injuries involving the head and neck: Clinical and anatomic aspects. In *Sports Injuries: The Unthwarted Epidemic*. Edited by PF Vinger and EF Hoerner. Littleton MA, PSG Publishing, 1981.

OVERTRAINING

W. Ben Kibler

Overtraining is the down side of athletic activity, competition, and conditioning. Overtraining is not one particular set of physical findings and one particular set of performance parameters, but is the result of overconditioning of the body, both psychologically and physically. Peak performance can be thought of as the top of a hill and conditioning is the process that brings the athlete to the top of the hill. The top of the hill is a very small area, however, and it does not take much to push the athlete over the top to the down side of the hill. The overtrained athlete will exhibit certain physical and psychological characteristics that will detract from performance and predispose him or her to injury, as well as make the athlete psychologically stale for further competition. Criteria for establishment of the diagnosis of overtraining are somewhat difficult because the manifestations may vary. Performance parameters associated with overtraining include alteration in mechanics of performing the athletic activity, increase in running or swimming times for the same distance, decrease in ability to achieve certain training goals, lack of motivation to continue workouts, and lack of goal planning in the workout sessions. It also includes irritability, inability to cooperate with teammates in practice and team situations, and decreased team play. Physical findings associated with overtraining include increased resting heart rate, easy fatiguability, insomnia, and metabolic changes including alterations in plasma cortisol level, thyroid hormone, and 24-hour epinephrine secretion.

The most common response of the athlete to the original manifestations of overtraining and decreased performance is to try to increase training intensity in order to restore performance levels to their previous peak. This training intensity, however, rebounds to increase the overtraining symptoms, thereby unleashing a vicious cycle of decreased performance in the face of increasing training intensity, which is both frustrating for the athlete and conducive to overload injuries.

Prompt recognition of the early symptoms of overtraining can lead to proper diagnosis and institution of treatment programs that will decrease the chances of psychological and physical overload. Because the symptoms of overtraining may vary, a high sense of awareness of the condition should be present in the sports medicine team. The use of periodization cycles can be very helpful in maintaining the volume of training below the level that would lead to overload and overtraining. The principles of periodization cycles should be carried out, both in terms of variety of activities with rest and recovery periods interspersed in the training cycles and in variation in the volume of the training as peak periods of athletic competition are approached. The athlete should not try to continue the preseason conditioning program while he or she is involved in in-season athletic competition. The volume of work will then be additive and will be too high for the individual to tolerate for a long period of time. Training programs should be addressed with these principles in mind so the training cycle will not be the source of the overtraining problem. Within the training and competition cycles, adequate time should be provided for rest and recovery cycles to allow physical and psychological recovery.

The diagnosis of an overtrained athlete is usually made retrospectively, and it is very important for the sports medicine professional to be involved in the athletic team so this diagnosis can be readily made in an early stage of development. A diagnosis is basically based on the clinical findings, which may be supplemented by laboratory evaluation of the plasma cortisol and urine excretion of epinephrine when needed. A major role should be played by proper education and warning of the athletes about the overtraining syndrome.

Competitive athletes usually tend to spend more time in training and intensity as competition progresses and they decrease the amount of rest and recovery that is necessary. The athlete should be warned of the possibility of overtraining, and it should be stressed that rest and recovery should be a normal component of any training program. In athletes who play several sports at the same time, the risks of overtraining should be stressed in these individuals as well. In high school and junior high school athletics, the athlete who is gifted usually plays several sports at a high-intensity level. This athlete is especially at risk of overtraining because of the constant demands for his or her athletic ability. The athlete in peak training should be shown how to take a resting heart rate in the morning so any abnormal elevation in heart rate can be noticed as an early warning sign of overtraining.

Overtraining can also be seen in athletes who are trying to condition too rapidly. The athlete who is in relatively poor shape and then tries to gain strength, aerobic endurance, or anaerobic endurance too rapidly will demonstrate the same type of overtraining symptoms. He or she will reach a plateau in improvement that is usually below the level of desired athletic conditioning. Further intensity of workouts will then lead to increased injury risk or no improvement in conditioning. Any athlete who presents with a series of nagging injuries that are usually the result of overload and that do not improve with normal therapy should be considered for the diagnosis of overtraining.

Treatment of overtraining syndrome is based on the diagnosis. After the diagnosis has been made, education of the athlete on the nature of the problem is the first course of treatment. Treatment should then be directed towards decreasing the volume of work and monitoring the relationship between the amount of conditioning and the amount of athletic activity. More rest intervals should be employed, and if the athlete is actually injured, physical therapy should be instituted to correct any muscle inflexibilities or weaknesses that result from the injury itself. The athlete should also be cautioned about trying to return to athletic competition at a high level immediately after the injury, because this will cause further problems with the injury itself and may result in recurrent overtraining symptoms. As with most athletic problems that are due to overload or overuse of the musculoskeletal system, the overtraining syndrome is best prevented rather than treated. A high index of suspicion, proper education of the athlete, and early institution of decreased intensity in volume of training are the best factors for keeping this from progressing to a frustrating situation for both the athlete and the sports medicine professional.

RECOMMENDED READING

Barron GL, Noakes TD, Levy W, Smith C and Millar RP: Hypothalmic dysfunction in overtrained athletes. *J Clin Endocrinol Metab* 60:803–806, 1985.

Kuipers H and Keizer HA: Overtraining in elite athletes. *Sports Med* 6:79–92, 1988.

Morgan WP, Brown DR, Raglin JS, O'Connor PJ and Ellickson KA: Psychological monitoring of overtraining and staleness. *Br J Sports Med* 21:107–114, 1987.

Ryan AJ, Brown RL, Frederick EC, Falsetti HL and Burke RE: Overtraining of athletes; a round table. *Phys Sportsmed* 11:93–110, 1983.

SPECIAL MEDICAL CONCERNS

GENDER SPECIFIC: FEMALE ATHLETE

Arthur J. Siegel

"Women cheerfully share with men hardships, toil and endurance, climb mountains, sail on the seas, face wind and rain and the chill gusts of winter, as unconcernedly as they once followed their quiet occupations by their firesides. . . . It is scarcely necessary nowadays to offer an apology for sport. . . . "

—Lady Greville, Equestrienne, 1894

"The only way to win at international cross-country races is to go out hard. Today my hard was harder than anyone else's."

—Lynn Jennings, Winner,
World Cross-country Championships,
Aix-les-Bains, France, March 24, 1990

The call to action by Lady Greville has been sounded by women of all ages and in all sports. As noted by Sally Fox in her documentary of the emancipation of the sporting woman, the female athlete in the 1990s has truly come of age. The ancient Greeks excluded women from competition and as spectators at the Olympic games. Women's footraces held to honor the goddess Hera were limited to 500 feet (160 meters), in contrast to inauguration of marathon competition (26.2 miles or 4200 meters) at the 1984 Olympic games in Los Angeles. The tough competitive spirit of Lynn Jennings after her recent victory in the world cross-country championships dramatically states the case that women's toughness in quest of the competitive edge is every bit equal to that of males of the species.

Women's sporting opportunities were severely limited from antiquity to the turn of the century, when women began to participate in active sports such as bicycling, field sports, court sports such as tennis, mountaineering, and skiing. Activities that involved strenuous exertion, physical contact, and intense competition remained reserved for men only until the last few decades. Lingering doubts

215

existed about the physiologic capability of women to undergo rigorous training and to survive the strain of competition on a scale with men. One has only to consult the daily press to appreciate the heights to which women have risen in sports performance in all areas. Items gleaned from three newspapers on Friday, March 16, 1990 relate the following remarkable sports accomplishments:

1. Harvard runner, Meredith Raney '90, breaks the 800-meter National Collegiate Athletic Association indoor track and field championship record in a time of 2:02:77 in Indianapolis. This shatters the earlier NCAA record, 2:09:9, set by Mary Decker in 1978 (*Harvard University Gazette 85*:1, March 16, 1990).
2. Leanne Fetter, a 20-year-old junior at the University of Texas, breaks the National Collegiate Athletic Association Women's 50-yard swimming record with a time of 21:92 seconds, breaking the 22-second barrier for the first time. (*New York Times* B27, Friday, March 16, 1990).
3. Lynn Jennings wins the Women's World Cross-country Championships, Aix-les-Bains, France (6 km) with a time of 19:21:2.
4. Susan Butcher wins her fourth victory in the 1158-mile Iditarod dog sled race across the Alaskan tundra (distance from Boston to Chicago) with a record time of 11 days, 1 hour, 53 minutes, and 23 seconds. She celebrated this fourth victory in 5 years in a tee shirt with the following slogan "Alaska, where men are men and women win the Iditarod."

These remarkable accomplishments establish women as equally capable as men in intensive high-performance sports at all extremes of strength, speed, and endurance.

The following sections detail some of the aspects of the evaluation and management of women athletes specific to their gender status. Health-care providers may be faced with various issues in providing comprehensive care to women who range from novice exercisers to elite athletes where special attention to women's needs may enhance enjoyment and performance in a variety of sports.

THE HUMAN (FEMALE) CONDITION: ONE BASIC PHYSIOLOGY OF EXERCISE

The connection between health and exercise pertains to the cardiovascular systems of women and of men equally. All evidence from exercise physiology suggests that the respiratory and cardiovascular systems of men and women are equally susceptible to incremental improvements in maximal oxygen uptake ($\dot{V}O_{2\ max}$) with endurance training. The physiologic benefits of exercise training pertain equally to women, who show an aerobic training effect at all ages and of proportional magnitude (incremental aerobic capacity by roughly 20%) to that in men.

Mounting numbers of epidemiologic studies also show that physical fitness confers protection from the common and chronic medical illnesses of later years such as coronary heart disease, hypertension, noninsulin-dependent diabetes mellitus, osteoporosis, obesity, and mental health problems. The recommendations of the United States Preventive Services Task Force for physical activity counseling for healthy adults as a primary preventive intervention endorse the efficacy of physical activity in disease prevention for these six major medical conditions. Although women enjoy a lesser incidence in severity of cardiovascular disease with aging, the benefits of physical fitness on hypertension and cardiovascular disease prevention apply equally to both sexes.

BODY COMPOSITION AND OPTIMAL HEALTH: ESTROGEN VERSUS ANDROGEN EFFECTS

Whereas men and women share a common exercise physiology, some differences in body composition are derived from the selective effects of estrogen versus androgen on peripheral tissues. Body composition parameters are under hormonal influence, which in turn affects skeletal or bone mass and lean body mass (muscle tissue, and reciprocally determines the percentage of body weight in fat tissue).

One differential model has been proposed by Behnke to reflect relative body composition differences for a "reference" or "idealized average" man and woman. These values show that the reference man is 4 inches taller and roughly 30 pounds heavier than the female, with half of this weight increment reflected in bone density and half in a larger muscle mass. "Reference" woman demonstrates a higher total percentage of body fat (15 to 17%) relative to males, with 10 to 12% derived from the differential hormonal effects.

These proportions are determined by the greater anabolic influence of steroids on bone muscle tissue with preferential and selective estrogen-regulated storage of peripheral adipose tissue. These signals in women are closely connected to central nervous system receptors, which in turn can guide gonadotropin and endocrine reproductive function. A minimum of 12% of "essential" fat as a proportion of total body weight is required to trigger and maintain the normal endocrine-reproductive cycle initiated at the hypothalamic level. A reduction in reserves of body energy stores below this level leads to menstrual dysfunction and irregularity, and ultimately to oligo- or amenorrhea.

The clinical evaluation in management of menstrual dysfunction in athletes requires a systematic approach to exclude causes other than the physiologic effects of athletic training programs on the menstrual cycle. Barring detection of underlying pathologic conditions, exercise-associated menstrual dysfunction can be put to the clinical test by reductions in training, which frequently allow adjustments in body composition in weight to trigger resumption of menses and/or ovulation. Therapy for hypoestrogenic amenorrhea can be tailored to clinical needs using cyclic estrogen/progesterone therapy, such as is available in oral contraceptive medication. The minimum estrogen dose shown to be effective in preventing bone loss is conveyed in these medications if they are administered together with calcium supplementation. Consultants can be introduced when special problems such as unusual delays in menarche or pro-ovulatory therapy need more in-depth assessment.

EXERCISE AND OSTEOPOROSIS

The beneficial effects of exercise on bone density depend on the adequacy of dietary calcium and the physiologic effects of estrogen on bone tissue. The efficacy of physical activity is perhaps most clear with respect to prevention and/or retardation of osteoporosis. Women may encounter obligatory loss of bone mass of up to 1% per year promoted by estrogen deficiency and inactivity. Multiple cross-sectional studies indicate that sports-active women have greater bone density than nonathletes. Several controlled intervention trials have suggested that postmenopausal women may retard bone loss by engaging in aerobic physical activity for 30 to 40 minutes up to 3 times per week. The critical role of estrogen in addition to activity is highlighted in studies of premenopausal women such as athletes encountering exercise-associated menstrual dysfunction. A combination of sports activity and estrogen support provides the most prudent preventive program for osteoporosis and its sequelae such as vertebral and perhaps hip fractures in later life. Calcium supplements may also be beneficial although perhaps not required when minimum calcium requirements are met by a balanced diet.

DOES RUNNING CAUSE OSTEOARTHRITIS?

High-impact-loading sports such as running expose joints to five to seven times the impact of body weight with each footfall. Concern has developed that participation in such stressful activities can lead to joint damage and chronic osteoarthritic changes. Research suggests that high-load-bearing exercise does not cause injury to normal weight-bearing joints, but that once injury occurs, heavy doses of exercise can hasten or accelerate damage in specifically injured joints. Intra-articular injuries in athletes should lead to reassessment of training and modification perhaps to different events to select nonimpact-loading exercise sparing specifically injured joints. Individuals with no evidence of joint injury or abnormality can exercise without fear that chronic exercise will lead to development of degenerative changes. Low-impact aerobic training and alternative exercises such as swimming or biking may be necessary once ankle, knee, or back injuries in runners are accompanied by objective signs of intra-articular injury leading to destructive changes.

SPORTS NUTRITION FOR WOMEN

Previous sections of this chapter have discussed specific needs for calcium requirements in women to maintain strong bones even with requisite estrogen availability. Sports-active women should consume at least 1000 mg dietary calcium daily to maintain calcium balance, whereas 1500 mg per day, with the addition of supplements to the diet, should be used if calcium intake is inadequate.

Evaluation of anemia in female athletes may be difficult because of the many factors that can influence iron balance in such individuals. The expanded blood volume of sports-active individuals may lead to a dilutional effect with an apparent decrease in hemoglobin suggesting a diagnosis of pseudoanemia. Recent reports, however, show that up to 80% of female athletes are iron deficient and warrant supplementation. Female athletes are especially vulnerable to iron deficiency from losses in sweat as well as during menstruation. The importance of iron in energy metabolism is clear because a low serum ferritin level can result in a decrease in exercise tolerance even in the absence of frank anemia. The conclusion is that female athletes with hemoglobin levels in the low-normal range may benefit from daily iron supplementation to ensure adequate reserves. When selected athletes encounter either gastrointestinal (GI) bleeding or hematuria during training, a medical workup should be undertaken to exclude a specific pathologic process in the lower GI tract or bladder by appropriate endoscopic examination. After an appropriate negative workup, such individuals can be monitored clinically and maintained on iron replacement to prevent cumulative or recurrent losses. Daily iron supplementation such as ferrous sulfate, 325 mg, may be ingested daily or even three times a week for maintaining adequate stores. That supplements of iron, calcium, and estrogen may specifically be required in women differentiates their needs nutritionally from male athletes. High carbohydrate requirements for prolonged aerobic activity such as cross-country skiing, long distance running, or swimming, are identical to muscle requirements for peak performance seen in men. Prior theories that women may have a selective benefit for prolonged strenuous exercise conferred by the higher percentage of body fat derived from estrogens miss the point. Women's skeletal muscle is susceptible to carbohydrate depletion and subsequent rhabdomyolsis from substrate depletion, as are muscles of men. Carbohydrate loading, adequate hydration during sports, and nutritional repletion during prolonged strenuous exercise are requirements common to both men and women.

PREGNANCY

The physiologic adaptations of healthy women during pregnancy permit ongoing safe sports participation not only without risk but also with possible benefits for well-being and fetal outcome. In contrast to the clear benefits of aerobic conditioning, caution should pertain during pregnancy to limit participation in sports involving direct trauma. In addition, the intensified hormonal changes of pregnancy may promote more rapid fluid loss and possibly increase the risk of heat-related injury. Pregnant women are advised to continue customary and usual aerobic sports but to avoid extremes of intensity and exertion. Studies have shown that regular aerobic exercise has no deleterious effects on pregnant women. Exercise that women have been conditioned to do before they become pregnant is fine for them to continue during pregnancy. Undertaking a new strenuous exercise program during pregnancy is inadvisable, however. In the past, many have been concerned about a "fetal steal syndrome" or shunting of oxygenated blood away from the placenta. Evidence to date does not suggest that this occurs. Indeed, many women have exercised right up to and through the third trimester without ill effects.

Some sporting activities such as scuba diving have definitive dangers. Accidental hypoxemia from equipment failure or accident may result in injury to mother and/or fetus. Judgment should be used to refrain from such activity until after pregnancy.

Exercise in the postpartum period offers physiologic and psychological benefits to women. Many female athletes including champions at speed skating, diving, and running have achieved their best performance levels in the years after childbirth. As a guideline, women may resume a characteristic sports activity such as swimming or cycling within 2 weeks of uncomplicated postpartum recovery. Incremental training should follow the guidelines of the American College of Obstetricians and Gynecologists for conservative exercise targets to allow reconditioning without injury or overuse sports-related complications. The lactating female has increased requirements for basic vitamins and nutrients during breast-feeding. Exercise should be tailored to take into account these additional nutritional needs and should be within comfortable limits to avoid acute overexertion or development of chronic fatigue.

EATING DISORDERS

Most athletes regard thinness as desirable in sports performance and share the notion with many coaches that "thinner is better, faster, more desirable." A female athlete's attention to training, caloric intake, and body composition may sometimes become obsessional, and thinness rather than training and sports performance may become the goal of exercise. Training may become so obsessional that no amount of exercise is enough, just as no weight on the scale can be too low.

Physicians must do a careful clinical review of dietary intake and exercise patterns in combination with physical findings related to muscle mass on clinical examination. Patterns of restrictive eating and intensive exercise may give rise to progressive weight loss below a physiologically appropriate weight range and into progressive loss of lean body mass. Patients may combine restrictive anorexia with severe exercise bulimia through a self-imposed rigid program of dietary restriction and intense physical activity. Progressive weight loss leads to menstrual dysfunction, amenorrhea, osteoporosis, and stress or fractures in patients who may perceive their problem to be an inability to maintain their training or exercise level. A sensitivity to the risk factor of endurance sports participation for development of an eating disorder deserves attention by athletes, coaches, and clinicians alike. Intensive training becomes a risk factor for development of an eating disorder only when coupled with predisposing psychological factors (e.g., low self-esteem). The astute clinician may be able to identify when sports participation moves from a health-promoting and wellness-oriented goal into a self-destructive illness pattern.

SUMMARY

Sports can offer women the same benefits as men in terms of preserving function, retarding illnesses of middle and later life, and enhancing enjoyment of life at all stages through regular fitness and sports participation. Differences between men and women relate to physiologic effects, estrogen versus androgen, differences that are far more a cause for celebration than for concern.

RECOMMENDED READING

Fox S: *The Sporting Woman: A Book of Days.* Boston: Bullfinch Press, Little, Brown, 1989.

Means RH and Siegel AJ: Women and sports. In *Sports Medicine in Primary Care.* Edited by RC Cantu. Lexington, MA: Collarmore Press, DC Health, 1982, pp. 91–101.

Hale RW: Factors important to women engaged in vigorous physical activity. In *Sports Medicine.* Edited by RH Strauss. Philadelphia: W. B. Saunders, 1984, pp. 250–269.

Haycock CE: *Sports Medicine for the Athletic Female.* Oradell, NJ: Medical Economics, 1980.

Siegel AJ: Medical conditions arising during sports. In *Women and Exercise: Physiology and Sports Medicine.* Edited by M Shangold and G Mirkin. Philadelphia: F. A. Davis, 1988, pp. 220–238.

Siegel AJ: Understanding abnromal lab values in the female athlete. *Contemp OB/GYN* 25:73–84, 1985.

THE MEDICAL BAG

E. Lee Rice

The team physician should ensure that proper equipment is present for handling on-the-field injuries as well as routine medical problems during travel. Planning and preparing are the keys to appropriate handling of athletic injuries. The physician should be prepared for every foreseeable occurrence, regardless of severity. It is unwise to count on necessary medical equipment or supplies being provided by others. Therefore, the constant presence of a well-stocked medical kit containing the supplies necessary to allow the team physician to properly care for emergencies is imperative.

The contents of the bag may vary depending on whether other sources of equipment are also available. In some cases, the trainer is responsible for certain types of field emergency or CPR equipment. Ambulances are often required to be present at certain types of events and generally are well equipped with CPR equipment. Regardless of how the equipment is organized, the team physician should have the ultimate responsibility of ensuring that all essential medical needs are provided for and that all equipment and supplies are present prior to the start of competition.

Listed here are what are considered to be minimum requirements for medical equipment and supplies. Each physician probably has his or her own preferences regarding some items, and the lists will need to be modified to reflect individual choices and practice methods. Requirements may also vary depending on whether the contest is "at home," "away," or "overseas."

After each event or trip, the supplies need to be restocked and updated and modifications made based on need. All too often, the equipment starts out the season in splendid form but by the end of the year the neglected bag suffers from disarray, empty containers, dead batteries, and used-up supplies. A consistent method of restocking with reference to a master list is advisable to prevent the foregoing scenario. It is often helpful to keep a notepad in the bag on which all opened or used supplies are recorded. Then it is a simple task to refer to this record when restocking the bag.

PHYSICIAN'S BAG

Air cast-type ankle brace
Alcohol and povidone-iodine
    (Betadine) swabs
Bandages, including
   elastic (Ace, Elastoplast)
   plastic strip (Band Aids)
Batteries and bulbs (extra)
Benzoin
Blood pressure cuff
Cotton swabs
Eye kit with eye chart
Finger splints
Forceps
Gauze
Hemostats
Ice
Irrigation kit
Measuring tape
Nasal packing
Notepad/Dictaphone
Otoscope/ophthalmoscope
Penlight
Prep razor
Prescription pad
Prewrap
Reflex hammer
Scalpel
Scissors
Scrub brushes
Slings
Splints
Sterile gloves
Sterile water
Steri-strips
Stethoscope
Suture kit
  disposable sutures
  nonabsorbable suture (4–0,
   5–0, 6–0)

Syringes and needles
Tape
Thermometer

FIELD EQUIPMENT

Air splints
Blankets
Bolt cutters
Cervical collar (rigid)
Crutches
Sandbags
Spine board
Stretcher

CPR EQUIPMENT

Airway/endotracheal tube
Bulb suction syringe
Cardiac monitor/defibrillator*
Catheters, 14- and 18-gauge
Crash cart with cardiac and
    anaphylactic medications
Esophageal obturator
Intravenous setups (5%
        dextrose in water and
        lactated Ringer's solution)
Laryngoscope
Oral and nasal oxygen with
    mask

MEDICATIONS

Analgesics
  Aspirin or acetaminophen
  Codeine or synthetic
    analgesic tablets
  Morphine sulfate or
    meperidine injectable

---

* Cardiac monitor/defibrillator, although not mandatory for basic CPR, is required for advanced cardiac life support (usually supplied by the ambulance).

Antibiotics
   Cephalosporin
   Erythromycin
   Quinalone (optional)
   Tetracycline
Cardiac Medications
   Atropine
   Beta blocker
   Bretylium
   Digoxin
   Dopamine
   Epinephrine
   Furosemide
   Lidocaine
   Nifedipine
   Nitroglycerine
   Sodium bicarbonate
   Verapamil
Dermatologics
   Antibiotic ointment
   Antifungal cream
   Insect repellant
   Silver sulfadiazine cream
   Steroid cream
   Sun screen
   Sunburn cream
   Zinc oxide powder
EENT Medications
   Antibiotic ophthalmic drops
   Pseudoephedrine
   Scopolamine patch
   Tetracaine ophthalmic drops
Gastrointestinal Medications
   Antacids
   Antidiarrheic (Lomotil)
   Antiperistaltic (Loperamide)
   Antispasmodic (Donnatol)
   Bismuth subsalicylate
      (Pepto-Bismol)
   Prochlorperazine
Miscellaneous
   Albuterol inhaler
   Aminophylline
   Anaphylaxis kit

Antimalarial/antiparasitic
  medications
Clove oil
Dental packing
Diazepam, injectable
Diphenhydramine
Insulin, regular, human
Ipecac
Naloxone
Xylocaine

C H A P T E R 2 5

THE CHILD ATHLETE

Lyle J. Micheli

The physician dealing with young athletes, in particular children still undergoing changes associated with growth and development, must be very cognizant of the physical and psychological implications of growth in association with sports activities. Growth and development in the child have a number of variables that affect the rest of the development of motor skills, height, and muscle mass in the child. These variables include genetic, nutritional, neurologic, and psychosocial determinants.

The basic chronology of growth entails a slow, progressive decrease in the rate of growth beginning in infancy and continuing through the cessation of growth in late adolescence. During this time the child may have brief, transient periods of increase in growth, and in every child a period of increased growth or increase in peak height velocity occurs in the early stages of adolescence. This so-called adolescent growth spurt and the less-dramatic growth spurts occurring during the prepubescent period in the child are periods of increased risk of injury to muscle-tendons, bones, and physes.

The special risks of sports injury to the child, as opposed to the fully mature adolescent or adult, are related to the presence of growth cartilage in the child, the growth process itself, and the variable levels of coaching skills in this age group.

Sports injuries in the child, as in the adult, may result from two different mechanisms: (1) single-impact macrotrauma, as in a direct blow or twist; or (2) repetitive microtrauma, as in repetitive impact of the foot against the ground in running or repetitive circumduction of the shoulder during throwing or swimming. Although previously extremely rare in the child and early adolescent, overuse injuries now account for the majority of problems encountered in these young athletes as a result of the repetitive training inherent in organized sport. Although overuse injuries were once thought to be associated with a component of degeneration of the tissue, partic-

228

ularly in the adult recreational athlete, it has now become evident that children may be at special risk for overuse injury because of the presence of the growth cartilage and the phenomenon of the growth process, as noted previously.

Recent studies of sports injuries in children suggest that children differ from adults in their susceptibility to both macrotrauma and microtrauma injuries in the sports setting.

MACROTRAUMA

Macrotrauma results from a single application of a major force and the subsequent breakdown of the body's tissues. The different patterns of injuries sustained by children and early adolescents as opposed to adults can be explained by the fundamental differences in skeletal anatomy, physiology, and biomechanics. Pediatric bone is more porous than adult bone and fails in both compression and tension. "Greenstick" fractures are an example of this increased elasticity of the pediatric bone as compared to the adult.

Macrotrauma applied to the joint of the child may actually disrupt ligamentous tissue in the prepubescent, whereas in the adolescent involved in a significant growth spurt, frank disruption through the physis may occur. This potential for physeal disruption is also joint specific and plate specific; thus, injuries to the distal femoral epiphysis seem to be associated with a much greater incidence of growth arrest.

The child's enhanced ability to heal rapidly and with significant remodeling may change the time course of immobilization requirements in the child, but it also may contribute to physeal overgrowth because of the increased vascularity from bony healing with resultant limb-length discrepancy.

MICROTRAUMA

Overuse injuries in the child, the result of repetitive microtrauma, were essentially unknown before the advent of repetitive training techniques in sports. Very rarely are overuse injuries encountered in the physical education or free-play situation. As a result, the physician dealing with sports injured children has a tremendous range of "new" overuse injuries, including "jumper's knee" in the adolescent basketball player, "Little League shoulder,"

"Little League elbow," and "swimmer's shoulder," as well as "swimmer's knee."

As in the general discussion of overuse injuries in Chapter 30, the physician responsible for the diagnosis and management of overuse injuries in the young athlete must be very aware of the risk factors inherent in any overuse injury. These, of course, include training error, muscle-tendon imbalance, anatomic malalignment, footwear, playing surface, and associated disease state, as well as nutritional factors and cultural deconditioning. In addition, however, growth is a definite associated risk factor for overuse injuries in the child.

The adolescent at the time of the adolescent growth spurt has both host factors and environmental factors contributing to potential for injury. The relative weakening of the bone, physes, and the relative tightness of the muscle-tendon units spanning these rapidly growing bones are additional risk factors. During periods of rapid growth spurt, the relative intensity and duration of training regimens for the young athlete should be decreased. In addition, at the onset of pain, a presumption of overuse injuries should be readily made in the child involved in rapid growth spurt and doing training. Do not label these "growing pains."

Growth cartilage is located at three sites in the child: the physis, the joint surface, and the apophysis. Macrotrauma and overuse injuries have now been demonstrated to occur at all three sites in children. As noted previously, the possibility of a physeal injury should be suspected in any joint injury in the child who still has open growth plates and, in particular, in the adolescent undergoing a growth spurt. Similarly, with the question of acute joint disruption, one should always bear in mind the possibility of articular cartilage injury, although this is relatively rare in the child who still has open growth plates. Much more commonly, an acute macrotrauma to the joint surface in the child will involve the underlying bone, because the relatively more elastic articular cartilage in the child transmits force to the bone and a bony lesion and secondary aseptic necrosis of the bone may occur, ultimately manifesting itself as osteochondritis dissecans. Finally, particularly in children with excessive tightness, one may see frank avulsions of the apophyses in the child that would normally manifest as muscle-tendon strains in the adult.

Similarly, we have now identified in sports-active children evidence of repetitive microtrauma to all three sites of growth cartilage. Reports of partial or sometimes complete physeal arrest at the wrist and, in particular, the distal radial epiphysis in young gymnasts confirm the possibility of this injury's occurring from repetitive impact. Although not yet documented for repetitive impact to the lower extremities, there must be putative concern for similar mechanisms of injury to the physes of the lower extremities of the child involved in excessive running. Overuse injuries or repetitive microtrauma to the joint surface in the child manifest themselves as osteochondritis dissecans. Once thought to be an osteochondromatosis of idiopathic origin, growing evidence now suggests that this is the result of repetitive trauma to the child. These injuries can occur, of course, at the knee, talus, hip, and elbow. Finally, repetitive microtrauma at the apophysis can result in such conditions as Osgood-Schlatter disease at the knee or Sever's apophysitis at the heel.

SPECIAL CONCERNS—CHILDHOOD INJURIES

HEAD AND NECK INJURIES

Cervical spine injuries in the child require special expertise in assessment and management. Radiographic interpretation of the child's cervical spine may be more difficult than in the adult. In particular, because of apparent increase in elasticity of the child's cervical spine, false-positive evidence of instability of the cervical spine on the flexion extension views, in particular at the C2 to C3 level, must always be borne in mind. In addition, severe disruption of the child's spine may occur without telltale fractures of the margins of the vertebral elements. Thus, complete displacement of the child's cervical spine, sometimes with only transient paralysis, may occur, the end result being a total segmental instability of the child that is not evident by plain radiographic assessment or neurologic assessment at the time of evaluation. Newer techniques of magnetic resonance imaging (MRI) and bone scans can be particularly helpful in assessing such injuries, as well as the carefully supervised flexion/extension x-rays of the cervical spine.

There appears to be an acquired increased lumbar lordosis in children and adolescents, particularly at the adolescent growth spurt. This is often associated with hip flexion contractures and tight hamstrings. This increased lumbar lordosis, which appears to be developmental in origin, may increase the risk of both disc injuries and posterior element injuries in the child who is also participating in vigorous sports training. We characteristically subdivide children with sports-associated back pain of the lumbar spine into mechanical back pain, which appears to be primarily associated with a fixed extension contracture or hyperlordosis; discogenic back pain, often without dramatic painful component but evidencing very tight hamstrings and occasionally neurologic deficit; and spondylolysis, particularly spondylolysis stress fractures (plain radiographs may be insufficient to diagnose these lesions adequately, but specialized techniques including SPECT bone scanning may now allow us to make early diagnosis and appropriate treatment of these lesions).

Finally, atypical Scheuermann's disease occurring at the thoracolumbar junction, apparently the result of repetitive flexion of the spine, may also be a source of back pain in the adult athlete. Interestingly, this lesion appears to be biomechanically most frequently associated with an abnormal structure of the spine with a very "flat back" alignment of both the thoracic and lumbar spine. The end result is both hypokyphosis of the thoracic spine and hypolordosis of the lumbar spine with a relatively neutral, or even kyphotic, posturing at the thoracolumbar junction.

Once a proper diagnosis of pain has been made, specific exercises to restore the full range of motion and strength of the spine, as well as appropriate back bracing, particularly antilordotic back bracing in injuries that appear to be associated in onset with hyperlordosis of the back, are usually effective in treating these conditions.

PELVIS AND HIP INJURIES

Injuries about the pelvis and hip in the young athlete are less common than other injuries, but may be a source of significant disability.

Most acute macrotrauma about the pelvis in the child consists of avulsion injuries at the apophyseal juncture. The apophyses at risk include the iliac margin, anterior superior iliac spine (insertion of the sartorius), ischium (insertion of the hamstrings), lesser trochanter (insertion of the iliopsoas), and anterior inferior iliac spine (insertion of the rectus). These avulsion injuries about the pelvis are often associated with acute pain and disability. Fortunately, they will most often heal if the patient is allowed to undergo a program of relative rest and subsequent rehealing. As occasionally discussed in the literature, acute reduction of large avulsions, such as at the ischium, may be considered. In addition, late resection of persistent painful sites, such as the rectus femoris or ischium, may also be considered.

Overuse injuries of the apophyses may also be encountered. These include the aforementioned apophyses. In particular, young distance runners or hurdlers may develop painful iliac crest apophyses that may be very slow in healing and may respond only to prolonged periods of rest.

Stress fractures may occur about the pelvis and involve the ischium, pubic ramus, proximal femur, including the neck of the femur, and distal femur. In addition, complaints of pain about the hip, pelvis, and even the knee in the athletically active child must always be carefully assessed to rule out the possibility of slipped capital femoral epiphysis, toxic synovitis, and infectious or neoplastic conditions that may become painful in coincidental association with athletic activities.

In addition, we have seen a number of cases, even in younger athletes, of osteitis pubis presenting itself as adductor spasm and pain. Sometimes plain radiographs may be diagnostic, but more commonly, as in stress fractures, technetium-99 bone scanning may be required to confirm the diagnosis. In general, cycling and swimming are, of course, good training alternatives during this period of healing.

The complaint of "snapping hip" may be encountered in young gymnasts and dancers. This is occasionally due to iliotibial band irritation over the greater trochanteric area with associated inflammation of the trochanteric bursa. Occasionally, it may represent tenosynovitis of the iliopsoas tendon running over the head and neck of the femur. A conservative stretching and strengthening program and postural realignment about the hip and pelvis are usually successful in alleviating symptoms. Occasionally, surgical decompression may be required.

KNEE INJURIES

Fractures

As noted previously, any complaint of macrotrauma about the knee in the child must always be carefully assessed to rule out the possibility of physeal injury to the distal femur or proximal tibia.

Fractures of the tibial tubercle should always be considered in any case of overuse pattern injury with a consistent complaint of pain.

Ligament Injuries

Ligament injuries in the child correspond to certain defined developmental patterns. In injuries to the collateral ligaments, conservative management is invariably successful.

Injuries of the cruciate ligaments, particularly the anterior cruciate ligament, are being identified with increased frequency. Our approach to midsubstance tears in the prepubescent consist of identification, sometimes with the use of arthroscopic technique. Bracing and exercise are then used, with definitive reconstruction recommended when the physes have closed; however, if the child remains symptomatic with intermittent effusions and progressive deterioration of the knee in response to function, I usually recommend an extra-articular reconstruction utilizing an iliotibial band in the over-the-top technique and then grooving the tibial portion of the knee. This is described to the family as a temporary procedure that will await final definitive ligamentous reconstruction when full growth has been attained.

I believe that tibial spine injuries have often been undertreated or inappropriately treated. Often these injuries are unstable, and plain radiographs cannot be trusted to show a true picture of relative stability of the knee. I also arthroscope these injuries to determine the relative stability of the fragment. If arthroscopic evaluation is carried out early, often a very simple reduction of the fragment under arthroscopic control can be performed with appropriate internal fixation, consisting either of cannulated screws or removable Kirschner wires. Subsequent stability of the knee is very reassuring following these repairs. In particular, I have observed that attempts to reduce these in full extension do not, in reality, cause a reduction of the tibial spine avulsion in its bed. Rather, full extension results in lifting of the fragment out of its bed, consistent with studies done of anterior cruciate tightness. As determined in studies of adult knees, the anterior cruciate is least tense in a position of approximately 30 to 40° of flexion of the knee. My practice has been to reduce these fragments in this posture of the knee and then to perform internal fixation.

In the adolescent with an injury to the anterior cruciate ligament of the knee, a number of recent studies have demonstrated that the long-term prognosis for this injury in this age group is really quite poor, and consideration should be given toward early ligamentous reconstruction in this group in particular.

Partial anterior cruciate ligament injuries in adolescents are not rare, in my opinion. I believe that many of the complete disruptions seen in this age group are actually second injuries, in which the first initial injury has not been diagnosed or appreciated. Diagnosis of this injury is difficult; often the best guide initially is physical examination, which demonstrates increased laxity when compared to the opposite extremity. In addition, ligamentous testing may be helpful to make this diagnosis. Unfortunately, MRI is not specific enough for the anterior cruciate to diagnose this lesion with certainty. In adolescents suspected of having sustained this injury who have undergone confirmatory laxity tests, my practice has been to proceed with arthroscopy to make the diagnosis definitively. I then will treat these ligaments with a 12-week period of knee bracing and crutch immobilization followed by progressive rehabilitation very similar to that employed after ligament reconstruction.

Internal Derangements

Internal derangements of the knee in the child and adolescent have a somewhat different pattern than in the adult. Meniscal lesions are really quite rare, although they certainly can be encountered in mid-to-late adolescence. In the younger child who complains of athletically associated knee pain, consideration should also be given to the possibility of a discoid lateral meniscus that has become manifest because of sports activity.

Osteochondritis dissecans may indeed be a source of knee pain in the child or adolescent. Diagnostic techniques, including bone scanning and MRI, have dramatically increased our ability to make the diagnosis of this lesion.

With early detection, simple immobilization may be sufficient to obtain healing of osteochondritis. In larger lesions or in lesions that remain symptomatic despite immobilization, transarticular drilling may also be successful in attaining healing in the underlying dead bone and subsequent stabilization of the articular cartilage superficial to this. Absorbable pin fixation of these lesions may also hold promise, but results have not been confirmed by prospective testing.

Extensor Mechanism

Most overuse injuries about the knee in the child or adolescent involve the extensor mechanism. In my experience, true chondromalacia is extremely rare in the articular cartilage of individuals with open growth plates. Patellofemoral stress syndrome appears to be a more appropriate diagnosis for parapatellar pain in this age group. The lateral and superior deviation of the patella at the time of the growth spurt may be a major anatomic contributor to the occurrence of this lesion in this age group.

Initial intervention in the case of patellofemoral stress syndrome may include directed physical therapy to stretch out the structures about the knee including the hamstrings, iliotibial band, and lateral retinaculum. I also characteristically employ a static progressive-resistive-exercise (PRE) straight-leg-raising or terminal-extension program and set as a goal 12 pounds of static PRE straight leg raising done in 3 sets of 10 repetitions with both legs. In my experience, 91% of a very large series of adolescents with parapatellar knee pain responded with complete cessation of symptoms and return to full function. My approach to the other extensor-mechanism overuse injuries is similar, including Osgood-Schlatter disease, Larsen-Jo-hansson, and quadriceps tendinitis.

Injuries to synovial plica about the knee may occur at this age and stage of development, either as a result of single-impact macro-trauma or repetitive microtrauma. Conservative treatment may often also be successful in relieving symptoms, although on occasion, re-section of the painful and fibrotic plica may be required.

FOOT AND ANKLE INJURIES

Foot and ankle injuries and complaints of pain in the young athlete are relatively common. Sprains of the lateral collateral ligament of the ankles can certainly occur, particularly in the pre-pubescent, although careful physical examination should always be done to ensure that there is no tenderness and pain at the physis. Radiographs must be obtained in such cases. If there is any doubt of a physeal injury to the distal fibular epiphysis or lateral tibial physis, cast immobilization for 3 weeks and then subsequent x-ray should be obtained.

Overuse injuries about the foot and ankle are common in this age group. Perhaps the most commonly encountered is Sever's disease, an apophysitis of the os calcis. This appears to occur particularly in children with tightness of the tendo Achilles and relative weakness about the foot and ankle, particularly of dorsiflexion inversion. There may be an associated pronation here at the foot. In my ex-perience, these children respond to a well-directed exercise program consisting of heel cord stretching and dorsiflexion strengthening, as well as possible transient heel lifts or accommodative orthotics if there are indeed biomechanical problems with the foot.

Adolescents in particular may be subject to unusual stress frac-tures about the foot and ankle. The stress fractures of the navicular metatarsals, including the second metatarsals and sesamoids, may be encountered with frequency. The team physician must be very certain not to attribute pain at the foot or ankle simply to a strain of the muscle-tendon units or ligamentous structures. Very careful assessment including physical examination and, if necessary, tech-netium-99 bone scanning to determine the possibility of a stress fracture must be undertaken.

Osteochondritis dissecans of the talus can occur as a result of macrotrauma (most commonly lateral lesions) or repetitive micro-trauma (most commonly medial lesions). Any vague complaints of ankle pain in this age group in which the ankle is stable and no other lesions are apparent should be carefully assessed for the possibility of osteochondritis dissecans. Initially, these lesions may not be apparent on plain radiographs because the underlying bone has not undergone necrosis. MRI imaging can be very helpful in these instances.

These lesions should be taken very seriously, and every attempt should be made to effect healing or, in the case of smaller medial lesions, to perform resection of the lesions

Peroneal tendon subluxations or dislocations may occur as a result of repetitive microtrauma or occasionally as overuse injuries. Unexplained pain about the lateral aspect of the ankle must always be assessed for this possibility. In my experience, these are rarely successfully treated using conservative techniques such as localized pads and braces. In an established painful subluxating peroneal tendon situation, surgical intervention is usually required.

SHOULDER INJURIES

Injuries about the shoulder can be encountered with increased frequency in this age group. These can be the result of acute macrotrauma or repetitive microtrauma overuse injury. It is important to remember that the shoulder joint consists of four separate components: the scapulothoracic, the glenohumeral, the acromioclavicular, and the sternoclavicular. All four components may actually be involved in the pathomechanics of a given condition. In particular, we are now finding that glenohumeral derangements, including impingements and anterior subluxations, may be associated with significant disruption of the normal function of the scapulothoracic mechanism with loss of muscle strength and coordination.

Instability of the shoulder may be encountered in a great variety of sports, including the throwing sports, swimming, and contact sports. It usually occurs when the forces involved in throwing or performing overhand sports exceed the passive mobility and stability of the glenohumeral joint. Both anterior subluxation and multidirectional instability have been recognized with increased frequency in this age group.

A further contributor in this age group is the generalized hyperelasticity in some of athletes that can contribute to the occurrence of instability. A repetitive pattern of overhand and abduction use of the arm may result in a relative scapulothoracic dyskinesis with relative weakness of the serratus anterior and tightness of the posterior glenoid humeral capsule with resulting anterior and superior subluxation of the humeral head with secondary impingement on the glenoid labrum or rotator cuff muscles anteriorly and superiorly. Although the patient may initially present with rotator cuff impingement-type signs very similar to those seen in the adult, the pathomechanics may be quite different, with the primary disorder an anterior subluxation.

In my experience, with early intervention in such cases, restoration of the normal biomechanics is quite possible. A tip-off on physical examination is a generalized loss of internal rotation of the involved shoulder and an often increased external rotation. Surgical intervention is rarely required in this age group, but if the shoulder symptoms are unresponsive to conservative management, an exact diagnosis must be obtained with the use of diagnostic techniques such as computed tomographic (CT) arthrography or MRI. Often the primary instability of the shoulder must be addressed in order to resolve symptoms. This age group does not sustain significant tears of the rotator cuff mechanism, and rotator cuff symptoms are usually secondary to the biomechanical instabilities of this mechanism.

Dislocations in this age group can be encountered. I have successfully treated them with a period of at least 4 weeks of immobilization. This is in contrast to the adult or professional athlete.

Acromioclavicular and Sternoclavicular Injuries

As with adults, acromioclavicular injuries in this age group are generally able to be treated quite satisfactorily conservatively and not operatively. Occasionally, a fracture of the distal physis of the clavicle may be encountered at this site, and it must be carefully identified by radiographic assessment. With severe displacement of this particular injury, operative reduction may be required to restore normal bone growth. On occasion, traumatic osteolysis may be seen after overuse or acute traumatic injury in this age group. Conservative management, including anti-inflammatory agents and relative rest, may be successful. In recalcitrant cases, I have used resection arthroplasty with great success.

Derangements of the sternoclavicular joint are also encountered in this age group. These may often be the result of repetitive microtrauma, and these injuries invariably are anterior subluxations that present as pain. In my experience, relative rest and a strengthening of the entire parascapular and shoulder mechanism may be successful in treating these disorders. On occasion, it has been necessary to perform operative resection arthroplasties in these sites.

As with other areas of the body, very careful attention should be given to the history of the onset of symptoms, and a careful physical examination will be helpful in diagnosing the condition.

"Little League shoulder," which is a traumatic injury at the proximal physis of the humerus, should always be entertained as a possible diagnosis of unresolved pain at this site. Plain radiographs may show widening of the physeal plate; the bone scan is usually positive at this site. The child will invariably become asymptomatic if allowed to rest and heal this lesion.

ELBOW INJURIES

Acute traumatic injuries to the elbow are one of the more serious areas of concern for children in general and athletic children in particular. In recent years, pediatric orthopedists have begun to recognize the importance of an exact anatomic reduction in the case of supracondylar fractures of the lateral condyle or medial epicondyles. The growing trend has been toward accurate and exact anatomic reduction and internal fixation even in the younger age groups. All medical personnel involved with the child must appreciate that an injury about the elbow with severe pain and swelling must be treated as an absolute emergency. The potential for neurovascular compromise, particularly with supracondylar injuries, is always present with subsequent and secondary ischemia of the muscles of the forearm. When in doubt about the possibility of a fracture at this site, comparative radiographs of the opposite extremity may be obtained. Once again, MRI may be extremely useful in helping to make the proper diagnosis.

Overuse injuries at the elbow have been dubbed "Little League elbow." These appear to be the result of repetitive overhand throwing, serving in tennis, or overhand throwing such as in javelin. They may occur in the medial aspect of the elbow with a medial epicondylitis or laterally with injuries to the capitellum articular surface or proximal radial physis. Any complaint of elbow pain or associated elbow flexion contracture and a sense of locking elbow must be examined very carefully for this lesion. Modern diagnostic techniques include not only plain radiographs but also MRI, which can enable us to make this diagnosis early nowadays.

If the condition is detected early, a relative rest program associated with specific therapy to stretch out the front of the elbow and strengthen the triceps and elbow extensors will be very effective. In cases where disruption of the articular cartilage of the capitellum has already occurred or where loose bodies are present, surgical intervention must be initiated to debride the joint and to restore normal mechanics to the joint.

PREVENTION OF INJURIES

The team physician has a pivotal role in the prevention of injuries in this age group. Particularly in community-based sports situations where athletic trainers and other support medical personnel are not present, careful attention to the complaints of pain associated with repetitive training and, in particular, attention to the increased susceptibility of the child during the growth spurt may be extremely helpful in preventing injury. Most overuse injuries in this age group are preventable with early detection and recognition. In addition, as the team physician becomes more experienced in dealing with the growing child, children who appear to be particularly susceptible to training injuries, such as the very tight or the hyperlax, should be put on specific exercise programs to restore normal strength and motion as well as stability. In cases where demands on tissues may be excessive and the child shares the common systematic deconditioning of all children that is occurring because of modern inactivity in our daily life, supplemental strengthening exercises in particular must be considered. The child who leads a uniformly sedentary existence throughout the week with rides to school, sitting in school, watching television after school, and playing Nintendo games is an absolute setup for injury if the parents decide to provide him or her with an exercise program consisting of 1 hour of organized sports training 4 days a week. This is the worst possible combination for occurrence of overuse injury.

RECOMMENDED READING

Bar-Or O: *Pediatric Sports Medicine for the Practitioner*. New York: Springer-Verlag, 1983.

Brown E and Branta CF (eds.): *Competitive Sports for Children and Youth: An Overview of Research and Issues*. Champaign, IL: Human Kinetics, 1988.

Micheli LJ: Pediatric and adolescent musculoskeletal sports injuries. *Scientific Foundations of Sports Medicine*. edited by CC Teitz. Philadelphia: B.C. Decker, 1989.

Micheli LJ: The exercising child: injuries. *Pedatr Exerc Sci* 1:329–335, 1989.

Micheli LJ (ed.): *Clin Sports Med 7*, 1988.

Micheli LJ: The traction apophysitises. *Clin Sports Med* 6:389–404, 1987.

Micheli LJ: Pediatric and adolescent sports injuries: recent trends. In *Exercise and Sport Science Reviews*. Vol. 14. Edited by K Pandolph. New York: Macmillan, 1986, pp. 359–374.

Micheli LJ (ed.): *Pediatric and Adolescent Sports Medicine*. Boston: Little, Brown, 1984.

Micheli LJ: Overuse injuries in children's sports: the growth factor. *Orthop Clin* 14:337–360, 1983.

Micheli LJ: Sports injuries in children and adolescents. In *Sports Medicine and Physiology*. Edited by RH Strauss. Philadelphia: W. B. Saunders, 1979, pp. 288–303.

Sewall L and Micheli LJ: Strength training for children. *J Pediatr Orthop* 3:13–30, 1986.

Sullivan JA and Grana WA (eds.): *The Pediatric Athlete*. Park Ridge, IL: American Academy of Orthopaedic Surgeons, 1990.

THE PHYSICALLY CHALLENGED ATHLETE

Donna B. Bernhardt

The emerging awareness of health promotion through sport and fitness has been extended to include not only the able-bodied, but also the physically challenged. Research has documented that an increase in strength, endurance, mobility, and cardiovascular fitness provides physiologic and psychological benefits for both groups of individuals, including a higher level of independence and self-satisfaction and greater self-esteem. Societal attitudes are changing with positive results in hiring, architectural accessibility, and socialization.

As a result of these realizations available athletic pursuits have expanded at both recreational and elite levels. Amateur and professional competition in individual and team sports is currently a goal of many physically challenged athletes. Technologic advances in the design and development of adaptive equipment have fostered participation. Although many aspects of the team physician's role are similar for all athletes, several additional considerations bear mention when working with a physically challenged athlete.

KNOWLEDGE OF THE SPORT

As with any athlete, the physician should understand not only the physiologic, musculoskeletal, and psychological requirements, but also the potential medical risks of a sport for the athlete. The physically challenged athlete may be prone to additional injury or illness secondary to his or her disability. For example, the loss of sensation in the athlete with a spinal cord injury may increase susceptibility to hypothermia, hyperthermia, or pressure sores.

Systems of classification exist for the type and severity of disability. The physician will be involved in determination of the phys-

242

ical or physiological level of function for classification level. Rules are often modified for the physically challenged athlete (e.g., the wheelchair is considered a part of the body in wheelchair basketball). Knowledge of rule alterations is helpful when performing preparticipation screening or injury/illness evaluation.

Amateur and professional sports have developed guidelines regarding permissible medications or drugs. The physician needs to be aware of these guidelines to screen current medications, prescribe medication, or conduct drug testing. If the athlete is taking medications related to his or her disability, the physician must check to see whether the drug is permissible, and if not, substitute an allowable medication.

MEDICAL EVALUATION

HISTORY

The history should include how and when the disability occurred and all medical management including surgery and rehabilitation. Also important is assessment of current occupation, athletic activities, and socioeconomic situation. Description of medical problems prior and secondary to the disability, or related to the sport, is vital. The physician should document previous athletic history (before and since disability) and specific goals for the sport. Releases from the athlete's physician and parental consent if the athlete is a minor are often required for training or competition. Releases for filming or pictures may be necessary for media purposes.

PHYSICAL EXAMINATION

During the interview, level of understanding, vocalization and communication abilities, and hearing are assessed and documented. In addition to the routine physical examination, several specific areas must be assessed by the physician, by a physical therapist, or by an athletic trainer.

Strength and endurance of the muscles required for the athletic endeavor must be evaluated. Manual testing or mechanical assessment may be used. The documentation of joint mobility and of musculotendinous length is important. Greater-than-normal mobility and muscle length might be necessary for athletic participation in certain sports. For example, the athlete with a spinal cord injury requires flexible hip joints for positioning in a sports wheelchair. Documentation of limb length and girth is also important.

Thorough assessment of all sensory systems is vital for both classification and safety. Documentation of auditory and visual abilities is necessary. All sensory abilities, including pain, temperature, touch, and pressure, should be charted. Examination of passive kinesthesia and of proprioception assists in training and safety programs. Determination of eye and hand dominance is necessary for certain sports such as archery, riflery, and field events. Documentation of the presence of abnormal muscle tone and primitive, protective, and pathologic reflexes is critical for participation in sports such as horseback riding, swimming, and gymnastics. Definitive evaluation of both segmental and eye-hand coordination is required to ensure both safe participation and successful training efforts.

Evaluation of skin condition and history of any skin problems is necessary in any athlete with alteration of sensation or with an orthotic/prosthetic device. Assessment of integrity and toughness of the skin (especially in areas of previous insult) is required. The proper fit of any device should be assessed. Hygiene education is frequently necessary.

Evaluation of sitting or standing posture and of balance as it pertains to participation in the sport and the preparatory activities is vital. The athlete who skis or competes in seated speed skating must have adequate trunkal posture and balance to negotiate turns. Similarly, the equestrian athlete must be able to balance on the saddle. Evaluation of athletic position either in a mock-up or actual situation is most desirable.

If the athlete is ambulatory, assessment of gait is mandatory. An analysis of the pattern and effectiveness of gait should be done as well. Any assistive or orthotic devices should be noted. If the athlete is nonambulatory, a description of the method of locomotion is required, with a notation of independence or assistance needed. An estimation of locomotor endurance should be included in the screening.

Assessment of gross and fine motor skills as appropriate to the sport and disability is indicated. These may include stair climbing, sit to stand, push-ups, sit-ups, hop or jump, heel or toe walking, toe touch, object manipulation, daily living skills, and combined motions such as knee bends with reciprocal arm movements. The assessment should include bilateral comparison and should be performed at various speeds. Grades should indicate whether the athlete is unable to perform, is partially able or needs assistance, or performs independently. Additionally, the timing and quality of the movement should be noted.

PHYSIOLOGIC ASSESSMENT

Assessment of physiologic status includes exercise testing, body composition evaluation, and nutritional analysis. In all situations the evaluation of body composition and of nutritional status is indicated as a baseline for further medical advice.

In athletes with cardiorespiratory disability or disease, specific assessment of respiratory and cardiovascular status is critical. Electrocardiography and spirometry are particularly indicated.

Evaluation of body composition can be easily accomplished with skinfold measurement. Skinfold calipers for the measurement of percentage of body fat are accurate in the hands of an experienced examiner. Nutritional status can be assessed by either a patient's report or a 24-hour nutritional log. Both can be utilized for behavioral alterations in exercise or eating habits designed to lower body fat or reduce dietary imbalances.

Exercise testing may be advisable for assessment either of cardiopulmonary functional capacity or of the efficacy of medications when necessary. Traditionally, treadmill and bicycle ergometry are the most frequently utilized exercise tests. Physically challenged individuals, however, might not be able to perform these tasks and may instead utilize arm-crank, wheelchair, or single-leg ergometry. Either maximal or submaximal testing can be conducted in a continuous or discontinuous manner. If submaximal testing is utilized, maximal cardiopulmonary capacity and heart rate will be predicted. Because less equipment is involved and any form of task-specific exercise can be adapted, submaximal testing is most readily accomplished in the field.

When field testing the following principles must be met. The initial exercise intensity must be below anticipated maximal capacity. Exercise intensity should be gradually increased in stages, with regular monitoring of heart rate, patient response and symptoms, perceived exertion (RPE), and blood pressure. All observations should be continued for 7 to 10 minutes following test completion to monitor the recovery phase.

PSYCHOLOGICAL ASSESSMENT

The team physician should ascertain the level of understanding and adjustment to the disability. An assessment of family and social support systems is very helpful, especially in the advent of an injury.

Available psychological tests may be helpful. Assessment of determination, discipline, stress control, toughmindedness, loci of focus (internal or external), and adaptation to risk might assist both the trainer and the coach in working with the athlete.

EQUIPMENT EVALUATION

With few exceptions the participation of the physically challenged athlete is intimately linked to technology and equipment, whether modified assistive devices such as wheelchairs, special orthotic and prosthetic appliances, or newly designed or adapted sports accessories. Hence, assessment of the effectiveness and safety of this equipment is part of the overall evaluation.

Wheelchairs have undergone much adaptation for sport (Fig. 26–1). Back height has been lowered for increased mobility. Seat width has been reduced, with snug molding of the chair to the body. Seat height has been lowered for stability and reduced wind resistance. The angle between back and seat is reduced so the knees are closer to the chest; this adaptation eliminates the need for trunk balance while preserving efficient breathing. Larger, 26-inch tires are now

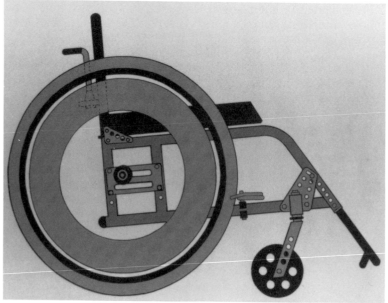

FIG. 26–1. Sports wheelchair.

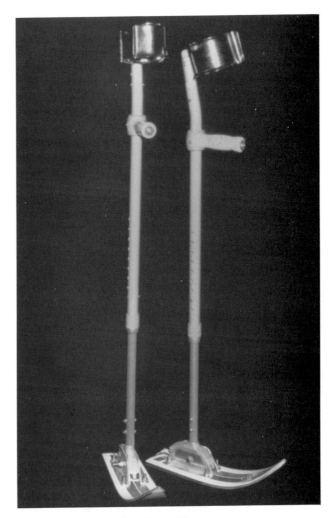

FIG. 26–2. Outriggers for alpine skiing.

allowable to permit greater distance per revolution and to place the wheel closer to the hand for a more effective stroke. Small, 5-inch front casters pivot more easily and provide greater clearance. Wheel camber adjustment with the tops slanted toward the chair increases stability, provides quicker turning, and allows greater access to the handrims for a down-out push. Finally, new materials (aluminum, titanium) significantly reduce the weight of the chair to below 20 lb.

One advance in prosthetics has been the development of a "peg leg," a modified socket with a removable distal portion. The leg can be used for locomotion when intact. When the athlete is participating in a sport, such as skiing, the peg can be removed. The remaining socket provides both warmth and protection to the residual limb. This limb is aligned ½ to 1 inch shorter than the remaining limb in the above-knee amputee to facilitate ambulation without a knee joint.

Adaptations of sports equipment are both numerous and ingenious. Shooting releases and release cuffs assist archers without wrist and finger function to shoot. Specially designed "outriggers" (forearm crutches with a ski tip affixed to the base) assist the skier with one lower limb or neuromuscular difficulties (Fig. 26–2). Sit skis make alpine skiing and speed skating possible for the athlete with a spinal cord injury.

The team physician should become familiar with the adaptations required by the disability and the sport. The equipment should be inspected for safety and adherence to rules of the governing sports administration. Finally, the equipment should be examined for correct fit and function to allay any secondary injury or medical problem.

RESTRICTION FROM PARTICIPATION

The physician is the final authority in any decision-making regarding participation. Although the criteria for safe participation are similar for any athlete, the physical or physiologic disability might alter medical considerations. Febrile illness might be more restrictive in an athlete with chronic obstructive pulmonary disease, as a pressure sore might be in the insensitive limb of a paraplegic. Discussions with the coach, athletic trainer, or physical therapist may determine whether modifications or protections can be designed to prevent further injury, or whether restriction is vital.

In the case of preparticipation screening, several medical conditions preclude active athletic participation at a high level. These include severe aortic or pulmonary stenosis, active myocarditis, cardiomyopathy, recent embolitic disease, third-degree heart block, acute pericarditis, valvular disease, atrial tachycardia or fibrillation, coarctation of the aorta, patent ductus arteriosus, rheumatic heart disease, uncontrolled metabolic or epileptic disease, and a serious systemic disorder such as mononucleosis or hepatitis.

SUMMARY

The role of the team physician in managing the physically challenged athlete is both interesting and challenging. These athletes possess the same motivation, discipline, and earnest intent as the able-bodied. The understanding of how the physically challenged athlete competes in his or her sport is an interesting and exciting educational experience.

SUGGESTED READING

American Academy of Pediatrics: Cardiac evaluation for participation in sports. *Phys Sportsmed* 7:102–108, 1978.

Athletes and exercise-induced bronchospasm. *Med Sci Sports Exec 18:* 314–334, 1986.

Bar-Or O: *Pediatric Sports Medicine for the Practitioner.* New York, Springer-Verlag, 1983.

Belman M and Wasserman K: Exercise training and testing in patients with chronic obstructive pulmonary disease. *Resp Care* 27:724–736, 1982.

Bernhardt D (ed.):Sports physical therapy. *Clin Sports Med 10,* 1986.

Bernhardt D (ed.): *Recreation for the Disabled Child. Physical and Occupational Therapy in Pediatrics.* Vol 4. New York: Haworth Press, 1985.

Biery M: Riding and the handicapped. *Vet Clin North Am* 15:345–354, 1985.

Bundgard A: Exercise and the asthmatic. *Sports Med* 2:254–266, 1985.

Byers P: Effects of exercise on morning stiffness and mobility in patients with rheumatoid arthritis. *Res Nurs Health* 8:275–281, 1985.

Caplow-Lindner E, Harpaz L and Samberg S: *Therapeutic Dance/Movement: Expressive Activities for Older Adults.* New York: Human Services Press, 1979.

Costill D, Miller J and Fink W: Energy metabolism in diabetic distance runners. *Phys Sportsmed* 8:63–71, 1980.

Coutts K: Heart rate of participants in wheelchair sports. *Paraplegia 26:*43–49, 1988.

Coutts K, Rhodes E and McKenzie D: Maximal exercise responses of tetraplegics and paraplegics. *J Appl Physiol* 55:479–482, 1983.

Curtis K and Dillon D: Survey of wheelchair athletic injuries: common patterns and prevention. *Paraplegia* 23:170–175, 1985.

Curtis K, McClanahan S, Hail K, et al.: Health, vocational and functional status in spinal cord injured athletes and nonathletes. *Arch Phys Med Rehabil* 67:862–865, 1986.

Dold H: Exercise and asthma in athletes. *Illinois Med J* 164:134–7, 1983.

Dreisinger T and Londeree B: Wheelchair exercise: a Review. *Paraplegia* 20:20–34, 1982.

Fletcher G, Lloyd A, Waling J, et al.: Exercise testing in patients with musculoskeletal handicaps. *Arch Phys Med Rehabil* 69:123–127, 1988.

Frank L: Organization and support for a handicapped ski program. *Am J Sports Med* 10:276–284, 1982.

Freeman G: Therapeutic horseback riding. *Clin Management* 4:20–25, 1984.

Gelb A, et al.: Exercise-induced bronchodilitation in asthma. *Chest* 87:196–201, 1985.

Gloag D: Rehabilitation in rheumatic disease. *Br Med J* 290:132–136, 1985.

Haas F, Pineda H, et al.: Effects of physical fitness on expiratory airflow in exercising asthmatic people. *Med Sci Sports Exerc* 17:585–592, 1985.

Helm P, et al.: Function after lower limb amputation. *Acta Orthop Scand* 57:154–157, 1986.

Hilbers P and White T.: Effects of wheelchair design on metabolic and heart rate responses during propulsion by persons with paraplegia. *Phys Ther* 67:1355–1364, 1987.

Hoffman M: Cardiorespiratory fitness and training in quadriplegics and paraplegics. *Sports Med* 3:312–330, 1986.

Holzer F, et al.: The effect of a home exercise programme in children with cystic fibrosis and asthma. *Aust Paediatr J* 20:297–301, 1984.

Horvat M, et al.: A comparison of the psychological characteristics of male and female able-bodied and wheelchair athletes. *Paraplegia* 24:115–122, 1986.

Jackson R: Sport for the spinal paralysed person. *Paraplegia* 25:301–304, 1987.

James U: Effect of physical training in healthy male unilateral above–knee amputees. *Scand J Rehabil Med* 5:88–101, 1973.

James U and Nordgren B: Physical work capacity measured by bicycle ergometry and prosthetic treadmill walking in healthy active unilateral above-knee amputees. *Scand J Rehabil Med* 5:81–87, 1973.

Kegel B: Physical fitness: Sports and recreation for those with lower K limb amputation or impairment. *J Rehabil Res Dev* 1:1–125, 1985.

Kegel B, Webster J and Burgess E: Recreational activities of lower extremity amputees: a survey. *Arch Phys Med Rehabil* 61:258–264, 1980.

Kofsky P, Davis G, et al.: Field testing: assessment of physical fitness of disabled adults. *Eur J Appl Physiol* 51:109–120, 1983.

LaMere T and Labanowich S: The history of sport wheelchairs: Part II. *Sports 'n Spokes* May/June, 1984. Part III. *Sports 'n Spokes* Jul/Aug, 1984.

Leach S, et al.: Exercise-induced asthma. *Compr Ther* 11:7–12, 1985.

Leung P: Persons with disabilities skiing, *J Rehabil* 54:10–13, 1988.

Madorsky J and Curtis K: Wheelchair sports medicine. *Am J Sports Med* 12:128–132, 1984.

Madorsky J and Madorsky A: Scuba diving: taking the wheelchair out of wheelchair sports. *Arch Phys Med Rehabil* 69:215–220, 1988.

Makisara G, et al.: Progression of functional capacity and work capacity in rheumatoid arthritis. *Clin Rheumatol* 1:117–125, 1982.

Mangus B: Sports injuries, the disabled athlete, and the athletic trainer. *Athlet Training* 22:305–310, 1987.

Marquardt E, et al.: Amputations and prostheses for the lower limb. *Int Orthop* 8:139–146, 1984.

Morrison J and Ursprung A: Children's attitudes toward people with disabilities: a review of the literature. *J Rehabil*, 45–49, 1987.

Nilsen R, Nygaard P and Bjorholt P: Complications that may occur in those with spinal cord injury who participate in sport. *Paraplegia* 23:152–158, 1985.

Orenstein D, Henke K and Cerny F: exercise and cystic fibrosis. *Phys Sportsmed* 11:57–63, 1983.

Oseid S and Edwards A (eds.): *The Asthmatic Child in Play and Sport*. Bath, England; Pitman Press, 1982.

Panush R and Brown D: Exercise and arthritis. *Sports Med* 4:54–64, 1987.

Pineda F, Haas F and Axen K: Treadmill exercise training in chronic obstructive pulmonary disease. *Arch Phys Med Rehabil* 67:155–158, 1986.

Rose K: Which cardiovascular problems should disqualify athletes? *Phys Sportsmed* 3:62–68, 1975.

Rourke L: Elements of archery: Part 3—Instruction. *Sports 'n Spokes Mar/Apr:*18–20, 1987.

Rourke L and Heer M: Elements of Archery: Part 2–Equipment. *Sports 'n Spokes Jan/ Feb:*11–14, 1985.

St Clair E, et al.: Therapeutic approaches to the treatment of rheumatic disease. *Med Clin North Am* 70:285–304, 1986.

Sasaki M and Pink M: Self protection/defense for persons with disabilities. *Clin Management* 4:6–11, 1984.

Shapiro W: Is medicine catching up with the wheelchair athlete? *Phys Sportsmed* 2:54–57, 1974.

Schleien S and Ray M: *Community Recreation and Persons with Disabilities.* Baltimore: Paul Brookes, 1988.

Shayevitz M and Shayevitz B: Athletic training in chronic obstructive pulmonary disease. *Clin Sports Med* 5:471–491, 1986.

Sloedefalke K, Balke B, Ryan A and Gale J: Effect of dynamic physical activity on handicapped university students. In *Exercise and Fitness.* Edited by D Franks. Chicago, IL: Athletic Institute, 1969.

Sonstroem R: Exercise and self-esteem. *Exer. Sport Sci Rev* 12:123–155, 1984.

Special problems and management of allergic athletes. *J Allergy Clin Immunol* 73, 1984.

Stewart N: Value of sport in rehabilitation of the physically disabled. *Can J Appl Sport Sci* 6:166–167, 1981.

Stotts K: Health maintenance: paralytic athletes and nonathletes. *Arch Phys Med Rehabil* 67:109–112, 1986.

Symposium on Asthma. *Clin Chest Med* 5:555–713, 1984.

Tahamount M, Knowlton R, Sawka M, et al.: Metabolic responses of women to exercise attributable to long term use of manual wheelchair. *Paraplegia* 24:311–317, 1986.

Taylor A, McDonell E and Brassard L: Effects of arm ergometer training programs on wheelchair subjects. *Paraplegia* 24:105–114, 1986.

Twenty-seventh Aspen Lung Conference. Asthma, *Chest* 87(*Suppl.*), 1985.

Valliant P, Bezzubyk I, Daley L, et al.: Psychological impact of sport on disabled athletes. *Psychol Rep* 56:923–929, 1985.

vanAlste J, et al.: Exercise electrocardiography using rowing ergometry suitable for leg amputees. *Int Rehabil Med* 7:1–5, 1985.

vanAlste J, et al.: Exercise testing of lower limb amputees. *Acta Orthop Scand* 57:154–157, 1985.

vanEysdem-Bessling M: The (non)sense of present-day classification system of sports for the disabled, regarding paralysed and amputee athletes. *Paraplegia* 23:288–294, 1985.

VanLoan M, McCluer S, Loften J, et al.: Comparison of physiological responses to maximal arm exercise among able-bodied, paraplegics and quadraplegics. *Paraplegia* 25:397–405, 1987.

Wicks J, Oldridge N, Camerson B, et al.: Arm cranking and wheelchair ergometry in elite spinal cord injured athletes. *Med Sci Sport Exerc* 15:224–231, 1983.

Wisecup L: Dance therapy. *Clin Management* 1:26–27, 1981.

BEHAVIORAL CONSIDERATIONS

Shane M. Murphy

Psychological issues surround the everyday work of the team physician. The psychological style that is chosen in interacting with an athlete will often determine the degree of treatment adherence and outcome. Psychology is used in calming the distressed athlete, and psychological awareness is necessary for successful interactions with coaches, administrators, and other personnel. In this chapter, three basic areas of psychology of primary importance to the team physician are covered: (1) the use of psychological principles to promote healing and recovery; (2) guidelines for successfully utilizing the services of a psychologist consultant; and (3) how to deal with common psychological problems encountered in the work of the team physician.

USING PSYCHOLOGY TO PROMOTE HEALING AND RECOVERY IN ATHLETES

Much of the work of the team physician revolves around treating injury and illness in athletes, so it is appropriate to begin with a discussion of the most important behavioral considerations in working with the injured or sick athlete. Much has already been written about the psychology of injury rehabilitation (Gordon, 1986; Wiese and Weiss, 1987, Yukelson, 1986). These authors have stressed the importance of such factors as clear communication with the athlete concerning the nature of the injury and the steps involved in the rehabilitation process, regularly checking with athletes to see whether they have understood what the treating physician has told them, understanding the common emotional reactions to injury (denial, anger, depression), and utilizing psychological interventions such as relaxation and visualization to deal with pain and frustration during rehabilitation.

In this section, two areas of behavior that can have a great impact on an athlete's recovery from injury are discussed. First, a description is provided of how an athlete can be most effectively helped to take responsibility for his or her rehabilitation. The use of goal-setting programs in conjunction with rehabilitation is discussed, and the main points for setting up an effective goal-setting program are summarized. Second, a discussion is provided of an area rarely mentioned in the sports medicine literature—the implications of psychoneuroimmunology for injury prevention and rehabilitation.

GOAL SETTING FOR EFFECTIVE REHABILITATION IN SPORTS SETTINGS

The team physician working with the injured athlete knows the value of having goals and striving to reach them. What may not be as well known is that the practice of setting goals and their effect on productivity have been well researched, initially in the business area (Locke and Latham, 1984) and more recently by sport psychologists (Weinberg et al., 1990). Some general principles have been established through research that help to ensure the optimum effectiveness of a goal-setting program (Locke and Latham, 1985). These principles are:

Principle 1: Involve the athlete in setting his or her own goals. The athlete's rehabilitation will proceed faster if he or she feels personally responsible for the outcome of the therapy program. Once the therapy regimen has been described, and appropriate outcome goals have been discussed, it is useful for the athlete to take responsibility for determining goals such as how often to come to therapy, how long to spend on a particular procedure, and what sort of exercises to perform at home. The physician can be the guide during this process, helping the athlete set reasonable goals that are neither too taxing nor too easy.

Principle 2: Goals should be written down in specific, measurable terms. Research has shown that individuals will show more commitment to their goals if they are made concrete and specific, rather than vague and general. My own experience suggests that athletes will be able to stick to their goals more easily if they write them down, for example in a notepad. The more concrete the goal, the better. A goal such as "I will come to the clinic for therapy 4 days a week for an hour" is better than a goal of "I will attend therapy regularly."

Principle 3: The athlete should receive regular feedback and reinforcement about his or her progress. Again, research has shown that for goal setting to be effective, the individual must be able to determine how he or she is doing in achieving his or her goals. If the goal is written in concrete terms, as previously suggested, it is usually a simple matter to keep track of how frequently required behaviors are performed, or the length of time involved. Some sort of reward system should be built into the program by the athlete. For example, if all the goals for a week are met, the athlete will reward himself or herself by going to the movies or engaging in some type of pleasurable activity. Although this suggestion seems simple, it is often the critical factor in determining the athlete's motivation over the long haul of therapy.

PSYCHONEUROIMMUNOLOGY: IMPLICATIONS FOR RECOVERY FROM TRAINING AND INJURY

The knowledge that psychosocial factors are involved in the disease process goes back many years, one of the best-known lines of research being that of Hans Selye (1946). Selye showed that stress was related to the onset of certain diseases through the "general adaptation syndrome." Also important to the field of sports medicine was the work of Holmes and Rahe (1967) and others, who showed a relationship between increased levels of psychosocial stress and higher levels of illness and injury. The study of the relationship between psychosocial factors and immune system functioning has come to be known as psychoneuroimmunology (PNI), and the field of PNI has seen much active research in recent years (Borysenko, 1984; Glaser et al., 1987; Kennedy, Kiecolt-Glaser, and Glaser, 1988).

PNI research has clear implications for the field of sports medicine. Because high stress levels have been shown to be related to compromised immune system functioning, those responsible for the health care of athletes must be aware of the general stress level of those athletes. Athletes under high stress levels (such as those on intense training schedules or those who are training and working under difficult conditions) are probably at increased risk of injury or illness. Often, the treating physician will become aware of this situation through seeing an athlete who is overtrained, or "burned out," or suffering from chronic injuries. A variety of emotional indicators (anxiety, frustration, depression) may accompany the overtraining or burnout states. Although rest and time away from training have been prescribed as the most appropriate treatments of chronic staleness in an athlete (Morgan et al., 1987), PNI research indicates that more active intervention techniques may speed the recovery process and may help to prevent stress-related disorders.

Although a variety of interventions intended to enhance immune system functioning have been described in the PNI literature (Heyman, 1989; Norris, 1989), several elements appear common to many of these interventions. One is the *deep relaxation* component. Relaxation can be taught in a variety of ways (autogenic relaxation, progressive muscle relaxation, diaphragmatic breathing, guided imagery, the Alexander method, biofeedback), but all these approaches share the outcome of teaching the patient how to deeply relax his body. Another component is that some *cognitive process* is usually prescribed along with the relaxation. This cognitive process might be meditation, visualization, or body awareness, but in some way the patient becomes actively involved in the self-healing process. The third component common to the various PNI strategies is the process of *self-control*. The patient becomes an active participant in the treatment program, is given responsibility, is required to learn new skills, and is expected to improve. There is no room for the patient to be a passive recipient of the therapy. Combining these three elements suggests that athletes involved in recovery from injury, or those who wish to optimize their recovery from intense training, learn and practice a relaxation technique that has an associated cognitive element. We have had promising results at the Olympic Training Center in Colorado Springs using such techniques with athletes who are engaged in very demanding and intense training programs. Further research needs to be done studying intervention results, but this promises to be a productive area for the sports medicine field. Active relaxation treatments can be employed by athletes, and taught by athletic trainers, in conjunction with more traditional therapies. In fact, they may help to promote a sense of self-control in the athlete recovering from injury.

UTILIZING A PSYCHOLOGIST IN A SPORTS CLINIC

Having available the services of a professional trained in clinical or counseling psychology is no longer the luxury it once was in the athletic clinic. Many universities and colleges are now putting athletic counseling programs in place, most professional teams have retained the services of a behavioral health consultant, and clinical/counseling psychologists are regular members of sports medicine teams provided by the United States Olympic Committee. It is still more common to be in the situation of *not* having a psychologist available to consult with, however, so in this section I both offer guidelines for working with a psychologist and also make some recommendations concerning appropriate referral procedures.

GUIDELINES FOR WORKING WITH A PSYCHOLOGIST IN A SPORTS SETTING

From experience, I have distilled some guidelines for the most effective utilization of the services of a psychologist. First, it is important to introduce the psychologist to the athlete in a way that minimizes a defensive response from the athlete and promotes the chances of establishing a good working relationship. For example, an introduction such as, "This is Dr. Smith; she will be working with you to help you with rehabilitation and make your therapy as effective as possible," sets up appropriate expectations and establishes a hopeful outlook for the athlete/patient. A less-effective introduction would be, "This is Dr. Smith, our psychologist. We expect you to have a difficult time with recovery, so we thought Dr. Smith could help you in talking about your problems." Immediately, negative expectations for recovery are introduced, and the chances for an effective consultation are probably lessened.

The first introduction example reflects a philosophy of team treatment that is well matched to the effective utilization of a psychologist. That is, the psychologist is a regular part of the sports medicine team and will be involved in treatment on a routine basis. If the psychologist is perceived by athletes as dealing only with severe emotional issues then it becomes a negative experience to be referred to the psychologist for evaluation or treatment. By the same token, it is important not to overemphasize the potential contribution of the psychologist. If the athlete is given reason to expect that the psychologist will provide a technique or treatment that will completely take away the pain, make rehabilitation compliance easy, or remove feelings of frustration, anger, or sadness, then the athlete will inevitably be disappointed, and the psychologist's credibility will be lessened.

GUIDELINES FOR REFERRAL OF AN ATHLETE TO A PSYCHOLOGIST

In some situations, the athlete client will have a presenting problem such that referral to a clinical/counseling psychologist or a psychiatrist will be most appropriate, e.g., an eating disorder, a substance abuse problem, or a depressive disorder. Naturally, the best situation is to have available a referral to a professional with whom you have worked in the past and in whom you have confidence. In seeking a new referral, some general guidelines can be suggested. First, the psychologist or psychiatrist should have some experience working with athletes or should be trained in athletic counseling techniques. This information usually can be obtained in a telephone interview. A check on how familiar the professional is with the field of sport psychology can be obtained by asking whether he or she is a member of either Division 47 (the Division of Sport and Exercise Psychology) of the American Psychological Association or of the Association for the Advancement of Applied Sport Psychology (AAASP). Both these organizations also have membership directories that can be obtained in order to assist with referrals.* The United States Olympic Committee also maintains a Registry of sport psychology professionals who have extensive experience with athletes.† Second, the psychologist should have a behavioral approach to assessment and intervention. This ensures prompt attention to problem resolution. Third, the psychologist should be willing to work with you in the athletic environment. In my experience, the psychologist will be most effective if he or she is available at times for the athlete in the athletic clinic, if he or she is willing to work closely with the athletic trainer and team physician, and if he or she is able to spend some time with the athlete at practice or in related sports settings. That is, the psychologist should be capable of establishing an effective relationship with the athlete in the athlete's environment.

COMMON BEHAVIORAL PROBLEMS ENCOUNTERED IN THE SPORTS SETTING

Naturally, various types of clinical behavioral problems are likely to be encountered in the sports setting with about the same frequency as they occur in the normal population. Over time, the team physician is likely to encounter the full range of behavioral problems, from anxiety disorders to personality disorders, from eating problems to familiar problems. This chapter does not attempt to discuss all the behavioral problems that might be encountered in sports, but focuses on two problems that for various reasons are more frequently encountered in sports settings: eating disorders and substance abuse problems. Discussion of the case-management is-

* Note, however, that both these organizations also have many members who are not licensed psychologists, but who are educators by training and profession.

† The USOC Registry can be obtained by writing to: Department of Sport Psychology, USOC, 1750 E. Boulder, Colorado Springs, CO, 80909.

sues encountered in treating these two problems will provide a prototype for the management of other behavioral problems.

EATING DISORDERS IN ATHLETICS

Health-care professionals working with athletes have reported encountering eating disorders with increasing frequency over the past several years. Research is equivocal, however, with respect to whether athletes as a population have a higher incidence of eating disorders than the general adolescent and young adult populations (Borgen and Corbin, 1987; Burckes-Miller and Black, 1988). What *does* seem clear is that a variety of pathogenic weight-loss techniques are utilized by athletes, and that many sports place a great emphasis on athletes' maintaining low weight and low body fat percentages. Whether these factors will result in more eating disorders in athletes after their competitive careers are over than would otherwise have been the case remains to be seen. This section briefly describes the pressures in sport that promote unhealthy eating behaviors, ways to recognize and diagnose eating disorders, and treatment.

Special Situations in Sport that Complicate the Eating/Weight Loss Habits of Athletes

Three main situations in sport focus a great deal of attention on the body weight and composition of athletes. First, a number of sports emphasize *lean body image* in the outcome of the competition. Sports that reward athletes for looking thin and svelte include gymnastics, rhythmic gymnastics, figure skating, diving, and synchronized swimming. Because females experience the highest frequency of eating disorders (female:male ratio is about 9:1), and because the onset is usually during adolescence, this emphasis on being thin in such sports is likely to cause the most problems for young women and girls entering puberty. Second, many sports employ *weight-class classifications* that encourage athletes to lose weight rapidly shortly before competition ("cutting weight"). Such sports include judo, boxing, wrestling, tae kwon do, and weightlifting. Not surprisingly, the use of pathogenic weight-loss techniques is common in these sports. Frequently reported techniques for weight loss include fasting, crash diets, dehydration, induced vomiting, diuretics, and laxative use. In these sports, men greatly outnumber women. Third, several sports emphasize *body leanness for optimal performance*. Although many athletes believe that "lean equals mean," the sports where this belief is most frequently encountered include distance running, swimming, and cross-country skiing. These three factors in sport are not likely to change in the near future and virtually ensure that a variety of eating/body image complications will continue to be seen in the sports medicine clinic.

Recognizing and Diagnosing Eating Disorders

Individuals with eating disorders frequently do not refer themselves for treatment. Often, the suspicion that an athlete has an eating disorder is voiced first by a teammate, a roommate, a coach, or a parent. Warning signs include: a reluctance to eat with the rest of the team (solitary eating); notable lack of caloric intake, or intake of a large amount of high-calorie food (binging); visits to the restroom immediately after eating, or long stays in the restroom (for purging); obsessive thoughts about weight; rapid mood swings rapid weight fluctuations; constant monitoring of weight; self-statements that indicate a large discrepancy between body image and actual weight; and dental problems, particularly with caries (from frequent exposure to digestive acids). None of these signs is an indicator of an eating disorder by itself, but each is a cause for concern. Unfortunately, many athletes share features common to eating-disordered individuals, which can make accurate diagnosis difficult at times. For example, features such as a preoccupation with diets, controlled consumption of calories, low body weight, almost obsessive exercise, and amenorrhea are found in many otherwise healthy athletes, but are also common to eating-disordered individuals.

The two most common eating disorders are *anorexia nervosa* and *bulimia nervosa*. Of these, anorexia is the less frequent (about 1% of the college population) and the most serious (approximately 10% of cases are fatal). As the name implies, anorexia is a starvation-type disorder. The chief criteria for a diagnosis of anorexia nervosa are: (1) an intense fear of becoming obese; (2) a disturbance of body image; (3) 15% or more weight loss; and (4) a refusal to maintain body weight. Bulimia, on the other hand, is characterized by binge eating and pathogenic weight-loss attempts. The chief criteria for a diagnosis of bulimia nervosa are: (1) recurrent binge eating; (2) at least three of the following—eating high-calorie food in binges, inconspicuous eating, sudden binge termination, pathogenic weight-loss attempts, and 10-pound or more weight fluctuations; (3) a fear of not being able to control one's eating behavior; and (4) depressed mood and guilt feelings. Unfortunately, it is not at all uncommon to encounter eating disorders that do not fit exactly into either category, and a mixture of features is common. Intense anxiety asso-

ciated with food, eating, and weight gain is the predominant feature
that should be assessed when an eating disorder is suspected.

Treatment Issues in the Athlete with an Eating Disorder

Sport may actually provide an advantageous context for the
detection of eating disorders, because it is difficult to hide an
eating disorder amid frequent social contacts. Referral for a thorough
assessment should be made if there is *any* question of an eating
disorder, because early detection and treatment are associated with
the best prognosis. The key to successful intervention with eating-
disordered athletes is to have a treatment *plan* and a treatment *team*
set up prior to the event. Treatment of eating disorders is multifaceted, and most treatment teams include specialists in medicine,
nutrition, psychotherapy, group therapy, and family therapy. The
team physician should work with administration to have a plan of
action drawn up for confrontation and referral of the athlete with a
problem. Hospitalization contingencies should be considered because inpatient treatment is often necessary for severe cases, particularly of anorexia nervosa.

Clearly, the coach is a crucial member of the referral and treatment
support network. Education concerning eating disorders, their nature, onset, and treatment, is therefore highly recommended for all
coaches and support staff, as well as for athletes.* Coaches need to
be sensitive to the role they can play in focusing undue attention
on weight and body image (such as through weekly team weighings
and so on), but even more important, they can be a valuable resource
during the treatment process. It is preferable for a therapist working
with an athlete in this situation to seek permission to be able to
consult regularly with the coach. Experience suggests coaches sometimes have a difficult time understanding that setting weight-loss
goals can be destructive to the recovery of a bulimic, even when
there are excellent performance-related reasons for setting such
goals. In these cases the physician or therapist can work with athlete
and coach to provide alternative means of achieving weight-related
goals (dietary considerations, appropriate weight training, and interval exercise programs, etc.). Coaches can also be instrumental in
discouraging the use by athletes of dangerous weight-loss techniques such as diuretics and dehydration. Education programs em-
phasizing nutrition-performance relationships and suggesting ef-

---

* The NCAA has produced an informative set of three videos and supporting documentation on eating disorders in sport.

fective and safe weight-management programs can help athletes to find alternatives to sudden weight loss.

The fundamentals of effective case management of a behavioral problem are illustrated in this example. Regular education efforts help greatly in increasing the awareness of this problem and in educating sports personnel on behaviors that can exacerbate the problem in predisposed individuals. Team planning that involves the coaching staff, health-care providers, and administration is valuable in determining when to confront an athlete, how to assess the situation, and what resources should be involved in providing treatment. Increased understanding of the course of this disorder helps all related individuals to provide appropriate assistance to the athlete during aftercare.

SUBSTANCE ABUSE PROBLEMS IN ATHLETICS

Many of the principles discussed previously, such as the important roles of education and prevention and the necessity of team planning for interventions, are also crucial to the effective treatment of substance abuse problems in sport. This section discusses the identification and treatment of substance abuse problems.

Identification of Substance Abuse Problems in Athletes

Again, the athlete with a substance abuse problem is seldom self-referred for treatment. Instead, the substance abuse problem often becomes an issue either through positive testing (e.g., for steroids or amphetamines) or through behavior problems related to substance use (driving under the influence, police arrest, etc.). From experience, it is highly desirable to distinguish between athletes who require treatment for the use of *performance-enhancement* drugs (e.g., steroids) and those abusing the so-called *recreational* drugs (alcohol, cocaine, etc.). These two "classes" of drugs are taken for very different reasons, and the implications of treating each are very different.

Within the performance-enhancement area of drug use, a distinction can be made between those drugs that are able to be detected through chemical analysis, such as steroids, and those that are not yet tested for, such as human growth hormone. Although the physician may occasionally encounter an athlete who "tests positive" and is therefore referred for treatment for use of substances such as steroids, an athlete is rarely referred for treatment for use of growth hormone or for blood doping. Detection of problems in this area therefore relies on advances in testing programs by sports authorities. Within the area of recreational drug use, a distinction can be drawn between the abuse of substances that are legal, such as alcohol, and those that are illegal, such as cocaine and marijuana. Although treatment of alcohol abuse offers choices between outcome goals of abstinence and controlled drinking, the final goal for treatment of illegal drugs is always abstinence.

Treatment of Athletes with Substance Abuse Problems

As discussed with regard to eating disorders, it is vital to have a planned intervention system ready and in place to deal with substance abuse problems as they occur. Little has been written about treatment of athletes who have been detected using performance-enhancing drugs. Because of the sanctions against the use of steroids and other substances, the emphasis has usually been on punishment rather than treatment. Although sanctions are necessary, it is unrealistic to expect athletes to refrain from using steroids without concerted education and interventional efforts from sports authorities. The most rational approach for an institution to adopt is a "no-use" policy, which is endorsed by administration, the coaches, and the players. Without the full support of the coach, a "no-use" policy is doomed to failure. In both education and treatment, the greatest challenge for the physician and other professionals is challenging the cognitive-belief system of the athletes (and frequently the coaches). Typical beliefs encountered in this area include, "everyone is using them," "the risk is worth it," "I will only achieve my goals by using drugs," "my performance is much better on steroids," and "steroids have no negative side effects." All these beliefs can and must be vigorously challenged if the health-care profession is to make any impact on this problem. Education efforts must balance information between the demonstrated benefits of the drug to performance and the serious consequences of use, including the long-term health issues, the overreliance on drugs as a crutch for achieving performance gains, the possible loss of career by detection, and the increasing information on the negative psychological side effects (e.g., Pope and Katz, 1990).

Alcohol abuse is the most common substance abuse problem encountered in athletics. A team or institution needs to have a clearly defined policy stating what steps will be taken to treat an athlete with a known problem. Again, education is invaluable in increasing the awareness of alcohol abuse as a behavioral problem that can be treated, rather than as a behavior that is always punished, without support for the punished individual. The physician can be instrumental in helping to shape the *philosophy* of the education program adopted and is usually the pivotal person in the development of a treatment-referral team. All key personnel in the sports setting need to know how to make a referral and what treatment options are available to the athlete. Prevention efforts must include education, but information alone has been shown to be ineffective in changing drinking patterns in college athletes. Instead, prevention programs must be multimodal, including a variety of components. Effectiveness is increased if the education efforts are long term, if the athlete's involvement in the program is emphasized (for example, athletes in college can be trained to be peer educators for high school athletes), and if coping skills are taught in the program. Much excellent information exists on the treatment and prevention of alcohol abuse in young people and in athletes (Asken, 1988; Carr, 1990; Miller and Hester, 1980, 1989).

Treatment of addiction and abuse of illegal drugs such as cocaine and marijuana should follow similar guidelines to treatment of alcoholism, especially with regard to the planned nature of the institutional response to the problem. Treating physicians and therapists need to be aware of special considerations related to these drugs, however. Information in this area is contained in Sheppard (1983) and Washton and Gold (1987).

SUMMARY

This chapter highlights some of the important psychological considerations in the work of the team physician. An awareness of some simple guidelines in the management of injury, the treatment of behavioral problems, and the referral of an athlete to a psychologist can increase the effectiveness of the physician's role with a team. Clinical issues in sport psychology are dealt with in more detail in works such as May and Asken (1987) and Nideffer (1981). This chapter does not deal with the use of psychological techniques to help the performance of athletes (e.g., visualization, stress management). Such issues have been excellently covered by Orlick (1990) and Williams (1986).

RECOMMENDED READING

Asken MJ: *Dying to Win: The Athlete's Guide to Safe and Unsafe Drugs in Sport.* Washington: Acropolis Books, 1988.
Borgen JS and Corbin CB: Eating disorders among female athletes. *Phys Sportsmed* 15:89–95, 1987.
Borysenko J: Stress, coping, and the immune system. In *Behavioral Health: A Handbook*

of Health Enhancement and Disease Prevention. Edited by JD Matarazzo, SM Wiss, JA Herd, NE Miller and SH Weiss. New York: John Wiley and Sons, 1984, pp. 241–260.

Burckes-Miller ME and Black DR: Male and female college athletes: prevalence of anorexia nervosa and bulimia nervosa. *Athlete Training* 23:137–140, 1988.

Carr C: Effective components of alcohol education and abuse prevention. Unpublished manuscript. Colorado Springs, CO: United States Olympic Committee, 1990.

Glaser R, Rin J, Sheridan J, Festal R, Stout J, Speicher C, Pinsky D, Kotur M, Post A, Beck M and Kiecolt-Glaser J: Stress-related immune suppression: Health implications. *Brain Behav Immun* 1:7–20, 1987.

Gordon S: Sport psychology and the injured athlete: a cognitive-behavioral approach to injury response and injury rehabilitation. *Sci Periodical Res Technol Sport* 1–11, 1986.

Heyman S: Psychoneuroimmunology: implications for clinical practice. In *Innovations in Clinical Practice. Vol. 8.* Edited by PA Keller and SR Heyman. Sarasota, FL: Professional Resource Exchange, 1989.

Holmes HT and Rahe RH: The social readjustment rating scale. *J Psychosom Med* 11:213–218, 1967.

Kennedy S, Kiecolt-Glaser R: Immunologic consequences of acute and chronic stressors: mediating role of interpersonal relationships. *Br J Med Psychol* 61:77–85, 1988.

Locke EA and Latham GP: The application of goal setting to sports. *J Sport Psychol* 7:205–222, 1985.

Locke EA and Latham GP: *Goal Setting: A Motivational Technique that Works.* Englewood Cliffs, NJ: Prentice-Hall, 1984.

May JR and Asken MJ: *Sport Psychology: The Psychological Health of the Athlete.* New York: PMA Publishing, 1987.

Miller WR and Hester RK: *The Handbook of Alcoholism Treatment Approaches: Effective Alternatives.* New York: Pergamon Press, 1989.

Miller WR and Hester RK: Treating the problem drinker: modern approaches. In *The Addictive Behaviors: Treatment of Alcoholism, Drug Abuse, Smoking, and Obesity.* Edited by WR Miller. Oxford: Pergamon Press, 1980.

Morgan WP, Brown DR, Raglin JS, O'Connor PJ and Ellickson KA: Psychological monitoring of overtraining and staleness. *Br J Sports Med* 21:107–114, 1987.

Nideffer RM: *The Ethics and Practice of Applied Sport Psychology.* Ann Arbor, MI: Mouvement Publications, 1981.

Norris PA: Clinical psychoneuroimmunology: strategies for self-regulation of immune system responding. 1989.

Orlick T: *In Pursuit of Excellence, 2nd Ed.* Champaign, IL: Leisure Press, 1990.

Pope HG and Katz DL: Homicide and near-homicide by anabolic steroid users. *J Clin Psychiatry* 51:28–31, 1990.

Selye H: The general adaptation syndrome and the disease process. *J Clin Endocrinol* 6:117–230, 1946.

Sheppard M: Development of a cannabis education program. *J Drug Educ* 13:115–117, 1983.

Washton AM and Gold MS (eds): *Cocaine: A Clinician's Handbook.* New York: Guilford Press, 1987.

Weinberg R, Bruya L, Garland H and Jackson A: Effects of goal difficulty and positive reinforcement on endurance performance. *J Sport Exerc Psychol* 12:144–156, 1990.

Wiese DM and Weiss MR: Psychological rehabilitation and physical injury: implications for the sportsmedicine team. *Sport Psychologist* 1:318–330, 1987.

Williams J: (Ed.). *Applied Sport Psychology.* Palo Alto, CA: Mayfield, 1986.

Yukelson D: Psychology of sport and the injured athlete. *Clinics in Physical Therapy.* Edited by DB Bernhardt. New York: Churchill Livingston, 1986, pp. 175–195.

MEDICAL MANAGEMENT OF ENDURANCE EVENTS: INCIDENCE, PREVENTION, AND CARE OF CASUALTIES

Bruce H. Jones and William O. Roberts

Over the last decade mass-participation endurance events such as marathons, triathlons, cross-country ski races, and bicycle road races have gained tremendous popularity. This chapter discusses the incidence and distribution of casualties at mass-participation endurance events and how this information can be used in organizing and planning prevention and treatment strategies for these events.

From a medical perspective mass-participation endurance events can be viewed as potential mass-casualty situations. Each type of endurance event has unique risks, but these events also share many common hazards and the approach to medical management is similar. The casualties at such events occur over a short period of time in a concentrated area, so careful planning is required to manage their care adequately.

Adequate advanced planning to prevent and treat casualties at mass participation endurance events requires information. Sound planning requires knowledge of the incidence and types of casualties that are likely to be encountered at a particular event. Medical organizers and staff also need to be familiar with the impact of environmental, biomechanical, and physiologic factors on the health and performance of event participants. Unfortunately, for many endurance events reliable information upon which to base preventive strategies, treatment protocols and medical logistics is either unavailable or scanty. Ultimately, the best information for future planning is information from the specific event being planned.

PURPOSE OF THE MEDICAL CARE SYSTEM

The primary purpose of the medical-care system at endurance events is to prevent serious injury and illness that might result in prolonged disability or death of participants. The prevention of all race-associated medical casualties is unrealistic because the nature of physical exertion under varied environmental conditions dictates that injuries will occur.

The event medical team is responsible for designing strategies to prevent injury and to identify, treat, and transfer casualties to minimize disabilities and fatalities. A properly functioning race medical system relieves local hospitals of the burden of masses of minor casualties. Serious casualties, however, should be evacuated to hospitals for definitive care. Tertiary care of serious casualties should not be an objective of the event's medical team. Although some race medical directors prefer treating all casualties at the race site, this is often impractical and unwise, unless emergency room transfer is not an option. Definitive treatment of serious casualties such as "heat stroke," myocardia infarction, and fractured limbs requires monitoring and diagnostic testing that usually cannot be provided at a race field hospital. Priorities for prevention and treatment protocols should be based on the frequency and potential severity of anticipated casualties.

INCIDENCE AND RISKS OF CASUALTIES

Estimates of casualty risks associated with mass-participation events are tabulated in Table 28–1. It is clear from available data that the incidence of casualties may vary widely even for the same type of event depending on a variety of factors. The factors having the greatest impact on the risks associated with endurance events are the distance of the event, the likely environmental conditions (temperature, humidity, wind speed, and solar radiation), and the type of event. The risk of constitutional complaints associated with cold exposure such s hypothermia and frostbite increases as temperatures decrease below an undefined critical temperature. Hypothermia occurs in distance runners at temperatures as high as 70° F (21° C) during and following marathon events.

The distance of an event has a significant impact on casualty rates at endurance events. For running events of marathon distance (42 km, 26.2 mi) or longer, the incidence of race casualties can be expected to be as much as 4 to 5 times higher than a shorter event of half marathon length or less held under similar environmental con-

TABLE 28–1. Range of Risks (%) of Participants of Endurance Events Becoming Casualties Needing First Aid or Medical Care

Type of Endurance Event (Distance of Event)	Environmental Risk* (Range of Risks, %)		
	Low (<65° F)	to	Moderate (65–73° F)
Running			
Marathons (42 km, 26.2 miles)	5		20
Road races (less than 21 km or 13.1 miles)	1		5
Triathlons			
Short (51 km, 31.6 miles: swim, bike, run)	2		5
Long, Ironman (225 km,139 miles: swim, bike, run)	15		30
Bicycle races (variable distances)		5(±4)†	

* Environmental risks based on ACSM guidelines.
† Estimates based on limited data.

ditions. Casualties at longer triathlons occur at similarly higher rates compared to shorter ones. Although data are limited or absent for other endurance events, it is reasonable to assume that casualty rates would be higher for longer events. This dose-response relationship between duration or distance of events and the incidence of casualties makes intuitive sense.

For running events it is well known that the incidence of heat injuries increases predictably as the ambient temperature increases. Figure 28–1 illustrates the high predictability of casualties at the Boston Marathon as a function of ambient temperature. At Boston all levels of race casualties from "dropouts" to those requiring intravenous fluids increase as temperature increases. The incidence of casualties in moderately warm weather can be expected to be two to five times higher than for cool weather, depending on factors such as previous warm weather, the fitness level of participants, and other such factors. Heat-associated casualty rates at other types of endurance events can be expected to increase in similar fashion.

Converse to heat injuries, the risk of complaints associated with exposure to cold weather, such as hypothermia and frostbite, probably increases as temperatures decrease. Hypothermia has been documented to occur with temperatures as high as 70° F (21° C). However, hyperthermia is not unusual in marathon runs when it is 40° F (4.5° C). Thus several points must be kept in mind when planning for endurance events when possible temperatures can range from cold to hot: heat-related casualty rates will increase as temperatures increase; cold injury rates will increase as temperatures decrease; and both types of injury will occur on the same day at the same event over a broad range of temperatures.

The type of event also has a large effect on the incidence and severity of casualties. The incidence of casualties is likely to be high and the relative severity of the casualties greater in an "ironman" triathlon competition than for a running event such as a marathon. Table 28–2 compares the overall incidence of casualties from the Boston Marathon with those from the Hawaii "Ironman" Triathlon. Although the overall incidence of casualties is only about twice as high for the triathlon as for the marathon, the incidence of those receiving intravenous therapy is about eight times as high. Such information is important in planning because it suggests that the triathlon casualties are more likely to require intensive care and thus has implications for staffing and supply requirements.

Knowledge of the specific types and relative frequency of casualties is important to medical planning. The types and frequency of casualties affect the focus of preventive strategies, the skills of staff recruited, and the inventory of supplies provisioned. The types of casualties likely to be experienced in association with an endurance event can be divided into three general categories: medical conditions, musculoskeletal injuries, and dermatologic complaints. A generic list of likely casualties associated with endurance events

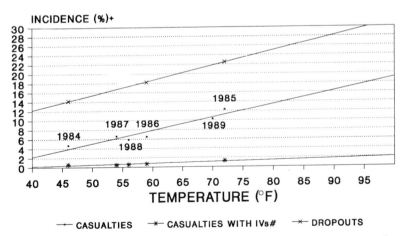

FIG. 28–1. Incidence of casualties and dropouts versus temperature on race day at the Boston Marathon, 1984 to 1989. Unpublished data. Incidence = (casualties/starters) × 100.

TABLE 28–2. Risk of Casualties and Need for Intravenous Fluid Therapy (IV) Associated With a Marathon and a Triathlon

Variable	Marathon[1]		Triathlon[2]	
	1984	**1985**	**1985**	**1986**
Temp. Dry Bulb	46° F	71° F	*	*
Starters (N)	6142	5038	1018	1039
Casualties (n)	290	596	192	249
Risk of casualties (% = n/N × 100)	4.7%	11.8%	17.7%	23.4%
IVs Started (n)	23	60	83	106
Risk (%) of IVs (% = no. IVs/N × 100)	0.4%	1.2%	8.1%	10.2%

[1] Adapted from unpublished data from the Boston Marathon.
[2] From data reported on the Ironman Triathlon in Hawaii by RH Laird in *Report of the Ross Symposium: Medical Coverage of Endurance Athletic Events.* Columbus, OH: Ross Laboratories, 1988, pp. 83–86.
* Temperatures not reported for specific year, but usual range is between 72 and 82° F.

is presented in Table 28–3. Tables 28–4 and 28–5 compare the incidence and relative frequency of common injuries from several road racing, triathlon, biking, and cross-country ski competitions.

Potentially serious medical complaints account for the majority of the casualties seen at marathons. At shorter running events minor musculoskeletal and traumatic injuries predominate (see Table 28–4). Available data indicate that serious musculoskeletal injuries account for a greater percentage of casualties associated with events such as cross-country ski races, bicycle races, and triathlons (see Table 28–5). The higher speeds achieved by participants who are skiing or biking increase not only the risk of injury, but also the severity of injuries. Planning for ski, bike, and triathlon races must consider the high incidence of musculoskeletal injuries and the risk of head injury. Data such as these reinforce the need for casualty data for specific types of events.

The most common and potentially serious medical complaints associated with all endurance events are caused or exacerbated by dehydration, metabolic disturbances, and impaired temperature regulation and may result in collapse. Casualties with symptoms of collapse on any given day may be hyperthermic, normothermic, or hypothermic over a wide range of ambient temperatures. Collapse is characterized by symptoms such as exhaustion, headache, lightheadedness, confusion, or nausea, and signs including vomiting, diarrhea, uncoordinated gait, muscle spasms, disorientation, inappropriate or combative behavior, and loss of consciousness. A common sign of collapse is the inability to walk without assistance. The core temperature determines whether a particular casualty is labeled hyper-, hypo-, or normothermic. All three types of collapse may occur at the same event on any given day.

At the Twin Cities Marathon over a period of 3 years, run at temperatures between 40 and 55° F (4.4 to 12.8° C), 81 cases of moderate-to-severe collapse were documented. Of these cases, 4.5% were hyperthermic, 68.0% were normothermic, and 27.2% were hypothermic. At the Boston Marathon 80 cases of collapse were observed on a single day when the temperature was 72° F. Of these 80 cases, 47.5% were hyperthermic, 47.5% were normothermic, and 5.0% were hypothermic. Thus, the medical team at many endurance events must be prepared to treat both hyper- and hypothermia.

Several low-frequency but severe conditions are of concern to medical-care providers at endurance events. These include cardiac arrest, severe asthmatic attack, and allergic or anaphylactic reaction. In our experience, only 1 cardiac arrest has occurred among approximately 100,000 starters over 8 years at the Twin Cities Marathon and Boston Marathon. At the "City to Surf" run in Australia, 3 cardiac arrests were documented among 145,000 starters over a 7-

---

TABLE 28–3. Casualties Likely to Occur in Association With Mass-Participation Endurance Events

---

Constitutional Conditions (Medical Complaints)

1. Hyperthermic collapse (temperature above normal, with symptoms and signs of collapse)
2. Hypothermic collapse (temperature below normal with signs of collapse)
3. Normothermic collapse/exhaustion (temperature normal with symptoms and signs of collapse)
4. Muscle cramps
5. Frostbite, emersion foot
6. Cardiac arrest
7. Asthma, and allergic/anaphylactic reactions
8. Other constitutional complaints

Musculoskeletal/Traumatic Injuries

1. Serious musculoskeletal injuries (fractures, dislocations, severe sprains, etc.)
2. Minor musculoskeletal injuries (mild sprains, strains, inflammations etc.)
3. Contusions
4. Head injuries/concussions
5. Other injuries

Dermatologic Conditions (Topical Complaints)

1. Abrasions/lacerations
2. Blisters
3. Chafing
4. Frostnip

TABLE 28–4. Average Incidence of Casualties (Number of Casualties/ 100 Starters) and Distribution (Average Percentage of Total Casualties) of Constitutional (Medical), Musculoskeletal, and Topical Complaints Associated with Running Events

Variable	Event		
	Road Race[1]	Road Race[2]	Marathon[3]
Distance	14 km	14 km	42 km
Years	1976–1979	1978–1984	1985–1987
Temperature (range)	48–59° F	53–64° F	56–72° F
Incidence of casualties	1.6/100	1.5/100	7.6/100
Distribution	(%)	(%)	(%)
		(% Total Casualties)	
Hyperthermia	10.5	9.0	4.9
Hypothermia	—	—	1.2
Collapse, exhaustion	—	13.0	10.7
Muscle cramps	3.6	(4.0)	31.2
Other medical	—	—	26.1
Total % Medical	14.1	26.0	74.1
Major musculoskeletal	0.7	0.7	0.1
Minor musculoskeletal	19.1	18.2	3.2
Lacerations/abrasions	9.9	9.7	—
Other musculoskeletal	4.5	—	7.2
Total % Musculoskeletal	34.2	29.3	10.5
Blisters	20.5	14.8	15.5
Chafing	31.2	24.0	—
Other topical	—	5.9	—
Total % Topical	51.7	38.8	15.5
Total %	100.0	100.0	100.0

1. Richards R, et al.: Reducing hazards in the Sydney Sun City-to-Surf Run, 1971–1979. *Med J Aust* 2:453–457, 1979.
2. Richards R, et al.: Exertion-related heat exhaustion and other medical aspects of the City-to-Surf Fun Runs, 1978–1984. *Med J. Aust* 8:799–805, 1984.
3. Unpublished data from Boston Marathon, 1985–1987.

TABLE 28–5. Average Incidence of Casualties (Number of Casualties/
100 Starters) and Distribution (Average Percentage
of Total Casualties) of Constitutional (Medical),
Musculoskeletal, and Topical Complaints Associated
with Cross-Country Skiing, Bicycle, and Triathlon Races

| | Event | | |
Variable	Cross-Country Skiing[1,2]	Bicycling[3]	Triathlon[4]
Distance	55 km		51 km
Years	1984	1983–1986	1984–1986
Temperature (range)	26° F	—	65–89° F
Incidence of casualties	4.4/100	6.4/100	3.1/100
Distribution	**(%)**	**(%)**	**(%)**
		(% Total Casualties)	
Hyperthermia	—	—	19.7
Hypothermia	15.5	—	9.6
Collapse, exhaustion	—	—	—
Muscle cramps	17.3	—	13.1
Other medical	—	—	7.6
Total % Medical	32.6	25.0	50.0
Major musculoskeletal	12.6	16.0	—
Minor musculoskeletal	—	6.0	16.2
Lacerations/abrasions	53.5	48.0	25.8
Head injuries	1.1	5.0	—
Total % Musculoskeletal	67.4	75.0	42.0
Blisters	—	—	8.0
Total % Topical			8.0
Total %	100.0	100.0	100.0

1. Gannon DM, et al.: The emergency care network of a ski marathon. *Am J Sports Med* 13:316–320, 1985.
2. Murphy P: Treating the wounded and the weary at a large cross-country ski marathon. *Phys Sports Med* 15:170–183, 1987.
3. McLennan JG, et al.: Accident prevention in competitive cycling. *Am J. Sports Med* 13:316–320, 1985.
4. Weinberg S: The Chicago Bud Light Triathlon. In *Report of the Ross Symposium: Medical Coverage of Endurance Athletic Events.* Columbus, OH: Ross Laboratories, 1988, pp. 74–78.

year period. This suggests that the occurrence of cardiac arrest in distance running events is rare, probably affecting less than 1 individual of 50,000 starters. Status asthmaticus and severe allergic reactions appear to occur with similar rarity.

Whereas medical planning of endurance events must include preparation to initiate care and stabilization of cardiac arrests and other emergencies, it makes the most sense to plan and arrange for rapid transfer of these athletes to nearby hospitals for definitive care. In some circumstances, this may require advanced life support with helicopter evacuation. Similar advice is appropriate for traumatic injuries such as fractures and head injuries. Splints and spinal stabilization devices should be available at the race site, but transfer to a facility that can perform x-rays and provide definitive care will be required.

Planning for medical care at a mass-participation event should begin with an estimate of the likely number of casualties to be treated. To estimate the number of casualties for an event one needs to know the number of participants anticipated and the expected incidence (risk, n/100) of casualties for the likely environmental conditions. Plots such as those of casualties versus temperature for the Boston Marathon (Fig. 28–1) or equations can be used to predict casualty rates. The estimated number of casualties can be calculated by multiplying the number of participants by the expected incidence of casualties. Once an estimate of the number of casualties, intravenous infusions to be started, and other factors has been made, projections of adequate staffing, supply, and equipment requirements can be established.

For initial planning of a new event, crude estimates of the number of casualties can be based on data from the existing literature and experiences from other events of the same distance. Once medical record, race participant, and weather data are available for more than 2 years when there was a difference in temperature, accurate estimates of the future number of casualties can be made (see Fig. 28–1). Race- or event-specific casualty data are the most valid foundation for estimating future rates because the ages and gender of participants and terrain of a source have a significant inpact on overall rates and these vary from event to event.

STAFF AND EQUIPMENT REQUIREMENTS

For the first-time race medical director, it is difficult to know how to estimate staff and supply requirements. Some general guidelines are provided by documents such as the American College

TABLE 28–6. Medical Staff and Bed (Cot/Stretcher) Requirements per Thousand Starters and per Hundred Casualties (Injuries) for Several Mass-Participation Events: Ratios Extrapolated from Footnoted References and the American College of Sports Medicine Guidelines and the Athletic Congress of the United States Guidelines for Running Races in Hot Weather

Event Type	Medical Staff (MD, RN, DPM, PT, AT, etc.)		Total Med. Staff (Med. Staff + Med. Support Staff)		Beds/Cots (Stretchers)	
	n/1000 Starters	n/100 Injured	n/1000 Starters	n/100 Injured	n/1000 Starters	n/100 Injured
Sydney[1] 14-km run	4/1000	24/100	7/1000	44/100	3/1000	18/100
Boston[2] 42-km run marathon	24/1000	24/100	39/1000	39/100	33/1000	33/100
Twin Cities[3] 42-km run marathon	6/1000	20/100	14/1000	50/100	7/1000	25/100
London[4] 42-km run	5/1000	17/100	20/1000	67/100	8/1000	25/100
Hawaii[5] triathlon	140/1000	46/100	—	—	—	—
Canada[6] 2225-km triathlon	92/1000	28/100	—	—	15/1000	8/100
Wisconsin[7] 55-km XC-ski race	7/1000	15/100	13/1000	29/100	—	—
ACSM[8]	6/1000	—	—	—	10/1000	—
TAC[9]	4–6/1000	—	10–12/1000	—	10/1000	—

1. Richards R, et al.: *Med J Aust* 8:799–805, 1984.
2. Boston Marathon unpublished data.
3. Twin Cities Marathon unpublished data.
4. Recommendations of a Consensus Conference: *Br Med J* 288:1355–1359, 1984.
5. Laird RH: In *Report of the Ross Symposium: Medical Coverage of Endurance Athletic Events.* Columbus, OH: Ross Laboratories, 1988, pp. 69–73.
6. Novak D: In *Report of the Ross Symposium: Medical Coverage of Endurance Athletic Events.* Columbus, OH: Ross Laboratories, 1988, pp. 69–73.
7. Gannon DM: *Am J Sports Med* 13:316–320, 1985.
8. ASCM: *Med Sci Sports* 19:529–532, 1987.
9. Robertson WO: *TAC Sports Medicine Manual for Long Distance Running.* Indianapolis: Athletics Congress of the USA.

of Sports Medicine's *Position Stand on the Prevention of Thermal Injuries at Distance Running Events* (1987). Most guidelines prescribe the amount and types of staff and supplies required on the basis of the number of participants or competitors. Ultimately, the number of casualties dictates the personnel and supplies that will be required for an adequate medical delivery system.

Data extrapolated from the published literature on the number of staff employed and beds needed to treat casualties at marathons, triathlons, and ski races are summarized in Table 28–6. Staff and bed ratios per 1000 participants vary widely for road races and other events. When the ratio of medical staff to casualties is calculated, however, the relative range in the number of staff required narrows considerably. This indicates that staffing can be more accurately predicted when based on estimates of casualties.

The experience of endurance events for which published data is available suggest that roughly 25 medical professional staff (physicians, nurses, podiatrists, athletic trainers, etc.) are required for every 100 casualties treated (Table 28–6). Additionally, for every medical professional at least one support staff member is usually necessary to assist with care, to retrieve dry clothing and beverages, and to perform other supportive tasks. With regard to equipment, most events will need to plan on having 20 to 25 beds or cots for every 100 casualties anticipated (Table 28–6). For marathon running events, data from the Boston Marathon indicate that as many as 1 in 10 casualties will require intravenous fluids to aid their recovery (Fig. 28–1). Guidelines such as these at best provide only crude estimates of the medical staffing, equipment, and supply requirements for endurance events. As such they should be used with caution and only until better information is available. After an event has been run several times, it can begin generating its own data on casualties rates, types, and treatments from which accurate estimates of future medical requirements can be made.

PREVENTION AND TREATMENT OF CASUALTIES

In addition to recruiting medical staff and procuring equipment and supplies, medical organizers must develop the policies, protocols, and methods for preventing and treating casualties. Most of what the event medical system does is primary or secondary prevention. Primary preventive measures aim to prevent the occurrence or reduce the incidence of different types of casualties. Secondary preventive strategies are designed to identify casualties early and to treat them before the injuries evolve into more serious disabling or fatal conditions.

With regard to primary preventive strategies, many measures necessary to prevent casualties involve factors over which the medical team does not have exclusive control on race day. For this reason, the race medical director should be involved in the planning of all aspects of race management that have an impact on the risk to participants. Areas into which the medical director should provide input include hazardous environmental conditions, traffic control, and safety aspects peculiar to specific events. Published guidelines do exist for many important aspects of race safety, but the race medical director may also need to establish his or her own safety policy and preventive strategies.

In general, preventive strategies that do not require cooperation from the potential casualties are most likely to succeed. These are termed passive strategies. Strategies that require the cooperation of or a behavioral change from the potential victim are less effective in preventing injuries and are termed active strategies.

For example, both passive and active strategies are employed to prevent hyperthermia at marathons. Passive strategies to limit heat exposure include running the race at a time of year when ambient temperatures are not likely to be too hot and at a time of day when temperatures and radiant energy (sunlight) are lowest. Picking a shaded course with minimum direct sunlight is another passive strategy. Active strategies include suggestions to competitors to slow their race pace if the weather is hot, drink adequate fluids, train adequately prior to racing, and acclimatize to heat before the race. The most effective way to prevent heat injuries is to schedule the race in a cool season during the early part of the day.

Several means can be employed to enhance the effectiveness of active strategies. Primary among these is the enforcement of safety advisories. At some ultramarathon events, fluid balance is deemed to be so important that fluid replacement is mandatory. Fluid replacement is enforced by having ultramarathoners weigh in at scheduled intervals. If their weights fall below a certain percentage of their prerace weight, they are required to rehydrate or drop from the race. Another enforcement strategy relates to training and experience. Although it is not possible to monitor the training of all competitors, it is possible to enforce entrance standards, requiring participants to provide documentation of having completed other events within specified time limits.

Because of the serious threat of heat injuries for running events, formal guidelines have been established to aid in assessing the risk of holding events at various temperatures. The *American College of*

Sports Medicine Position Stand on Prevention of Thermal Injuries During Distance Running (1987) categorizes risks from low to high based on ranges of wet-bulb black-globe (WBGT) temperature readings (Table 28–7). The WBGT readings account for temperature, relative humidity, wind speed, and radiant energy (sunlight) simultaneously. Ambient temperature and humidity are the factors of most concern in warm and hot weather. In general, distance running events, especially the longer ones, should not be scheduled when the anticipated environmental conditions exceed the moderate risk range for heat injury. Guidelines on heat exposure such as those established by the ACSM for running have yet to be established for other events.

In cold weather, risks of hypothermia and frostbite are complicated more by increasing wind speed than by humidity. The Federation Internationale de Ski cancels or postpones Nordic ski events at −20° C (−4° F). Cold-weather endurance events should not be started or continued when the wind chill is below the moderate risk range on a wind-chill chart. In estimating risks associated with cold-weather events, remember that wind chill is exacerbated by the speed at which competitors are traveling. This can be a significant factor on the downhill portions of cross-country ski races and bicycle races. Contingency plans should be established to alter, postpone,

TABLE 28–7 **Level of Risk for Thermal Casualties by Wet-Bulb Black-Globe Temperature (WBGT) Range as Suggested by the American College of Sports Medicine, and Comparable Dry Bulb (Ambient) Temperatures (Tdb) at Different Percents of Relative Humidity (%RH) with Color Codes for Each Category of Risk Provided**

Level of Risk (Hyperthermia)	WBGT (Tdb at %RH = 100%)	Temp db %RH = 75%	Temp db %RH = 50%	Color Code (Flag)
High	73–82° F (23–28° C)	77–85° F (25–29° C)	82–92° F (28–33° C)	Red
Moderate	65–73° F (18–23° C)	68–77° F (20–25° C)	75–82° F (24–28° C)	Amber
Low	<65° F (<18° C)	<68° F (<20° C)	<75° F (<24° C)	Green
Low (with risk of Hypothermia)	<50° F (<10° C)	— —	— —	White

See American College of Sports Medicine Position Stand: Prevention of thermal injuries during distance running. *Med Sci Sports* 19: 529–533, 1987.

or cancel any event if conditions become hazardous because of severe heat, cold, rain, ice, or lightning.

Another source of serious casualties associated with endurance events is collision with motor vehicles, pedestrians, and other objects on the race course. This is particularly true for bicycle and cross-country ski races where speed is a greater factor. Good traffic control and course design can minimize these hazards. Steep downhill slopes at the start and finish should be avoided. Downhill stretches and narrow roads can be particularly hazardous in larger events when masses of competitors are trying to get off to a fast start. Sharp turns at the bottom of downhill stretches can be especially dangerous in bike, ski, and wheelchair races. Obstacles such as trees and utility poles near the course or at the bottom of slopes should be avoided.

Some endurance events require special safety regulations that should be enforced. Wearing approved hardshell helmets should be requirement for participation in all bicycle and wheelchair events. Requiring wet suits for the swim portion of triathlons when water temperatures are cold may help reduce the incidence of hypothermia.

Safety policies and preventive strategies for mass-participation endurance events should target conditions for prevention on the basis of their frequency and severity and the modifiability of associated risk factors. Priorities for prevention should be predicated on sound, scientifically valid information for the specific event being managed or similar events. Caution should be exercised in implementing strategies that have not been proven to be effective, since many hypothetically sound preventive strategies do not work in practice. Although safety of participants is a primary concern, instituting measures in the name of safety that turn out to be ineffective only erodes the credibility of and confidence in the medical organization and medical professionals. In this regard, it is worth remembering that passive preventive strategies that do not require individuals to modify their behavior are more likely to be effective, especially in the near term.

Although primary prevention is important, the major focus of the event medical team is secondary prevention or treatment. The objectives of secondary prevention are the early detection of injury or illness and the provision of intervention to stop progression of the condition before irreversible injury or disability occurs. To meet these objectives the organization of medical operations should begin well in advance of the event, and special triage and treatment protocols should be devised for both usual and worst-case conditions. Elements of medical operations are outlined in Table 28–8. Planning should make provisions for not only triage and treatment of casualties but also transportation, communications, and records.

TABLE 28–8. Functional Elements of the Race Medical Organization

1. Identification and triage of casualties
2. Transportation of casualties to appropriate treatment facilities quickly
    aid stations
    field hospitals
    local hospital emergency rooms
3. Treatment of casualties promptly at all levels of care
    first-aid stations
    race field hospital(s)
    hospital emergency rooms
4. Communication
    with the race medical organization
    with the race administration
    with transportation and ambulance services
    with hospital emergency rooms
5. Maintenance of medical records
    to document the occurrence of casualties for medicolegal purposes
    to assist in planning and organization of future events
    to monitor the effectiveness and treatment protocols of preventive strategies

The first concern of medical care is identification of casualties. A system of spotters may be necessary to facilitate early identification and treatment of casualties along the course. Spotters should be located at and between aid stations, particularly over the later portions of the race course where casualties are most likely to occur. Spotters should be able to communicate with the transportation and treatment elements of the medical organization.

In warm weather spotters and race officials should be alert for participants who develop hyperthermia and become obviously symptomatic. These casualties may appear visibly weak and ataxic, they may be visibly disoriented, and they may have difficulty staying on the course. On questioning, the responses of such individuals may be confused, inappropriate, or belligerent. In cool weather the slower participants and those hobbled by injury may not be exercising at levels adequate to maintain a metabolic rate to sustain their normal body temperature, and they may become hypothermic. The symptoms of hypothermia are similar to those of hyperthermia. In addition, hypothermic casualties may appear lethargic, delirious, or intoxicated and they may or may not be shivering. Spotters and other race officers should be educated to recognize the significance of these symptoms and signs for thermal casualties in both cool and warm weather. Because the judgment of such casualties may be impaired, the race medical director may want to reserve the right to disqualify individuals who are at risk of serious harm if they continue.

Transportation of casualties and "dropouts" can take many forms.

On the race course ambulances and vans can convey injured participants and competitors who have dropped out to an aid station, the field hospital, an emergency room, or simply to the finish area. Near the finish line, field hospital, or aid stations on the course, transportation may be as simple as a shoulder to lean on. Longer events should have an ample supply of stretchers and wheelchairs to transport collapsed participants to the race medical care facilities. Another important element of the medical transportation system is a trail vehicle to pick up the ambulatory casualties and stragglers. Arrangements should be made in advance to have adequate ambulance service to transport serious casualties to local community hospitals.

Identifying casualties in the finish area where most become symptomatic requires special organization. A triage team should be located in the chutes and postchute areas. Spotters may be needed in the changing areas, and "sweep teams" may be necessary to comb the finish area for runners who collapse after they complete the race. It is not uncommon for runners who finished the race feeling strong to become dizzy and even faint 10 to 20 minutes after completing the race. In cool weather participants may be unable to maintain normal body temperatures and may begin shivering uncontrollably or may even suffer hypothermia 20 or 30 minutes after finishing, even though they had been warm immediately at the finish line. Competitors may develop severe muscle cramps after marathons in all weather conditions. These leg cramps can be excruciatingly painful and may prevent the individual from walking without assistance. All immediate and delayed casualties should be transported to a treatment facility where they may need IV fluids, active warming or cooling, or energy replacement to facilitate recovery.

It is important to have the medical system of larger and longer events linked by a communications network. Communications are needed to summon help to transport casualties on the course, to warn treatment areas that casualties are being transported, and to make decisions about triage, treatment, and disposition of casualties at outlying areas. Communications should link all elements of the medical-care system: spotters, aid stations, transport vehicles, triage, and the field hospital. The race medical system should also have communications with local ambulance services, hospitals, and police to arrange for evacuation and transfer of casualties to hospital emergency rooms.

The treatment of casualties at endurance events usually takes place at two types of facilities, aid stations, and larger field hospitals. The aid stations along the course are the front line of the medical treatment system. These stations should provide first aid and comfort measures along with appropriate shelter from environmental exposure in hot and cold weather. Aid stations should be located every 2 to 3 miles along the course and perhaps more frequently in the last half of longer events. Each aid station should be staffed by at least one individual capable of administering first aid and basic life-support measures, several other individuals to provide assistance, and a communications volunteer. Aid stations should have radio communication with the finish line and emergency transport systems. When the last runner has passed the earlier stations, it may be helpful to transport the staff to later stations where more casualties are likely to occur.

The primary race treatment facility should be located in the finish area, 50 to 100 yards beyond the finish line, because a majority of the casualties collapse beyond the actual finish point. The field hospital should provide shelter appropriate for the existing environmental conditions. Medical care actually begins at the finish line where trained medical personnel are needed to triage and transport the competitors who collapse shortly after completing an event. A second line of triage should take place just inside the entrance to the field hospital. All casualties entering the race treatment area should be triaged to specific areas within the facility depending on the type of care they need. The medical treatment area can be divided into skin care, musculoskeletal care, medical care, and possible evacuation sections to facilitate the rapid evaluation and treatment of casualties. Staff with appropriate skills should be assigned to specialty areas in proportion to the estimated numbers of different types of casualties.

At all endurance events, medical staff should be alert for and knowledgeable about thermal injuries (hyperthermic, hypothermic, and normothermic exercise-associated collapse). Individuals in a state of collapse may be nauseated or vomiting. They are characteristically confused, disoriented, or stuporous and many have severe muscle cramps. Persistent tachycardia and hypotension are strong indicators of a need for rehydration. Although some debate exists about the role of dehydration in physiologic collapse of competitors, most competitors in events of marathon length or longer are dehydrated.

A common focus of treatment for all cases of collapse should be adequate hydration. The administration of 500 to 2000 ml IV fluids is advisable in all prostrate casualties with symptoms and signs of collapse who are unable to take fluids by mouth within 15 minutes of finishing. Severe muscle cramps are probably due to metabolic and electrolyte imbalances and also appear to respond quickly to the administration of IV fluids. Our experience is that most collapsed athletes recover quickly after the administration of 500 to 1500 ml 5% dextrose and .5 normal saline (D5 ½ NS). Usually recovery occurs within half an hour of fluid replacement. Individuals who do not respond to the administration of 1000 ml IV fluids or who do not improve after an hour of observation should be considered for evacuation to nearby hospitals. In events of 4 hours duration or longer, it may be advisable to administer normal saline because of the potential risk of exacerbating hyponatremia, which is documented to occur in ultradistance events. Casualties should not be allowed to leave the medical area until they are alert, well oriented, and can walk without assistance.

Collapsed athletes should be treated for hyperthermia or hypothermia as indicated by their rectal temperature. Oral temperatures are unreliable after vigorous exercise and may read in the hypothermic range in persons who are actually hyperthermic. The primary emphasis should be placed on identifying victims of collapse who are hyperthermic. Rapid cooling of core temperature to 102° F (38.9° C) may be crucial in preventing progression of thermal damage to vital organs such as the brain, liver, and kidneys. Great concern must be taken with any victim with temperatures above 105° F (40.6° C) or who demonstrates signs of central nervous system dysfunction. Active cooling should be initiated on casualties with high rectal temperature and for CNS signs. One simple means of lowering temperatures is to place ice packs over the major arteries in the groin, axilla, and neck. Tub immersion techniques may also be considered for hot-weather races, but are cumbersome.

Hypothermic casualties of distance running events are not usually severely hypothermic. Rectal temperatures are usually in the range of 90 to 95° F. The primary care needed for recovery of such mild casualties is usually shelter in a warm place, dry clothes, and assistance with walking. More severe cases of hypothermia are a concern in skiing and cold-water swimming events. Severe hypothermic casualties should be handled gently because of the potential for precipitating cardiac arrhythmias. Rewarming measures should be initiated, but should not delay prompt transfer to an emergency facility for active rewarming and cardiac monitoring.

Although thermal injuries are common concerns for all mass participation endurance events, other important types of casualties deserve attention depending upon the type of event and its duration. As mentioned, traumatic injuries occur frequently and pose a serious problem for participants and medical care providers at biking and cross-country skiing events. Race medical directors and staff must identify potential sources and types of casualties likely to occur at their event. Such information should be the foundation for developing preventive strategies, protocols for triage and treatment of casualties, recruiting appropriate staff, and procuring sufficient equipment and supplies.

MAINTENANCE AND UTILIZATION OF MEDICAL RECORDS

The best data for event planning are the documentation of past experience at a particular event through the use of medical records. The simplest means of ensuring that records are maintained on all casualties is to attach a medical record to each casualty as he or she enters the medical area and to retrieve a completed record from each casualty exiting the treatment area. Tabulation and summarization of records provides information useful for future planning.

At first glance, maintaining medical records may seem like a simple matter, but it is a complex, energy-intensive endeavor if complete and reliable records are to be maintained. Roughly one medical-records technician is needed for every five or six medical-care personnel. The primary task of these records technicians is to make sure each casualty has a record and to document baseline demographic and administrative information on the record. Medical data—symptoms, signs, diagnosis, treatment, and disposition—are recorded on the record by the medical treatment staff. Recording medical data is facilitated by use of checklist-type records that list the most common symptoms, signs, and diagnoses encountered at the event. Space on the record should be available for documenting observations and information not listed in the check-off sections.

Medical records are extremely important from several perspectives. Medical records serve as medicolegal documentation of diagnosis and treatment, help to predict future casualty rates, assist in estimating staff, equipment, and supply requirements, and aid in identification of risk factors for casualties. Medical planning for many mass-participation events is based largely on guesswork. Medical records and race participation data can be utilized to generate good estimates of casualty risks and staff and supply requirements.

SUMMARY

The very nature of competition and prolonged physical exertion dictate that casualties will occur in association with mass-participation endurance events. It is the responsibility of the event's medical organization to prevent and to treat these casualties.

The major objectives of the event's medical organization are primary and secondary injury prevention. The focus of primary prevention is the identification of modifiable risk factors for event-associated injuries and the development of strategies to prevent such injuries. The objective of secondary preventive care is the early identification of casualties and the treatment of these to prevent progression of injury and disability.

The medical organization planning should be based on estimates of the numbers and types of casualties likely to occur in association with a particular type of event, under the expected environmental conditions of the race. The best source of information for future planning of an event is past medical and participant data from the specific event itself.

Only over the last decade has medical care become a routine part of large endurance events. Experience demonstrates that it is possible to provide mass care at such events. One of the next challenges for race medical care systems is to develop methods of maintaining complete and accurate medical records. The information in medical data bases can then begin to provide sound recommendations for the future prevention and treatment of casualties.

RECOMMENDED READING

Adner MM, Scarlet JJ, Casey J, Robison W and Jones BH: The Boston Marathon medical care team: ten years of experience. *Phys Sportsmed* 16:99–106, 1988.

American College of Sports Medicine: Position Stand on the Prevention of Thermal Injuries During Distance Running. 1984. *Med Sci Sports* 19:529–533, 1987.

Gannon DM, Derse AR, Bronkema PJ and Primley DM: The emergency care network of a ski marathon. *Am J Sportsmed* 13:316–320, 1985.

Hansen P: Marathon medicine. *Emerg Med* 17:62–90, 1985.

Jones BH, Rock PB, Smith LS, Teves MA, Casey JK, Eddings K, Malkin LH and Matthew WT: Medical complaints after a marathon run in cool weather. *Phys Sportsmed* 13:103–110, 1985.

McLennan JG, McLennan JC and Ungersma J: Accident prevention in competitive cycling. *Am J Sportsmed* 16:266–268, 1988.

Murphy P: Treating the wounded and the weary at a large cross-country ski marathon. *Phys Sportsmed* 15:170–183, 1987.

Richards R and Richards D: Exertion-induced heat exhaustion and other medical aspects of the City-to-Surf Fun Runs, 1978–1984. *Med J Aust* 8:799–805, 1984.

Richards R, Richards D and Whittaker R: Method of predicting the number of casualties in the Sydney City-to-Surf Fun Runs. *Med J Aust* 8:805–808, 1984.

Roberts WO: Exercise-associated collapse in endurance events: a classification system. *Phys Sportsmed* 17:49–55, 1989.

Robertson JW: Medical problems in mass participation runs. *Sports Med* 6:261–270, 1988.

Recommendations of a Consensus Conference: Popular marathons, half marathons, and other long distance runs: recommendation for medical support. *Br Med J* 288:1355–1359, 1984.

Report of the Ross Symposium: Medical Coverage of Endurance Athletic Events. Columbus, OH: Ross Laboratories, 1988.

C H A P T E R   2 9

DRUG USE AND ABUSE*

Richard H. Strauss

Certain drugs and other substances are used by some athletes in an attempt to "get the edge," that is, to improve performance. The taking of such substances (also called doping) is officially condemned by virtually every major sports organization in the world. Nevertheless, the practice persists. In this section, an attempt is made to summarize the effects of several classes of drugs on both athletic performance and health.

Maximal performance depends highly on psychological factors. Administration of a physiologically inert substance may, in fact, help to improve performance if the athlete believes that this is likely. Thus, the placebo effect, rather than a pharmacologic effect, may be responsible for improvements in performance attributed by athletes to substances such as bee pollen and vitamin injections.

ANABOLIC STEROIDS

Testosterone is the natural male hormone produced by the testes in men. The increase in testosterone production at puberty is largely responsible for increased muscle size and strength as well as the appearance of secondary sexual characteristics such as beard growth and sexual maturation. Anabolic steroids are closely related to testosterone in structure and function. The term "anabolic" means "tissue building." These hormones are also masculinizing, or "androgenic," so their full name is anabolic-androgenic steroid hormones.

Anabolic steroids are used by athletes in many sports at all levels who wish to improve their muscular strength—by football players, weight lifters, and even female high school runners. In a study of

* Portions of this chapter adapted from Strauss RH: *Sports Medicine*. Philadelphia: W.B. Saunders, 1984.

male high school seniors, 6.7% admitted to using anabolic steroids at some time. Of these users, 27% did so to improve their physical appearance rather than to improve athletic performance.

Anabolic steroids are generally used in "cycles"—that is, taken for a period such as 8 weeks and then not taken for several weeks or months or taken in lower doses. Up to five types of anabolic steroids may be used simultaneously, a method called "stacking."

MECHANISMS OF ACTION

Anabolic steroids are available as oral or injectable preparations. They travel from the circulation, through cell walls, into the cytoplasm. Cytoplasmic receptors for testosterone and related male hormones exist in different types of cells and determine the cell's response to anabolic steroids by controlling the production of messenger RNA by DNA in the nucleus. In muscle cells, anabolic steroids have been shown to stimulate the production of muscle protein. In addition, anabolic steroids can block the catabolic effect of corticosteroids that are released during stress, thereby decreasing the loss of muscle protein. In addition, both the increased aggression often associated with anabolic steroids and the placebo effect may lead to more strenuous physical training.

In certain cells, male hormones stimulate secondary sex characteristics such as beard growth and thickening of the vocal cords. Once the cytoplasmic receptors are saturated, higher concentrations of anabolic steroids probably have no further physiologic effect. Thus, the huge doses of anabolic steroids currently in use appear to represent overkill.

EFFECTS IN MEN

Do anabolic steroids help to increase muscle size and strength in men? The answer is "yes"—when the individual is performing strenuous strength training concurrently and is well nourished, including sufficient protein. Although anabolic steroids may help to increase hemoglobin concentration, no scientific evidence indicates that they enhance aerobic capacity or endurance.

Do anabolic steroids affect health adversely? The answer is clearly "yes," and these side effects discourage many athletes from using steroids. The use of anabolic steroids results in decreased production of testosterone by the testes. Sperm production falls. A decrease in the size and firmness of testes is observed with extended use of anabolic steroids. These effects appear to be reversible over several months after steroids are stopped. Abnormal sperm may persist for months, so men planning to father a child would be wise to avoid anabolic steroids for a number of months beforehand.

Commonly, sex drive increases when steroids are begun and may decrease to normal or below normal after several weeks of use. When steroids are stopped, sex drive usually falls below normal for several weeks or months until the testes resume production of testosterone.

Human chorionic gonadotropin (HCG) is sometimes injected concurrently with anabolic steroids to prevent testicular atrophy or afterward to promote quicker resumption of testosterone production by the testes.

Gynecomastia develops in a minority of men who use anabolic steroids because a small amount of these androgens are metabolized to estrogens. Gynecomastia appears as a small, firm, tender mass of breast tissue under one or both nipples. Occasionally, the breast tissue is removed surgically for cosmetic reasons, but scarring may be visible.

Acne commonly appears or is made worse with steroid use. Loss of scalp hair and balding are accelerated in men who have inherited a tendency for baldness.

Increased aggressiveness and irritability are common with steroid use. Some athletes consider this an advantage because they "attack the weights" more aggressively. Problems with interpersonal relationships often occur, however. Transient psychotic episodes and criminal activities such as arson and murder have been associated with the use of anabolic steroids in a few cases. Depression sometimes follows the cessation of anabolic steroid use, not only because of possible chemical dependence, but also because the previously high levels of strength and muscularity are difficult to maintain. The user's peer group, and the user himself, respond negatively to such changes.

When anabolic steroids are used, HDL cholesterol decreases in plasma and low-density lipoproteins sometimes increase, suggesting a greater risk for cardiovascular disease. Myocardial infarctions have occurred in a few young men who had used anabolic steroids for several years. Steroid use exacerbates high blood pressure in individuals with hypertensive tendencies.

Liver tumors, both benign and malignant, have been linked with the administration of anabolic steroids as therapy for patients with serious diseases such as aplastic anemia. The 17-alpha-alkylated anabolic (oral) steroids, in particular, were implicated. Peliosis hepatis, in which liver tissue dies and is replaced by blood-filled cysts, also has been observed.

In healthy young athletes who used steroids, two cases of liver cancer (hepatocellular carcinoma) have been reported. In addition, two deaths have occurred from malignant kidney tumors (Wilms' tumor) in steroid users. It is possible that these occurrences were due to chance rather than to steroid use.

Moderate elevations of the common liver-function tests SGOT and SGPT do not necessarily indicate liver disease in persons who are training with heavy weights. Small amounts of these enzymes are released from the stressed skeletal muscles.

The use of shared needles for the injection of anabolic steroids is associated with the transmission of diseases such as hepatitis B and AIDS.

EFFECTS IN WOMEN

Many of the differences in secondary sexual characteristics between men and women are determined by testosterone. Therefore, it is not surprising that women who take anabolic-androgenic steroid hormones gradually develop masculine secondary sexual characteristics. Women athletes who take anabolic steroids do so because they wish to increase their strength or muscle size. Both these effects can occur when women train concurrently with weights. In contrast, women who train with weights but do not take steroids can increase their strength significantly without noticeably increasing muscle size.

Side effects of anabolic steroids in women include growth of facial hair, increased body hair, deepening of the voice, enlargement of the clitoris, and coarsening of the skin. These effects appear to be permanent. Effects that seem to return to normal after the male hormones are stopped include menstrual cessation or irregularity, increased libido, increased aggressiveness, and acne. Menopause may be reached sooner in women who have a long history of anabolic steroid use. Additional long-term risks discussed previously for men also apply to women.

EFFECTS IN BOYS

Teen-age boys often wish to gain strength or weight. The boy who tries anabolic steroids during training may, in fact, increase his strength or weight. This occurs largely because he has accelerated his rate of maturation, reaching a level of muscularity that may well have occurred anyway, but has occurred sooner. The drawback is that if the boy has not reached his full height, he may stunt his growth. Anabolic steroids tend to close the growth plates at the ends of bones sooner than normal, permanently decreasing further growth. In our society, height is an advantage. Most boys do not wish to be shorter than they normally would be.

GROWTH HORMONE

Human growth hormone (HGH, somatotropin) is not a steroid but a polypeptide hormone produced by the pituitary gland. Synthetic growth hormone is now manufactured in several countries and is available on the black market. In the past few years, athletes have injected human growth hormone in an attempt to increase muscular strength. Some users think it is effective and some do not. No scientific studies are available to evaluate this question.

As the supply of synthetic growth hormone becomes more readily available, adults may use sufficient amounts to become acromegalic. In acromegaly, height does not increase because growth plates are fused, but bones and connective tissue thicken so victims can no longer wear their rings or shoes. Facial features become coarser, sometimes grotesque, because of overgrowth of the brow, the jaw, and soft tissues. The heart, lungs, and liver may double in size. Longstanding acromegaly is characterized by muscular weakness, joint laxity, and cardiac disease. Growth hormone is diabetogenic.

During childhood, insufficient quantities of growth hormone result in dwarfism, whereas overproduction causes gigantism. Parents have been known to ask for growth hormone for a child, to make him or her a taller basketball player or a larger football player and thus increase the child's chances for a college scholarship. Although the administration of growth hormone to a child may result in an ultimate increase in height, the questionable safety and ethics of this practice make it inadvisable.

BLOOD DOPING AND ERYTHROPOIETIN

Hemoglobin concentration has been increased artificially by autotransfusion (blood doping) to see whether performance improves. Approximately 900 ml of blood are taken from the subject and frozen as packed red cells 4 to 10 weeks preceding the exercise test or contest. The subject's hemoglobin and training levels return to normal over the intervening time. A day or so before the exercise test, the red blood cells are reinfused into the donor, increasing the hemoglobin concentration. Several controlled studies found that maximal aerobic performance and endurance were increased by this method. Studies using lesser amounts of blood found no such effect.

Athletes in endurance sports, including long-distance running, cross-country skiing, and cycling, have been accused of blood doping but the charges were unsubstantiated because no test exists to detect blood doping. After the 1984 Olympics, however, several members of the United States cycling team admitted to having used blood doping for their Olympic races. These athletes were infused with the blood of other persons, a practice that presents the dangers of transfusion reactions and transmission of diseases such as hepatitis and AIDS.

Erythropoietin is a naturally occurring substance that is produced by the kidneys and acts on the bone marrow to stimulate the production of red blood cells. Recently, synthetic erythropoietin has become available and has been used to treat the anemia associated with chronic kidney disease. Injections of this substance are capable of raising the hemoglobin concentration of healthy individuals well above normal levels. Thus, the effects of blood doping can be achieved without the dangers of transfusion. As the concentration of red blood cells rises, however, the blood becomes more viscous. The dangers of too high a red blood cell concentration are well known from the disease polycythemia. High concentrations can lead to clot formation, stroke, hypertension, and congestive heart failure. Currently, no test exists for erythropoietin doping.

STIMULANTS

The amphetamines constitute a class of central nervous system stimulants that are sympathomimetic and related in structure to epinephrine. They are thought to stimulate the central nervous system by enhancing the release of neurotransmitters, particularly norepinephrine, from nerve terminals. Amphetamines were used as oral preparations during World War II to decrease the feeling of fatigue among military personnel, and since that time these drugs have been used for similar purposes by athletes, students, truck drivers, and the general public. When injected intravenously, amphetamines such as methamphetamine result in intense stimulation of relatively short duration. Methamphetamine is also smoked in a form called "ice."

Most athletes try to get themselves "psyched up" before an important contest. That is, they deliberately stimulate the sympathetic nervous system. A few use oral sympathomimetic drugs in an attempt to boost or sustain performance. The use of amphetamines during games has been recognized as a problem among football players and occurs in other sports in which maximum force or aggression is desired, such as weight lifting, shot-putting, and hockey. Amphetamines also are sometimes used by athletes such as jockeys and wrestlers for appetite suppression during attempts to lose weight.

Do amphetamines help to improve athletic performance? Older literature indicates a small improvement in running, swimming, and weight throwing by athletes using amphetamines in double-blind experiments. More recently, amphetamine use was associated with increased time to exhaustion while running and with increased knee-extension strength among male college athletes. When using amphetamines, athletes sometimes feel that their performances are outstanding, only to find afterward that such was not the case. Such optimism is apparently a result of mood elevation by the drug.

Signs of acute toxicity include restlessness, tremor, confusion, assaultiveness, anorexia, hypertension, and cardiac arrhythmias. At least one death—in a world-class cyclist—has been associated with amphetamine use. Chronic users may become psychologically dependent on the drug.

Cocaine, an alkaloid related to caffeine and nicotine, is used medically as a topical anesthetic and vasoconstrictor, particularly in the upper respiratory tract. When absorbed in sufficient quantities, cocaine also acts as a stimulant of the central nervous system and as a sympathomimetic. The coca leaf has been chewed for centuries by natives of the Andes Mountains to increase endurance and to promote a sense of well-being.

The use of cocaine by professional basketball and football players has received widespread attention. The drug appears to be used not only in an attempt to enhance athletic performance but, also, more often, as part of the individual's life style. Although studies of the effects of cocaine on athletic performance have not been done, the effects probably are similar to those of the amphetamines. Deleterious effects of cocaine include psychosocial problems, dependency, and sometimes damage to the tissue through which the drug is absorbed, such as the nasal mucosa.

Use of cocaine has caused the sudden death of several athletes due to cardiac arrhythmias. The use of crack, a pure form of cocaine that is smoked, is particularly associated with sudden death. When smoked, the drug reaches the blood almost instantly and causes the effects to be sudden and extreme in nature. The intense euphoria reinforces habitual use.

Ephedrine and phenylpropanolamine are sympathomimetic amines that are widely included in nonprescription cold medications as decongestants. They are mild stimulants, have no significant effects on athletic performance at normal doses, and are not often used as ergogenic aids. At high doses, adverse effects may include irritability, tachycardia, and mild hypertension.

Caffeine is a central nervous stimulant found in coffee, tea, and many soft drinks as well as in tablets sold to combat drowsiness. It has been used by runners, cyclists, swimmers, and other athletes to diminish feelings of fatigue. Older literature suggested that caffeine could increase the capacity for muscular work in humans but that motor skills could be affected adversely. More recent evidence has shown that caffeine can improve work production by promoting metabolism of lipids during exercise and thus sparing glycogen in muscle, the loss of which can limit exercise. Toxic effects of caffeine include restlessness, tremor, and irritability. At very high doses, seizures may occur.

DEPRESSANTS

Alcohol has been used by contestants in shooting events in an attempt to decrease intrinsic tremor and improve accuracy. The use of alcohol has been banned in some competitions. Diazepam (Valium) and other tranquilizers also have been used to decrease tremor but are not banned in competition. Alcohol is not generally used by other athletes to improve performance because it impairs judgment and motor skills. The recreational use of alcohol by athletes may create problems and often reflects usage by the athletes' peers.

Beta-adrenergic blockers, such as propranolol, are not depressants but sometimes are used to blunt the "stage fright" or fight-or-flight response associated with sports that require fine motor control such as figure skating, ski jumping, and shooting, as well as musical performances. Beta-blockers can cause a decrease in maximal heart rate, cardiac output, and work capacity and therefore are contraindicated when maximal work is required. Their use is banned in Olympic competition.

Sleeping medications such as the benzodiazepines (e.g., Dalmane) are used occasionally by athletes to induce sleep but are not taken to improve performance directly. The sleep induced by such medications may include a shorter rapid-eye-movement (REM) phase than is normal, and the user may not feel as rested as usual the following day. The drug may have a long enough effect to cause a "hangover" the next day. Thus, individuals should be cautious about experimenting with a sleeping medication the night before an important contest. The user may slip into a cycle of taking a medication to aid sleep and later a stimulant to become aroused in order to perform at a maximal level.

Narcotics degrade judgment and motor skills and are not used to enhance performance. They are banned at some international contests because they may mask significant pain and may contribute to further injury. Antidiarrheal medications that contain a narcotic (e.g., paregoric) should not be used at such contests.

OTHER DRUGS

The common cold has many remedies, none of which work well. Many prescription and over-the-counter cold medications contain both an antihistamine and a sympathomimetic decongestant. Antihistamines have the potential to degrade performance because they cause drowsiness. The decongestants probably do not affect performance but are banned where drug testing is carried out.

Asthmatics who require sympathomimetic bronchodilators may be treated with inhaled albuterol or terbutaline, which are currently allowed at the Olympic Games.

The so-called recreational drugs, such as marijuana and the hallucinogens, have the potential to degrade skills, judgment, and performance. Marijuana has been used occasionally by athletes to combat the boredom of practice.

DRUG CONTROL

Why do athletes take drugs? Because athletes are highly motivated to win, they think that certain drugs may help them to win, and they are willing to risk possible deleterious side effects. The arguments against using drugs fall roughly into the following, sometimes, conflicting, categories:

1. No drugs improve performance.
2. Some drugs improve performance and thus provide an unfair advantage to the user.
3. Such drugs are dangerous to health.
4. Drug use is cheating.

Perhaps the most important aspect of drug control is the education of the athlete. Scare tactics are not useful, but physicians can help their athlete patients to be aware of any potentially harmful side effects of drugs to which they may be exposed.

Techniques of drug testing are too complex to be discussed in this space. Physicians caring for athletes who may be subjected to drug testing should be careful not to prescribe medications that may lead to disqualification, however. In particular, sympathomimetics should be avoided, even in over-the-counter cold remedies, nose drops, and eye drops.

RECOMMENDED READING

Strauss RH: Drugs in sports. In *Sports Medicine*. Edited by RH Strauss. Philadelphia: W.B. Saunders, 1991.

Wadler GI and Hainline B: *Drugs and the Athlete*. Philadelphia: F.A. Davis, 1989.

C H A P T E R 3 0

OVERUSE INJURIES

Angela D. Smith

Overuse injuries are characterized by repeated microtrauma to a region of the musculoskeletal system, causing disruption of the normal tissue structure. An overuse injury begins as a microscopic tear of soft tissue or a microscopic fracture of bone. The injured tissues can heal if the stress that caused the injury is not repeated for a sufficiently long period of time. If sufficient stress is applied again before the microscopic injuries heal, however, then more soft tissue fibers or bony trabeculae are injured. Eventually, the injury may progress to a frank rupture or fracture.

Most sports participants notice overuse injuries of their soft tissues during the inflammatory phase. The painful swelling leads most injured people to decrease their level of activity. If the amount of healing exceeds the amount of new injury over a given period of time, then the injury heals. If there is no decrease in activity level, then the microscopic injuries increase in number and may affect such a large portion of the structure that the injured region cannot function normally. Continued stress may cause complete rupture of the soft tissue structure.

Overuse injuries of the bone may be recognized at an early point in the progression of the injury, when only the periosteum is inflamed. Many athletes do not feel enough discomfort to decrease their activity however. These sports participants do not consult a physician until so may bony trabeculae are disrupted that the bone is structurally weakened.

Almost all overuse injuries from athletic activities eventually resolve if the participant ceases the inciting activities. At best, the injured athlete generally loses training time; however, he or she may be forced to miss a major competitive event or may even develop a permanent disability. It is therefore important for the team physician to understand the factors that may cause overuse injuries in order to help the athlete avoid them. If an athlete does develop an injury from repetitive microtrauma, the team physician should be able to prescribe appropriate limitations of the athlete's activity and design a rehabilitation program tailored to the individual athlete's needs.

CAUSES OF OVERUSE INJURIES

ANATOMIC FACTORS

Congenital Malalignment. Athletes with rotational or angular malalignment of the lower extremities are vulnerable to overuse injuries. Those with increased femoral anteversion (increased inward rotation of the femur, causing the knee to face more medially than usual) have an increased incidence of patellofemoral symptoms. People with excessive genu valgum, or knock-knees, also are vulnerable to patellofemoral pain and medial knee symptoms. Athletes who have excessive genu varum, or bowlegs, are more likely to develop lateral knee pain because the iliotibial band rubs across the bony prominences of the lateral side of the knee.

The shape of the foot and the degree of pronation are also factors in the development of overuse injuries. The high-arched cavus foot is rigid and absorbs shock poorly. Athletes with cavus feet therefore have a greater chance of sustaining impact-related lower extremity injuries, such as stress fractures. They also may develop plantar fasciitis or Achilles tendinitis. Flat feet are usually flexible and absorb shock well; however, most people with flat feet have excessive pronation of the foot with each step. Excessive pronation can be related to the development of stress fractures, posterior tibial tendinitis, and exertional compartment syndrome.

Muscle Imbalance. An athlete's muscles should be strong, but flexible. If the strength or the flexibility of a muscle group is too different from the strength and flexibility of its antagonist muscle group, then an overuse injury may occur. One of the most frequent examples of this is patellofemoral pain syndrome. Many of the athletes who suffer from this disorder have weakness of the quadriceps muscles compared with the hamstrings, and tightness (decreased flexibility) of the hamstrings compared with the quadriceps.

Even a well-trained athlete may develop a muscular imbalance. Among skeletally immature participants, muscle groups tend to lose flexibility during each growth spurt unless special attention is paid to stretching them. An athlete of any age may develop a muscular imbalance during vacation time from sport or treatment for an injury.

TRAINING ERROR

Training errors probably are the direct cause of most overuse injuries. A training error can occur when a change in the training regimen is made too rapidly, or when a change of technique is too drastic. An overuse injury may result from an increase in the *length of time* of workouts. Increasing the *frequency* of training sessions may lead to similar problems. Increasing the *intensity* of the workout may also cause overuse injuries; this includes such changes as increasing speed, changing stride length or stroke length, adding hill training, or increasing the amount of sprint training.

An athlete may change his or her technique to improve performance. These changes often occur when the athlete switches from one coach to another. The new technique may require alterations in the coordination and usage of the muscle groups. If the stresses on a particular musculoskeletal structure change too drastically, then an overuse injury occurs.

CHANGE OF EQUIPMENT

Changes of equipment may lead to the development of overuse injuries. Determining the change that caused an injury sometimes requires subtle detective work, such as discovering that the running shoes have been worn so much that the cushioning effect of the sole has been lost. Other changes are more obvious: the tennis player's new racquet, the soccer player's move to an indoor surface, or the skater's new boots.

GENERAL PRINCIPLES OF TREATMENT

PREVENTION

One half or more of all overuse injuries could probably be prevented by appropriate attention to the development of the strength and flexibility required for a specific athletic activity before the athlete begins the activity. Ideally, each athlete should undergo a preparticipation history and physical examination before embarking on a new activity, followed by examinations at regular intervals. The musculoskeletal portion of this examination should include a thorough history of previous injuries, a functional examination of the joints, and strength and flexibility testing of the major muscle groups. The injury-prevention preparticipation examination is tailored to be as sport specific as possible.

Additional overuse injuries could be prevented by ensuring that the athlete and the coach have a good understanding of the body's methods of adaptation to physical stress and apply those principles to training program design. The team physician aids greatly in the development of their knowledge base by participating in coaching seminars, team meetings, and individual counseling sessions. Unfortunately, the most powerful time for providing such instruction is during the athlete's rehabilitation from an injury. The injured athlete becomes a captive audience for tips on injury prevention and improved training methods.

RELATIVE REST

An athlete who has sustained an overuse injury usually must decrease or stop the portions of his or her training program that caused the injury. When the cause is a change of equipment, the injury may still be severe enough that a period of decreased athletic activity is advisable in addition to addressing the equipment problem. During the time of decreased activity, the athlete should continue to participate in as much of the training program as the team physician determines to be appropriate. If a segment of the training program (or all of it) is deemed unsafe for the injured athlete, then the physician should assist the athlete and coach in designing a program of substitute activities that resemble the athlete's usual sporting activities as closely as possible. The substitute activities prescribed during this period of relative rest should utilize as many of the same muscle groups used in the sporting event as possible and use them in a manner that resembles the event as closely as possible. For example, a speed skater wearing a below-knee cast gains more sport-specific benefit from a workout on a stationary bicycle at speeds chosen to resemble skating training than from a similar-length session on a cross-country skiing machine.

During the healing phase, the athlete should work to improve the strength and flexibility of other, uninjured musculoskeletal structures. Other muscles may be required to compensate for injured regions once the athlete returns to full activity, and these muscles must have sufficient strength to do so. Additionally, because the injured athlete is not performing his or her usual training regimen, uninjured structures frequently become weak or inflexible unless a specific program is designed to allow the athlete to prevent this unnecessary sequela to an injury.

ANTI-INFLAMMATORY THERAPY

Both local and systemic anti-inflammatory therapies may be effective in the treatment of most overuse injuries. The local application of ice to the injured region for 15 to 20 minutes, four times each day, seems to help decrease the pain from an overuse injury and may speed the healing process. Cryotherapy is also useful for the injured athlete who is continuing to participate in sports despite the injury. The application of ice immediately following activities that exacerbate the injury reduces the severity of new inflammation and resultant edema.

New evidence seems to suggest that systemic nonsteroidal anti-inflammatory medications (NSAIDs) may increase the healing rate of acute muscle strains, and perhaps of fractures as well. These medications may also be useful in the treatment of overuse injuries. Injured athletes report decreased discomfort, increased ability to train, and increased ability to perform therapeutic exercise programs when they take NSAIDs.

Because competitive athletes may be overzealous, the physician should caution the athlete who is using local or systemic anti-inflammatory agents. When the injured young or recreational athlete is in the healing phase, it is usually inadvisable to recommend anti-inflammatory medications immediately before a competitive event, or even before a competitive practice session. The anti-inflammatory agent masks discomfort, and the athlete may risk further, more severe, overuse injury without realizing the excessive level of stress on the injured structure. Of course, an athlete may be willing to risk further injury for the chance to compete in a major tournament. The final caution concerns the prescription of NSAIDs for children. The use of aspirin by children has been associated with Reye's syndrome, a serious disorder that may be fatal. Other NSAIDs should not be considered safe from a similar association. Fortunately, most children and young adolescents with overuse injuries respond very rapidly to relative rest and local ice application, so NSAIDs are not necessary.

SPLINTING IF NECESSARY

On occasion, an overuse injury may be so severe that immobilization, or even surgery, is appropriate treatment. Scientific studies from the past decade have shown, however, that most soft tissue injuries heal better if some motion of the affected region is allowed. Articular cartilage requires motion of its joint for proper nutrition. The musculature crossing an immobilized joint loses strength and flexibility. If possible, any splint for treating an overuse injury should be removable, so gentle therapeutic stretching and strengthening exercises can be performed.

Some areas of tendinitis (such as tendinitis near the wrist) respond well to brief periods of immobilization. Osgood-Schlatter disease and osteochondritis dissecans in the adolescent athlete may require temporary immobilization if improvement of symptoms is inadequate with the use of relative rest and local ice application. Some athletes who have sustained stress fractures require immobilization. These are generally athletes who have not responded to relative rest without immobilization, or those who have difficulty complying with the principles of relative rest.

Two musculoskeletal conditions related to overuse may require internal splinting by surgical procedures. Osteochondritis dissecans of the knee, ankle, or elbow can cause osteochondral fragments or flaps of articular cartilage to interfere with the normal mechanics of the joint. Frequently, these fragments can be replaced surgically and held in place with pins. The other relatively common condition that requires internal splinting is a stress fracture of the femoral neck. Although some athletes prefer to let the fracture heal without surgery, the risk of displacement of a nondisplaced complete femoral neck stress fracture is sufficiently great that many orthopedic surgeons recommend internal fixation of the fracture.

CORRECTION OF DEFICITS

Before the athlete returns to full activity, any deficits of strength or flexibility should be determined and addressed. Equipment may need to be changed to decrease the chance of recurrent injury. Shoe inserts or other orthotic devices should be prescribed if appropriate. The training program should be examined and any necessary changes recommended.

PROGRESSIVE RETURN TO ACTIVITY AS TOLERATED

Unless the athlete's injury has been very minor and the period of decreased activity very brief, the return to full activity must be planned carefully and monitored frequently. Both the injured and the uninjured musculoskeletal structures are at risk for injury if the physical demands of the sporting activity greatly exceed the demands of the rehabilitation program. The progressive return to activity also should allow the athlete to redevelop the proprioceptive input and coordination patterns needed for the sport.

SPECIFIC INJURIES

FOOT, ANKLE, AND LOWER LEG

Inflammatory Processes. *Achilles tendinitis* is an inflammation of the tendon that connects the gastrocnemius and soleus muscles to the calcaneus. It may be related to decreased flexibility of those muscles.

Plantar fasciitis affects the strong fibrous tissue that helps to support the longitudinal arch of the foot, connecting the calcaneus to the metatarsal heads. It occurs most frequently in cavus feet. It may also be related to tight calf muscles.

Calcaneal bursitis, usually caused by improperly fitting shoes rubbing against the posterior aspect of the heel, may be associated with achilles tendinitis.

Anterior ankle area tendinitis usually results from pressure from shoes or boots.

Peroneal tendinitis occurs more frequently in athletes with bowlegs or with cavus feet—those athletes who tend to run on the lateral aspects of their feet. Some peroneal tendinitis is caused by direct pressure, for example, from an ill-fitting boot.

Posterior tibial tendinitis most frequently occurs in runners with flat feet. The posterior tibial muscle provides a significant proportion of the support for the arch in a flat foot and helps to prevent excessive pronation. The pain along the posteromedial border that is caused by this disorder is often referred to as "shin splints."

Compartment Syndrome and Stress Fracture. *Exertional compartment syndromes* affect the lower leg most frequently. Recurrent, exercise-related compartment syndrome occurs when an exercising muscle group becomes so enlarged or "pumped up" that the small blood vessels within the fascial compartment become compressed. Lack of sufficient circulation causes pain and weakness, and perhaps even sensory loss. If the pressure within the compartment is high, and if it persists, then permanent damage to the nerves and muscles within the compartment results. Fortunately, permanent damage is rare among athletes with the recurrent exertional form of compartment syndrome.

Stress fractures of tibia, fibula, metatarsals, and navicular result from recurrent impact to the lower extremity. They may occur more frequently in athletes with rigid cavus feet and in those who wear footgear that has little cushioning. Athletes with stress fractures may have had pre-existing symptoms of tendinitis, but continued repetition of the injuring forces finally leads to fracture. The new fracture is often diagnosed by a change in the athlete's pain from diffuse tenderness to point tenderness and by the finding of pain on gentle three-point loading of the bone. Stress fractures may not be evident on plain radiographs, but are apparent on a radionuclide bone scan.

KNEE

Inflammatory Processes. *Patellofemoral pain syndrome* is irritation of the undersurface of the patella. In older athletes, the patellar articular cartilage may become softened or fibrillated (chondromalacia patellae). Participants with increased femoral anteversion, genu valgum, or flat feet seem prone to this disorder. Almost all young athletes who have patellofemoral pain syndrome resolve their pain by strengthening their quadriceps (particularly the vastus medialis obliquus) and stretching their hamstrings.

Patellar tendinitis is another disorder of the extensor mechanism of the knee, sometimes related to tight quadriceps muscles. Some jumping athletes develop this problem despite normal flexibility, however, and these athletes usually respond to treatment only slowly.

Iliotibial band friction syndrome results from the band's repeated rubbing against the prominent lateral femoral condyle. Athletes who suffer from this injury often have varus knees (bowlegs), cavus feet, or tight tensor fasciae latae muscles. In addition to stretching of the tight musculature, shoe inserts to decrease the apparent varus are useful.

Jumper's knee occurs in the same groups of athletes who are vulnerable to patellar tendinitis. This inflammation at the inferior pole of the patella is usually related to tight quadriceps.

Osgood-Schlatter disease is inflammation at the insertion of the patellar tendon into the tibial tubercle of the skeletally immature child or adolescent. It is often caused by tight quadriceps, but it may be precipitated by recurrent blunt trauma to the region.

Other Disorders. *Osteochondritis dissecans*, as an overuse injury, generally is found among adolescents. The lesions in the articular cartilage and subchondral bone of the femoral condyles may be developmental or may be related to recurrent microtrauma. Treatment is determined by symptoms.

THIGH AND HIP

Greater trochanteric bursitis is caused either by blunt trauma or by the rubbing of the tensor fasciae latae and iliotibial band over the trochanter.

Adductor strain usually affects the adductor longus muscle. It may occur secondary to another injury around the hip.

Iliopsoas tendinitis is generally diagnosed only in gymnasts and ballet dancers, and it is often related to inflammation of the bursa that overlies the lesser trochanter.

Avulsion fracture of pelvis may follow a period of apophysitis or inflammation of the growth plate at the insertion of a tendon. If the adolescent athlete ignores the symptoms, a sudden strong contraction of the muscle may avulse its bony attachment from the rest of the pelvis.

Femoral neck stress fracture occurs not only in osteoporotic non-menstruating women, but in men as well. It should even be included in the differential diagnosis of groin pain in young adolescent athletes.

SPINE AND RIBS

Spondylolysis is generally a developmental defect of the bony arch of the spine, but it may begin to cause pain because of increased activity, especially in the athlete who has tight hamstrings, tight hip flexors, and tight lumbodorsal fascia.

Rib stress fracture has been reported in young, osteoporotic, non-menstruating female runners.

SHOULDER

Impingement syndrome should be considered in athletes who participate in overhead activities (swimming, tennis, etc.) and have shoulder pain. This inflammatory condition results when the supraspinatus tendon is compressed between the humeral head and the acromion.

Rotator cuff strain usually affects the supraspinatus muscle, but other rotator cuff muscles may be involved.

Subluxation may cause symptoms similar to those of impingement syndrome, but subluxators have demonstrable instability. Swimmers frequently complain of this problem.

Biceps tendinitis is inflammation of the tendon in its groove on the humeral head.

Subacromial bursitis causes point tenderness over the bursa.

ELBOW

Lateral epicondylitis (tennis elbow) produces painful forearm supination and wrist extension.

Osteochondritis dissecans (Little League elbow) may also affect adults. Loose bodies in the joint may result.

Medial epicondylitis may also occur in young pitchers. It causes painful forearm pronation and wrist flexion.

WRIST AND HAND

Wrist strain, as an overuse injury, often refers to stretching and inflammation of the capsular and tendinous structures about the wrist.

Kienböck's disease, or osteonecrosis of the lunate, can be caused by repeated loading or vibration of the lunate.

Carpal tunnel syndrome may occur in relationship to repetitive flexion maneuvers of the wrist.

Premature physeal closure of the distal radius has been reported among young gymnasts. Some seem to have stress fractures of the growth plate.

INDEX

Page numbers in *italics* indicate figures; page numbers followed by t indicate tables.

Abdominal emergency(-ies), 146–147
Acetazolamide (Diamox), for mountain
        sickness prevention, 112
Achilles tendon injury, 184, 303
    taping for, 134, *136*
ACLS. *See* Advanced Cardiac Life
        Support
Acquired immunodeficiency syndrome
        (AIDS), in steroid users, 290
Acromegaly, 291
Acromioclavicular joint separation, 164
    bracing for, *139*, 140
    treatment of, 165
Adaptation, in training, 34
Adductor longus strain, 305
Adenosine triphosphate (ATP), as
        energy source, 5t, 27–29
    regeneration of, 3–6
Adolescent(s). *See* Child(ren)
Adolescent growth spurt, 228
    increased lumbar lordosis at, 231
    overuse injury during, 230–231
Advanced Cardiac Life Support
        (ACLS), arrhythmia treatment
        in, 144
    equipment for, 225
Aerobic power, maximal. *See* Maximal
        aerobic power
Aerobic training, 36–37
Agility, assessment of, in
        preparticipation examination,
        77
Aid station(s), at endurance events,
        281–282
AIDS (acquired immunodeficiency

syndrome), in steroid users,
        290
Air pollution, 112–117, 116t
Air quality standard(s), 116t
Air splint(s), for ankle or foot injury,
        128, *129*, 186
Airway management, in emergency
        care, 143
Albuterol, 295
    for exercise-induced asthma, 56
Alcohol, 294
    abuse of, 262–263
    as recovery drink, 64
    performance and, 69
Alkaline salt(s), 68
Allergic reaction(s), severe, 146
    at endurance events, 274
Altitude, 109–112
    acclimatization to, 110
    acute physiologic responses to,
        109–110
    illness due to, 111–112
    training adjustments at, 110–111
Amenorrhea, 218
American Academy of Pediatrics
        (AAP), recommendations for
        participation in competitive
        sports, 77, 78–79t
    sports classification system, 77, 80t
American Psychological Association,
        Division of Sport and Exercise
        Psychology of, 257
Amino acid(s). *See* Protein
Amphetamine(s), 69, 292–293
Anaerobic threshold, 37–38
    training to raise, 38

Anaerobic training, 38–39, 39t
Anaphylaxis, 146
  at endurance events, 274
Anemia, 48–49
  iron-deficiency, 48–49
    due to gastrointestinal bleeding, 50
    in female athletes, 219–220
Aneurysm, intracerebral, rupture of,
    148, 149
Ankle, fractures of, treatment of, 187
  injury to, in children, 236–237
    limb-threatening, 157–158
    overuse, 236–237, 303–304
    recognition and evaluation of,
      185–187
    return-to-play criteria after, 204
  physical examination of, 185–186
  sideline screening examination of,
    161
  sprains of, bracing, splinting, and
    taping techniques for, 127–128,
    129, 130
    in children, 236
  treatment of, 187
Ankle corset(s), 127, 128, 129
Ankylosing spondylitis, hip pain due
    to, 175
Anorexia nervosa, 221, 259
Anterior cruciate ligament, injury to,
    178
  in children, 233–235
  tests of, 177–178
Anterior drawer test, 177–178
Anterior tibial artery, injury to, 157
Antidiarrheal medication(s), narcotic-
    containing, 295
Antihistamine(s), 295
Apophysitis, chronic, of pelvis, 172,
    232
  Sever's, 231, 236
Apprehension test, in shoulder
    examination, 164
Arrhythmia(s), emergency treatment
    for, 144
Arteriovenous malformation,
    intracerebral, rupture of, 148,
    149
Arteriovenous oxygen difference

$(a - \bar{V}_{O2})$, in response to
    exercise, 11–15, 12–13
  training's effect on, 20–21
Artery(-ies), injury to, 155
  with shoulder injury, 164–165
Arthritis, infectious, of hip, 175
  running and, 218–219
Articular cartilage injury, in children,
    230
Aspirin, Reye's syndrome and, 301
Association for the Advancement of
    Applied Sport Psychology
    (AAASP), 257
Assumptions of risk. *See* Release(s)
Asthma, adverse effects of sulfur
    dioxide inhalation in, 117
  drugs for, 295
  exercise-induced, 55–56
  severe attack of, at endurance events,
    274
Asystole. *See* Cardiac arrest
Athletic pseudonephritis, 51–52
ATP. *See* Adenosine triphosphate
Avascular necrosis of femoral head, 175
Avascular necrosis of lunate, 168, 306
$a - \bar{V}_{O2}$. *See* Arteriovenous oxygen
    difference
AVPU system, for emergency
    neurologic evaluation, 144
Avulsion injury(-ies), in children, 230
  of knee, in children, 234
  of lesser trochanter, 174
  of pelvis, 172, 173, 305
    in children, 232
Axillary nerve neurapraxia, with
    shoulder injury, 164

Back pain, 305
  in children, 231–232
Balance, assessment of, in
    preparticipation examination,
    77
Beck's triad, 145–146
Bee sting allergy, 146
Behavior, 252–265. *See also* Substance
    abuse
  steroid use and, in men, 289
    in women, 290

Benzodiazepine(s), 294–295
Beta-blocker(s), 69, 294
Biceps tendon, inflammation of, 165, 306
rupture of, 165
Bladder, "jogger's," 52
Bleeding. See Hemorrhage
Blood doping, 68, 291–292
Blood flow, in response to exercise, 11, 12–14
Blood pressure, in response to exercise, 11, 14
Body composition, assessment of, in physically challenged athlete, 245
in preparticipation examination, 75
eating disorders due to emphasis on, 258–259
sex differences in, 217–218
Body temperature, regulation of, 101–102
Bohr effect, 15
Bone, overuse injury to, 297
training's effects on, 22
Boxers' fracture(s), 170
Brace(s). See Bracing
Brachial artery laceration, 156
Brachial plexus injury, with shoulder injury, 164
Bracing, of lower extremity, 127–134, 132–134
of upper extremity, 137–139, 137–140
Bradycardia, emergency treatment for, 144
Breastfeeding, 221
Bronchodilator(s), 295
Bulimia nervosa, 221, 259
Bursitis, calcaneal, 303
greater trochanteric, 174, 305
iliopsoas, 174
pes anserinus, 182–183
subacromial, 306

Caffeine, 69, 294
Calcaneal bursitis, 303
Calcium, requirements for, 219
supplemental, for osteoporosis prevention, 218, 219

Carbohydrate(s), as energy source, 7, 7, 35
exercise duration and, 24–25, 26
exercise intensity and, 24, 26
in postcompetition eating, 63
in precompetition meal, 60
requirements for, in female athletes, 220
Carbohydrate loading, 67
Carbon monoxide (CO), 113, 113–114, 116t
Carboxyhemoglobin (COHb), blood levels of, maximal aerobic power and, 113, 113–114
Cardiac arrest, at endurance events, 271–274
emergency treatment for, 144
Cardiac dysrhythmia(s), emergency treatment for, 144
Cardiac output (Q̇), in response to exercise, 9, 12–13
maximal aerobic power and, 8, 31
maximal capacity for oxygen transport and, 31
training's effect on, 19, 20
Cardiac tamponade, 145–146
Cardiopulmonary resuscitation (CPR). See also Advanced Cardiac Life Support
equipment for, 225
Cardiovascular system, detraining's effects on, 23
disease of, steroid use and, 145, 289
sudden death risk in, 144
responses of, to exercise, 9–16, 12–14
abnormal, 12–13, 15, 15–16
regulation of, 11–15, 13, 14
training and, 19–21, 19t
Carpal tunnel syndrome, 306
Cerebral edema, high-altitude, 112
Certification, of sports medicine practitioners, 118–119
Cervical spine injury, 149–150
in children, 231
return-to-play criteria after, 207–208
shoulder pain due to, 163
Cervical traction, helmet use for, 151
Chest, flail, 145

Child(ren), 228–241
  growth hormone administration to, 291
  injury in, ankle and foot, 236–237
    elbow, 239
    hip and pelvis, 232–233
    knee, 233–236
    mechanisms of, 228–229
    prevention of, 240
    shoulder, 237–239
    spinal, 231–232
  muscular imbalance in, 298
  precautions in nonsteroidal anti-inflammatory drug use for, 301
  steroids' effects in, 290–291
  training for, aerobic, 37
    anaerobic, 39
    power, 45
    strength, 43
    threshold, 38
Childbirth, resumption of exercise after, 220–221
Chondromalacia patellae, 304
  in children, 235
Circulation, changes in, in response to exercise, 11, 12–14
  management of, in emergency care, 144
Clavicle, fracture of, 164
  in children, 238
Clearance, 77
  for physically challenged athlete, 248
Clinical judgment, 161
Clipping, prophylactic knee braces for prevention of, 131–132
Coach, role of, in eating disorder treatment, 260–261
Cocaine, 144, 263, 293
Cold, 106–109
  acclimatization to, 107
  injury due to, 107–109. See also Hypothermia
    at endurance events, 268, 278
    limb-threatening, 153–154
    prevention of, 108–109, 278
    treatment of, 109
  physiologic responses to, 106–107
  stress index for, 107, 108t, 278

  therapeutic use of, 193
Cold medication(s), 295
Collapse, at endurance events, 270–271
  treatment of, 282–283
Communications, at endurance event, 281
Compartment syndrome, 155
  exertional, 157, 303
  of arm, 156
  of lower leg, 157, 184
  of thigh, 156
Competition phase, 141–187
  return-to-play decision during, 199–201
Compression, in ankle and foot injury management, 186
Concussion, classification of, 206t
  return-to-play criteria after, 205–207, 206t, 207t
Conductance, in response to exercise, 11, 12–14
Congenital heart disease, sudden death risk in, 144
Contraceptive(s), oral, for hypoestrogenic amenorrhea, 218
Cool-down, in training, 46
Coronary artery disease (CAD), steroid abuse and, 145, 289
  sudden death risk in, 144
Corticosteroid(s), for exercise-induced asthma, 56
  oral, for musculoskeletal injury, 193
Counseling, 255–257
  on substance abuse, legal issues in, 122
CPR (cardiopulmonary resuscitation). See also Advanced Cardiac Life Support
  equipment for, 225
Crack, 293
Cramp(s), heat, 53–54, 103–104
  muscle, after endurance event, 281
Creatine phosphate (phosphocreatine, CP), as energy source, 4, 5t, 27–29
Cromolyn sodium, for exercise-induced asthma, 56

Cycle ergometer, maximal aerobic power measurement on, 8

Dalmane (flurazepam hydrochloride), 294–295
Death, sudden, 144–145
Decongestant(s), 295
Dehydration. *See also* Fluid replacement
collapse and, 282
in heat injury, 104
Delayed-onset muscle soreness, causes of, 45
Depressant(s), 69, 294–295
Detraining, 22–23
Diabetes mellitus, growth hormone and, 291
Diamox (acetazolamide), for mountain sickness prevention, 112
Diazepam (Valium), 294
Diet. *See* Nutrition
Disabled athlete(s). *See* Physically challenged athlete(s)
Dislocation(s), Lisfranc, 157
of elbow, 166
taping for prevention of, *138*, 139–140
of hip, 174–175
of knee, 156–157
of patella, 180
bracing for prevention of, 128–130, *132*
of peroneal tendon, 237
of shoulder, 156
in children, 238
taping for prevention of, 140
Diuretic(s), 70
Doping, 68–70, 287–296. *See also* Steroid(s), anabolic; Substance abuse
blood, 68, 291–292
testing for. *See* Drug testing
Dorsalis pedis pseudoaneurysm, 157
Drink(s), sports. *See* Sports drink(s)
Drug(s), therapeutic. *See* Medication(s)
Drug profile, 98
Drug testing, 98, 296
in international competition, 99
legal issues in, 122
Drug use. *See* Doping; Steroid(s), anabolic; Substance abuse
Duodenal hematoma, intramural, 146–147

Eating disorder(s), 221, 258–261
Edema, high-altitude cerebral, 112
high-altitude pulmonary, 112
Ejection fraction (EF), in response to exercise, 16
Elbow, bracing, splinting, and taping techniques for, *138*, 139–140
dislocation of, 166
taping for prevention of, *138*, 139–140
fracture of, 166
in children, 239
injury to, in children, 239
limb-threatening, 156
overuse, 239, 306
recognition and evaluation of, 166–168, *167*
return-to-play criteria after, 202
"Little League," 168, 230, 239, 306
sprains of, 166–167
"tennis," 168, 306
Electricity, therapeutic use of, 193
Electrolyte replacement, 64
Electromechanical dissociation, emergency treatment for, 144
Elevation, in ankle and foot injury management, 187
Embolism, pulmonary, 146
Emergency(-ies), ABCs of care for, 143–144
abdominal, 146–147
drills in preparation for, 96, 143
life-threatening, 143–150
immediate response to, 162
limb-threatening, 153–158
neurologic, 147–150
organization for response to, 95–97, 97t
in international competition, 99
sideline equipment for, 97t
thoracic, 145–146

Endurance, assessment of, in
   preparticipation examination,
   76
  training for. *See* Endurance training
Endurance event(s), aid stations at,
   281–282
  casualties at, identification of,
   280–281
   incidence and risks of, 267–274,
    268t, *269*, 270–273t
   predicting numbers for, 274
   prevention of, 276–279
   transportation of, 280–281
   treatment of, 281–284
   types of, 269–274, 271–273t
  communications at, 281
  field hospital at, 282
  maintenance and use of medical
   records for, 284
  medical management of, 266–286
   functional elements of, 280t
   purpose of, 267
   staff and equipment requirements
    for, 274–276, 275t
Endurance training, 43–44, 43t
  adjustments in, for heat stress, 103
  cardiovascular adaptations to, 19–21,
   19t
  respiratory system's adaptations to,
   18–19
  skeletal muscle's adaptations to, 20t,
   21
Energy, sources of, immediate, 27–29,
   28
   nonoxidative, 29
   oxidative, 30–31
  stores of, 5t
Energy metabolism, 3–8
  aerobic, 5, 6, 30–31, 35
  anaerobic, 4–6, *5*, 27–29, 35–36
  ATP regeneration in, 3–6
  exercise duration and, *5*, 6, 24–25,
   26, 28
  exercise intensity and, 24, *25, 26*
  substrate utilization in, 7, *7*, 31–32
Environmental condition(s), 101–117.
   See also Air pollution; Altitude;
   Cold; Heat

casualties in endurance events and,
   267, 268–269, *269*
  limb-threatening emergencies due to,
   153–154
Ephedrine, 294
Epicondylitis, 167–168, 306
Epidural hematoma, 147–148
Epiphysiolysis, 168, *170*
Equipment, athletic, for physically
   challenged athlete, *246,*
   246–248, *247*
   overuse injury due to change in,
    299
  medical, 223–227
   for emergency care, 97t
   for endurance events, 274–276,
    275t
   for sideline use, 159–160
Ergogenic aid(s), 66–70. *See also*
   Doping; *specific aids*
  ethical issues involving, 70
  mechanical, 66
  nutritional, 67
  pharmacologic, 68–70
  physiologic, 67–68
  psychological, 67
Erythrocythemia, induced (blood
   doping), 68, 291–292
Erythropoietin, 292
Esophageal reflux, 50
Estrogen, body composition and,
   217–218
  bone density and, 218
  for amenorrhea, 218
Ethical issue(s), of ergogenic aids, 70
Examination. *See* Preparticipation
   examination
Exercise. *See also* Training
  aerobic vs. anaerobic metabolism in,
   5, 6
  cardiovascular response to, 9–16,
   12–14
   abnormal, *12–13, 15*, 15–16
   regulation of, 11–15, *13, 14*
   training and, 19–21, 19t
  duration of, energy metabolism and,
   5, 6, 24–25, *26, 28*
  eating during, 62

efficiency of, 24
endocrine response to, 32
intensity of, energy metabolism and,
    24, 25, 26
metabolic response to, 24–33
    factors affecting, 24–29
osteoarthritis and, 219
osteoporosis and, 218
supramaximal, energy metabolism in,
    8
transition to, from rest, 27, 28
ventilatory response to, 9, 16–18, 17
    training and, 18–19
Exercise physiology, 3–23
    defined, 3
    for women athletes, 216–217
Exercise testing, of physically
        challenged athlete, 245
Extradural hematoma, 147–148

Fasciotomy, for compartment
        syndrome, 155
Fat, as energy source, 5t, 7, 7, 32, 35
    exercise duration and, 25, 26
    exercise intensity and, 24, 26
    training and, 25–27, 26
Female athlete(s), 215–222
    body composition of, 217–218
    exercise physiology for, 216–217
    nutrition for, 219–220
    steroids' effects on, 290
Femoral artery laceration, 156
Femur, anteversion of, overuse injury
        and, 298
    fracture of, 156, 175, 176, 180
    osteoid osteoma of, 175
    slipped capital epiphysis of, 175
    stress fracture of, 175, 176, 305
        in children, 232–233
        internal fixation for, 175, 302
Ferritin, serum, performance and,
        48–49, 219
Fetal steal syndrome, 220
Fibula, fracture of, 157
    stress fracture of, 183, 303–304
Fick equation, 8
Field hospital, at endurance events, 282
Finger(s), fractures of, 170–171

overuse injuries of, 171
return-to-play criteria after injury to,
    203
taping of, 137–139
Finger tip crush injury, 171
First aid, 159–162
Fitness, aerobic, measurement of, 8
    training for, 36–37
    energy, 34, 35
        training for, 36–41
    muscular, 34
        training for, 41–46
    physical, benefits of, 217
    retention of, during rehabilitation,
        193–194
Flail chest, 145
Flexibility, assessment of, in
        preparticipation examination,
        75
Fluid consumption, before exercise, 60
Fluid replacement. See also Dehydration
    after exercise, 63–64
    for collapse, 282–283
    mandatory, in ultramarathons, 277
Flurazepam hydrochloride (Dalmane),
        294–295
Food. See also Nutrition
    psychological value of, 61
Foot, cavus, overuse injury and, 298
    flat, overuse injury and, 298
    fracture of, treatment of, 187
    injury to, in children, 236–237
        limb-threatening, 157–158
        overuse, 236–237, 303–304
        recognition and evaluation of,
            185–187
    physical examination of, 185–186
Forearm, limb-threatening injury to,
        156
Fracture(s), avulsion. See Avulsion
        injury(-ies)
    boxers', 170
    "greenstick," 229
    Jones, 187
    of ankle, treatment of, 187
    of clavicle, 164
        in children, 238

Fracture(s) (*Continued*)
  of elbow, 166
    in children, 239
  of femur, 156, 175, 176, 180
  of foot, treatment of, 187
  of hand, 170–171
  of humerus, 156, 164, 166
    treatment of, 165
  of knee, 180
    in children, 233
  of leg, 157
  of shoulder, 164
    treatment of, 165
  of tibial eminence, 180
  of wrist, 168, *169*
  stress. *See* Stress fracture(s)
Fracture board, 151
Frank-Starling mechanism, 11
Frostbite, 107, 153–154
  treatment of, 109
Frostnip, 153

Ganglion cyst(s), of wrist, 169–170
Gas gangrene, 154
Gastrointestinal bleeding, 50–51
  in female athletes, 219
Gastrointestinal problem(s), 49–51
Gender-specific concerns. *See* Female
    athlete(s)
Genu valgum, overuse injury and, 298
Genu varum, overuse injury and, 298
Glenoid, fracture of, 164
  treatment of, 165
Glucose, as energy source, 29, 31
  metabolism of, aerobic, 6
    anaerobic, 4
    regulation of, during exercise, 32
Glycogen, as energy source, 4, 5t, 29,
    31–32, 35–36
Glycogenolysis, 29
Glycolysis, 29
Goal-setting, principles of, 253–254
Greater trochanteric bursitis, 174, 305
"Greenstick" fracture(s), 229
Growth cartilage, 230–231
Growth hormone (HGH), 291
Growth plate(s), injury to, 229, 230

premature closure of, due to overuse,
    230, 306
  due to steroids, 291
Growth spurt. *See* Adolescent growth
    spurt
Gynecomastia, due to steroid use, 289

Hamstring injury, return-to-play criteria
    after, 203
Hand(s), fracture of, 170–171
  injury to, overuse, 306
    recognition and evaluation of,
      168–171
    return-to-play criteria after, 203
HCG (human chorionic gonadotropin),
    use of, with steroids, 289
Head injury, 147–149
  return-to-play criteria after, 205–207,
    206t, 207t
Heart disease, congenital, sudden
    death risk in, 144
  steroid use and, 145, 289
  sudden death risk in, 144
Heart rate (HR), in response to
    exercise, 10, 11, *12–13*
  training's effect on, 19, 20
Heat, 101–106
  acclimatization to, 102
  endurance training adjustments in,
    103
  illness due to, 53–54, 103–106. *See
    also* Hyperthermia
    at endurance events, 268, *269*
    prevention of, 104–105, 105t,
      277–278, 278t
    risks of, during pregnancy, 220
    treatment of, 105–106
  physiologic responses to, 101–102
  stress index for. *See* WBGT index
  therapeutic use of, 193
Heat cramp(s), 53–54, 103–104
Heat exhaustion, 54, 104
Heat stroke, 54, 104
Helmet, removal of, 151
  traction applied with, 151
Hematoma, duodenal, 146–147
  epidural, 147–148
  intracerebral, 148–149

subdural, 148
Hematuria, 51–52
  in female athletes, 219
Hemorrhage, gastrointestinal, 50–51
    in female athletes, 219
  intracranial, 147–149
  subarachnoid, 149
Hemothorax, 145
Hepatitis B, in steroid users, 290
HGH (growth hormone), 291
High-altitude cerebral edema, 112
High-altitude pulmonary edema, 112
Hip, anatomy of, 173–174
  dislocation of, 174–175
  injury to, in children, 232–233
    overuse, 305
    recognition and evaluation of,
      173–175
  "snapping," 174, 233
History. *See* Medical history
HR. *See* Heart rate
Human chorionic gonadotropin (HCG),
    use of, with steroids, 289
Humerus, fracture of, 156, 164, 166
  treatment of, 165
  limb-threatening injury to, 156
  osteochondritis dissecans of, *167*, 168
Hydration. *See also* Dehydration; Fluid
    replacement
  monitoring of, 64
Hyperthermia, at endurance events,
    268, 270–271
  identification of, 280
  prevention of, 277–278, 278t
  treatment of, 283
Hypertrophic cardiomyopathy, sudden
    death risk in, 144, 145
Hyponatremia, heat cramps and, 53
Hypothermia, 55, 107
  at endurance events, 268, 270–271
    after finish, 281
  identification of, 280
  treatment of, 283
  in distance runners, 267
  treatment of, 109

"Ice" (methamphetamine), 292
Icing, 162, 186

for overuse injury, 301
Iliopsoas bursitis, 174
Iliopsoas tendon, hip "snap" due to,
    174, 233
  inflammation of, 174, 305
Iliopsoas tenosynovitis, in children, 233
Iliotibial band friction syndrome, 182,
    304
Iliotibial band irritation, hip "snap"
    due to, 233
Immobilization, deleterious effects of,
    192
  for ankle or foot injury, 186
  for overuse injury, 301–302
  for transportation, 151–152
  surgical, for overuse injury, 302
Impingement sign, in shoulder
    examination, 164
Impingement syndrome, 165, 305
Individual response, to training, 41
Information disclosure, 121–122
Informed consent, 121–122
Injury rates, 143, 159, 191
Injury surveillance, 98
Insect sting allergy, 146
Insulin, in regulation of glucose use
    during exercise, 32
International competition, team
    physician's responsibilities in,
    99
International Olympic Committee
    (IOC), drug policy of, 68–69
Interval training, 38–39, 39t
Intracerebral aneurysm, rupture of,
    148, 149
Intracerebral hematoma, 148–149
Intracranial hemorrhage, 147–149
Ipratropium bromide, for exercise-
    induced asthma, 56
Iron, dietary sources of, 49
Iron deficiency. *See under* Anemia
Isokinetic device(s), for power training,
    44–45

Jet lag, 99
"Jogger's bladder," 52
Joint injury. *See also under specific joints*
  exercise after, osteoarthritis and, 219
  in children, 229

Jones compression bandage, 186
Jones fracture, 187
"Jumper's knee," 229, 304

Kenny-Howard splint, *139*, 140
Kienböck's disease, 168, 306
Knee. *See also* Patella
  anatomy of, 176
  bracing, splinting, and taping
    techniques for, 128–134,
    131–135
  dislocation of, 156–157
  fracture of, 180
    in children, 233
  injury to, in children, 233–236
    limb-threatening, 156–157
    overuse, 180–183, 235–236, 304
    recognition and evaluation of,
      176–183
    return-to-play criteria after, 203
  "jumper's," 229, 304
  malalignment of, *181*
  sideline screening examination of,
    160
  sprains of, 177–178
    bracing, splinting, and taping
      techniques for, 130–131
    treatment of, 178
  stress tests of ligaments of, 177–178
  "swimmer's," 230
Knee immobilizer, 128, *131*
Knee sleeve(s), 134

Lachman test, 177
Lactate shuttle, 31–32
Lactate threshold, 37–38
  training to raise, 38
Lactation, 221
Lactic acid, accumulation of, fatigue
    and, 29
  ventilatory threshold and, 18
  muscle uptake of, 32
Larsen-Johansson disease, treatment of,
    236
Laryngoscope(s), 143
Lateral epicondylitis, 167–168, 306
Leg, injury to, limb-threatening, 157
  overuse, 183, 303–304

recognition and evaluation of,
    183–184
Legal issue(s), 118–126
Legg-Calvé-Perthes disease, 175
Life-threatening emergency(-ies),
    143–150
  immediate response to, 162
Ligament(s), of knee, stress tests of,
    177–178
  training's effects on, 22
Limb-threatening emergencies, 153–158
Lipid(s). *See* Fat
Liquid meal(s), 60
Lisfranc dislocation, 157
"Little League elbow," 168, 230, 239,
    306
"Little League shoulder," 229, 239
Liver disease, steroid use and, 289–290
Locked-arm technique for
    transportation, 151–152
Lower extremity, bracing, splinting,
    and taping techniques for,
    127–134, *128–136*
  injury recognition and evaluation in,
    172–184
  malalignment of, overuse injury and,
    298
Lumbar spine pain, in children,
    231–232

Macrotrauma, in children, 229
Marathon(s). *See also* Endurance
    event(s)
  casualties during, 267–268, 268t, 270t,
    272t
Marfan's syndrome, sudden death risk
    in, 144, 145
Marijuana, 263, 295
Maximal aerobic power ($\dot{V}O_{2max}$), 7–8
  altitude's effects on, 110–111, *111*
  carboxyhemoglobin levels and, *113*,
    113–114
  measurement of, 8, *10*
Maximal ventilatory capacity, 16–17
Maximal voluntary ventilation (MVV),
    16–17
Medial epicondylitis, 167–168, 306
Medical bag. *See* Equipment, medical

Medical history, in orthopedic
    screening examination, 94
  in preparticipation examination,
    72–73, 74t
  of physically challenged athlete, 243
Medical record(s), 98
  at endurance events, 284
Medical-legal issue(s), 118–126
Medication(s). *See also specific drugs and
    classes of drugs*
  for physician's bag, 225–227
  guidelines for, for physically
    challenged athletes, 243
  provision of, to athletes, legal issues
    in, 122–123
Medicine, sports. *See* Sports medicine
  unauthorized practice of, 123
Meniscus injury, *179*, 179–180
  in children, 235
Menstrual dysfunction, 218
Methamphetamine, 292
Microtrauma. *See* Overuse injury(-ies)
Mitochondrion(-a), in oxidative energy
    system, 30–31
  respiratory control and, 27, *27*
Moderation, in training, 47
Motion, in rehabilitation, 192–193
Mountain sickness, 111–112
Movement time, 45, 46
Movie theater sign, 181
Muscle, training's effects on, 20t,
    21–22, 42
Muscle action, types of, 3
Muscle cramp(s), after endurance
    event, 281
Muscle imbalance, overuse injury and,
    298
Muscle soreness, delayed-onset, causes
    of, 45
Musculoskeletal injury, return-to-play
    criteria after, 196–204
Myoglobinuria, exertional, 53

Narcotic(s), 295
Neck injury. *See* Cervical spine injury
Neck profile, 208
Needle-sharing, by steroid users, 290

Nerve(s), peripheral, injury to,
    154–155, 164
Neurologic emergency(-ies), 147–150
Neurologic evaluation, emergency, 144
Nitrogen dioxide (NO_2), 115
Nitrogen oxide (NO_x), 115
Nonsteroidal anti-inflammatory drug(s)
    (NSAIDs), 193
  for overuse injury, 301
Nutrition, 58–65
  assessment of, in physically
    challenged athlete, 245
  during exercise, 62
  ergogenic aids involving, 67
  for female athletes, 219–220
  postcompetition, 62–64
  precompetition, 58–62

Olecranon fracture(s), 166
Olympic Committee, International
    (IOC), drug policy of, 68–69
  United States (USOC), registry of
    sport psychology professionals
    of, 257
Organization, 95–100
Orthopedic screening examination,
    77–80, *81–93*, 94
Osgood-Schlatter disease, 231, 304
  immobilization for, 302
  treatment of, 236
Osteitis pubis, 233
Osteoarthritis, running and, 218–219
Osteochondritis dissecans, 231
  immobilization for, 302
  internal splinting for, 302
  of elbow, *167*, 168, 306
  of knee, 182, 304
    in children, 235
  of talus, in children, 236–237
Osteoid osteoma, of femur, 175
Osteoporosis, 218
Outrigger(s), for alpine skiing, *247*, 248
Overload, in training, 42
Overspeed training, 46
Overtraining, 209–211
  hazards of, 46–47
  stress reduction techniques for,
    254–255

Overuse injury(-ies), 297–306
  causes of, 298–299
  in children, 228–229, 229–231
  of ankle and foot, 303–304
    in children, 236–237
  of bone, 297
  of elbow, 306
    in children, 239
  of fingers, 171
  of knee, 180–183, 304
    in children, 235–236
  of pelvis, in children, 232–233
  of shoulder, 165–166, 305–306
  of wrist, 168–170, *170*, 306
    in children, 230, 306
  prevention of, 299–300
    in children, 240
  treatment of, 300–303
Oxygen consumption ($\dot{V}_{O_2}$), exercise
    intensity and, 24, *25*
  limitations to, during exercise, *4*
  maximal. *See* Maximal aerobic power
Oxygen deficit, 6, *6*
Oxygen extraction, tissue. *See*
    Arteriovenous oxygen
    difference
Oxygen transport, altitude's effects on,
    110
  maximal capacity for, factors limiting,
    31
Ozone, 114–115

Paregoric, 295
Paroxysmal supraventricular
    tachycardia, emergency
    treatment for, 144
Patella, dislocation of, 180
  bracing for prevention of, 128–130,
    132
Patellar stabilization brace, 128–130, *132*
Patellar tendinitis, 182, 304
Patellofemoral pain syndrome, 181–182,
    304
  anatomic factors in, 298
  in children, 235–236
Peaking, 40
"Peg leg," 248
Pelvis, injury to, in children, 232–233

recognition and evaluation of,
    172–173, *173*
Performance testing, preparticipation,
    75–77
Periodization cycle(s), 210
Peroneal artery pseudoaneurysm,
    157–158
Peroneal tendon, dislocation or
    subluxation of, 237
  inflammation of, 303
Peroxyacetylnitrate (PAN), 115
Pes anserinus bursitis, 182–183
Pes cavus, overuse injury and, 298
Pes planus (flatfoot), overuse injury
    and, 298
Phenylpropanolamine, 294
Phosphate(s), high-energy, 4, 5t, 27–29.
    See also Adenosine
    triphosphate
Phosphocreatine (creatine phosphate,
    CP), as energy source, 4, 5t,
    27–29
Photochemical oxidant(s), 114–115, 116t
Photography, of physically challenged
    athlete, permission for, 243
Physeal closure, premature, due to
    overuse, 230, 306
  due to steroids, 291
Physeal injury, 229, 230
Physical examination. *See*
    Preparticipation examination
Physical modalities, in rehabilitation,
    193
Physically challenged athlete(s),
    242–251
  equipment for, *246*, 246–248, *247*
  medical evaluation of, 243–246
  psychological assessment of, 245–246
  restriction of, from participation, 248
Physician. *See* Team physician
Physiologic control theory, 9
Physiology. *See also* Exercise physiology
  defined, 3
Pivot shift test, 178
Placebo effect, 287
Plantar fasciitis, 303
Plyometrics, 45

Pneumatic antishock garment (PASG), 144, 146
Pneumothorax, open, 145
  tension, 145
Popliteal artery injury, 156–157
Postcompetition phase, 189–211
  eating during, 62–64
Posterior tibial tendinitis, 303
Posteromedial tibial stress syndrome, 183
Power, assessment of, in preparticipation examination, 76
  training for, 44–45
Precompetition meal, 58–62
  liquid meal for, 60
  psychological value of, 61
  sugar in, 60–61
  timing of, 59–60
Precompetition phase, 1–140
  eating during. *See* Precompetition meal
  examination in. *See* Preparticipation examination
Pregnancy, 220–221
Preparticipation examination, 71–94, 196, 199
  clearance in, 77
  frequency of, 72, 75
  legal issues in, 121
  medical history in, 72–73, 74t
  objectives of, 71
  of physically challenged athlete, 243–246
  orthopedic screening in, 77–80, 81–93, 94
  performance testing in, 75–77
  physical examination in, 73–75, 76t
  station-type, 72, 73t
  timing of, 72
  type of, 72
Prescription(s), legal issues in, 122–123
Progression, in training, 37
Propranolol, 294
Protein, as energy substrate, 7
  exercise intensity and, 24
Proteinuria, 51
Pseudoanemia, 48

in female athletes, 219
Pseudoaneurysm, with ankle injury, 157–158
Pseudonephritis, athletic, 51–52
Psychological issue(s), 252–265. *See also* Behavior; Substance abuse
  assessment of physically challenged athlete, 245–246
  in rehabilitation, 252–255
Psychologist(s), using services of, 255–257
Psychoneuroimmunology, 254–255
Pubic ramus, stress fractures of, 172–173
Pulmonary edema, high-altitude, 112
Pulmonary embolism, 146
Pulmonary system. *See* Respiratory system

$\dot{Q}$. *See* Cardiac output
Quadriceps injury, return-to-play criteria after, 203
Quadriceps tendinitis, treatment of, in children, 236

Radius, fracture of, 166, 168
  premature physeal closure of, 230, 306
Raynaud's disease, frostbite in, 107
Reaction time, 45
Record keeping, 98
  at endurance events, 284
Reentry to play. *See* Return to play
Rehabilitation, 191–195
  accuracy of diagnosis in, 192
  for overuse injury, 302–303
  goals of, 191–192
  goal-setting for, 253–254
  psychological issues in, 252–255
  return-to-play decision after, 194, 202
Relaxation technique(s), 255
Release(s), 124
  for physically challenged athletes, 243
Renal abnormalities, 51–53
Renal failure, exertional, 52–53
Resistance, in muscular fitness training, 42

Respiratory rate (RR), in response to exercise, 16, *17*
Respiratory system, responses of, to exercise, 9, 16–18, *17*
   training and, 18–19
Rest. *See also* Immobilization
   relative, for overuse injury, 300
Retroperitoneal injury(-ies), 146–147
Return to play, criteria for, 194
   after cervical spine injury, 207–208
   after head injury, 205–207, 206t, 207t
   after musculoskeletal injury, 196–204
   after overuse injury, 302–303
   after rehabilitation, 194, 202
   during competition, 199–201
   decisions about, clinical judgment in, 161
   legal issues in, 121
Reye's syndrome, 301
Rhabdomyolysis, exertional, 53
Rib(s), overuse injury of, 305
RICE principle, 162, 186
Rotator cuff injury, 165, 305
   in children, 238
"Runner's trots," 49–50
Running, osteoarthritis and, 218–219

Scheuermann's disease, 232
Seizure(s), after head injury, 149
   due to cocaine toxicity, 144
Sever's apophysitis, 231, 236
Shoulder, bracing, splinting, and taping techniques for, *139*, 140
   dislocation of, 156
     in children, 238
     taping for prevention of, 140
   fractures of, 164
     treatment of, 165
   injury to, in children, 237–239
     limb-threatening, 156
     overuse, 165–166, 305–306
     recognition and evaluation of, 163–166
     return-to-play criteria after, 202
     treatment of, 165
   "Little League," 229, 239

   physical examination of, 163–164
   sprains of, 140. *See also* Acromioclavicular joint separation
   subluxation of, due to overuse, 305
     recurrent, 165
   "swimmer's," 230
Sickle cell trait, exercise death in, 52–53
   exercise-related hematuria and, 52
Situational awareness, 160
Sleeping medication(s), 294–295
Slipped capital femoral epiphysis, 175
"Snapping hip," 174, 233
Somatotropin, 291
Specificity, of training, 35
Speed, assessment of, in preparticipation examination, 76
   training for, 39–40, 45–46
Spinal injury. *See also* Cervical spine injury
   in children, 231–232
   overuse, 305
Spleen, ruptured, 146
Splint(s), air, for ankle or foot injury, 128, *129*, 186
   Kenny-Howard, *139*, 140
Splinting, for lower extremity, 127–134, *129*
   for overuse injury, 301–302
   for upper extremity, *137–139*, 137–140
   internal, for overuse injury, 302
Spondylolysis, 231–232, 305
Sports, classification of, for clearance, 77, 80t
   incidence of catastrophic injuries in, 143
   injury rates for, 159, 191
Sports anemia, 48
   in female athletes, 219
Sports drink(s), at precompetition meal, 60
   during exercise, 62
   for heat stress prevention, 54
   in postcompetition eating, 63–64
Sports medicine, certification in, 118
   definition of, 118

practitioners of, regulation of,
118–119
unauthorized practice of medicine
charges against, 123
standards of care in, 120, 124
Spotter(s), at endurance events, 280,
281
Sprain(s), of ankle, bracing, splinting,
and taping techniques for,
127–128, *129, 130*
in children, 236
treatment of, 187
of elbow, 166–167
of fingers, taping for, *137,* 137–139
of great toe, taping for, 127, *128*
of knee, 177–178
bracing, splinting, and taping
techniques for, 130–131
treatment of, 178
of shoulder, 140. *See also*
Acromioclavicular joint
separation
of wrist, 168
Sprint(s), acceleration, 40
hollow, 40
Sprint training, skeletal muscle's
adaptations to, 20t, 21–22
"Stacking," 288
Staff, of sports medicine program,
regulation of, 118–119
unauthorized practice of medicine
charges against, 123
requirements for, for endurance
events, 274–276, 275t
Standards of care, in sports medicine,
120, 124
Status asthmaticus, at endurance
events, 274
Sternoclavicular joint, derangements of,
in children, 238
Steroid(s). *See also* Corticosteroid(s)
anabolic, 69–70, 287–291
effects of, 288–291
mechanisms of action of, 288
premature coronary artery disease
due to, 145, 289
prevention of use of, 262
Stimulant(s), 69, 292–294

Sting allergy, 146
Strength, assessment of, in
preparticipation examination,
75
training for, 42–43, 43t
skeletal muscle's adaptations to,
20t, 22, 42
Stress, immune function and, 254–255
Stress fracture(s), immobilization for,
302
of ankle and foot, 303–304
in children, 236
of femur, 175, 176, 305
in children, 232–233
internal splinting for, 175, 302
of lower leg, 183, 303–304
of pelvis, in children, 232–233
of pubic ramus, 172–173
of rib, 305
of vertebrae, in children, 231–232
of wrist, 168
Stroke volume (SV), in response to
exercise, 9–10, 11, *12–13*
training's effect on, 19, 20
Subacromial bursitis, 306
Subarachnoid hemorrhage, 149
Subclavian vessel(s), injury to, 156
Subdural hematoma, 148
Subluxation, peroneal tendon, 237
shoulder, 305
recurrent, 165
Substance abuse, 261–263. *See also*
Doping; Steroid(s), anabolic
counseling on, legal issues in, 122
identification of, 261–262
of performance-enhancing drugs,
261–262
of recreational drugs, 262–263, 293,
295
prevention of, 262, 263, 295–296
sudden death and, 144–145
testing for. *See* Drug testing
treatment of, 262–263
Sudden death, 144–145
Sugar, pre-exercise, 60–61
Sulcus sign, in shoulder examination,
164
Sulfur dioxide (SO_2), 116–117, 116t

Supraventricular tachycardia, paroxysmal, emergency treatment for, 144

SV. *See* Stroke volume

"Swimmer's knee," 230

"Swimmer's shoulder," 230

Synovitis, transient, of hip, 175

Tachycardia, paroxysmal supraventricular, emergency treatment for, 144

ventricular, emergency treatment for, 144

Taper, 41

Taping, for Achilles tendon injury, 134, 136

of ankle, 128, *130*

of elbow, *138*, 139–140

of fingers, 137–139

of great toe, 127, *128*

of knee, 134, *135*

of shoulder, 140

of thumb, *137*, 139

of wrist, *137*, 139

Team physician, certification for, 118

provision of continuous care by, 97–98

responsibilities of, 95, 199

in international competition, 99

Tendinitis, Achilles, 184, 303

anterior ankle area, 303

biceps, 165, 306

iliopsoas, 174, 305

immobilization for, 302

of lower leg, 183–184

of wrist, 169

patellar, 182, 304

peroneal, 303

posterior tibial, 303

quadriceps, treatment of, in children, 236

"Tennis elbow," 168, 306

Tenosynovitis, iliopsoas, in children, 233

of wrist, 169–170

Terbutaline, 295

Testosterone, 287

Theophylline, for exercise-induced asthma, 56

Thigh, injury to, limb-threatening, 156

overuse, 305

recognition and evaluation of, 176

return-to-play criteria after, 203

Thoracic emergency(-ies), 145–146

Threshold training, 38

Thumb, return-to-play criteria after injury to, 203

taping of, *137*, 139

Tibia, fracture of, 157, 180

stress fracture of, 183, 303–304

Time zone shift, 99

Toe(s), fracture of, treatment of, 187

sprains of, taping for, 127, *128*

Traction, cervical, helmet use for, 151

Trainer(s), certification for, 118–119

emergency care training for, 143

Training, 34–47, *35*

adaptation to, 34

adjustments in, at altitude, 110–111

aerobic, 36–37

anaerobic, 38–39, 39t

during treatment of overuse injury, 300

effects of, on cardiopulmonary system, 18–21, 19t

on high-energy phosphate storage, 28–29

on metabolic response to exercise, 25–27, *25–27*

on mitochondrial material, 30

on nonoxidative energy system, 29

on skeletal muscle, 20t, 21–22, 42

endurance. *See* Endurance training

errors in, overuse injury due to, 299

for energy fitness, 36–41

individual response to, 41

injuries in, frequency, intensity, and time and, 159

interval, 38–39, 39t

long-term, 46

moderation in, 47

overload in, 42

power, 44–45

principles of, 34–47

progression in, 37

resistance, 42
reversal of, 22–23
seasons of, 40, *41*
specificity of, 35
speed, 39–40, 45–46
sprint, skeletal muscle's adaptations
    to, 20t, 21–22
strength, 42–43, 43t
    adaptations to, 20t, 22, 42
threshold, 38
variation in, 37
warm-up and cool-down in, 46
Tranquilizer(s), 294
Transportation, 151–152
at endurance events, 280–281
Treadmill, maximal aerobic power
    measurement on, 8, *10*
Treppe effect, 11
Triathlon(s). *See also* Endurance event(s)
    casualties during, 268, 268t, 269,
        270t, 273t

Ulna, fracture of, 168
United States Olympic Committee
    (USOC), registry of sport
    psychology professionals of,
    257
Upper extremity, bracing, splinting,
    and taping techniques for,
    137–139, 137–140
injury recognition and evaluation in,
    163–171

$\dot{V}$ (ventilation volume), 16–18, *17*
Valium (diazepam), 294
Variable-resistance device(s), for power
    training, 44–45
Variation, in training, 37
Vascular conductance, in response to
    exercise, 11, *12–14*
Vascular resistance, peripheral,
    training's effect on, 20–21
Ventilation, maximal voluntary (MVV),
    16–17

Ventilation volume ($\dot{V}$), 16–18, *17*
Ventilatory response. *See under*
    Respiratory system
Ventilatory threshold (VT), 18
Ventricular ectopy, emergency
    treatment for, 144
Ventricular fibrillation, emergency
    treatment for, 144
Ventricular tachycardia, emergency
    treatment for, 144
Vertebral injury. *See* Spinal injury
$\dot{V}O_2$. *See* Oxygen consumption
$\dot{V}O_{2max}$. *See* Maximal aerobic power
Volar plate injury(-ies), 171
Volkmann's ischemic contracture of
    forearm, 156
Von Willebrand's disease, hematuria
    in, 52
VT (ventilatory threshold), 18

Waiver(s). *See* Release(s)
Warm-up, in training, 46
WBGT index, 103
application of, 104–105, 105t, 278,
    278t
Weight-class classifications, eating
    disorders and, 258
Wet bulb globe temperature. *See* WBGT
    index
Wheelchair(s), sports, *246*, 246–248
Wind-chill index, 107, 108t
competitors' speed and, 278
Women. *See* Female athlete(s)
Wrist, bracing, splinting, and taping
    techniques for, *137*, 139
fractures of, 168, *169*
injury to, overuse, 168–170, *170*, 230,
    306
    recognition and evaluation of,
        168–171, *169*, *170*
    return-to-play criteria after, 202
sprains of, 168
strain of, 306